ALLE · ZEIT · WACH · 1842

BG Chemie

Toxicological Evaluations

4 Potential Health Hazards of Existing Chemicals

Springer-Verlag
Berlin Heidelberg New York
London Paris Tokyo
Hong Kong Barcelona
Budapest

Berufsgenossenschaft
der chemischen Industrie
Gaisbergstraße 11

W-6900 Heidelberg 1, FRG

ISBN 3-540-54984-6 Springer-Verlag Berlin Heidelberg New York
ISBN 0-387-54984-6 Springer-Verlag New York Berlin Heidelberg

Library of Congress Cataloging-in-Publication Data. (Revised for volume 4). Toxicological evaluations. Includes bibliographical references and index. 1. Toxicity testing. I. Berufsgenossenschaft der Chemischen Industrie. [DNLM: 1. Hazardous Substances – toxicity. WA 465 T7549] RA1199.T678 1990 615.9'07 90-10020
ISBN 3-540-54984-6 ISBN 0-387-54984-6 (alk. paper)

Typesetting, printing and bookbinding:
Brühlsche Universitätsdruckerei, Giessen
51/3130-5 4 3 2 1 0 – Printed on acid-free paper

Preface

As part of its programme for the prevention of health hazards caused by industrial work substances, the Berufsgenossenschaft der chemischen Industrie (BG Chemie) began in 1977 to investigate the toxicity of those substances which are widely used, have many different applications and are suspected of being dangerous to health, in particular those having long-term effects on health. The investigations consist of a literature search and – depending on the results – commissions of experimental studies. It is hoped by means of this testing to close gaps in our knowledge and to increase the scientific validity of the required risk assessments. The results of the toxicological investigations carried out by BG Chemie, and the resulting substance assessments have been published in German since 1987 in the form of "Toxikologische Bewertungen" ("Toxicological Evaluations").

In order to make this useful information internationally available, the BG Chemie began in October 1990 to publish them as a book series in English, of which the fourth volume (containing 13 individual evaluations) is presented here. Because of the short time between publishing volume 1, 2 and 3, printing of "Introduction" (consisting of a general overview of the programme, lists with names of people involved as well as substances under investigation) was abandoned in volumes 2 and 3. In this volume a revised "Introduction" is published presenting more detailed information about the ongoing work.

The publication of further individual evaluations and, if necessary, reassessments of previously published evaluations is planned.

BG Chemie hopes that, for many people working in the chemical industry, this information will be of practical help in assessing hazards to health at the workplace.

Contents

Introduction

The European inventory of existing commercial chemical substances (EINECS) has shown that, at present, about 100 000 existing chemicals are marketed for various purposes. Only a small proportion, however, of these 100 000 existing chemicals are of technical significance. According to a survey made by the Chemical Industry Association (VCI)[1] of the Federal Republic of Germany (FRG), only about 4600 substances are produced in quantities greater than 10 tons annually. Most of the remaining substances are laboratory chemicals or products manufactured or delivered in response to individual orders.

Whereas substances which, since 1981, have been placed on the market for the first time ("new chemicals") are required by the Act on Chemicals[2] to be submitted to evaluation under special conditions, this is necessary only in certain cases for existing chemicals if specific regulations are established.

The Employment Accident Insurance Fund of the Chemical Industry – Berufsgenossenschaft der Chemischen Industrie (BG Chemie) – was already concerned with the testing of industrial substances for health-endangering properties long before the Act on Chemicals came into force.

In 1977 the management of the BG Chemie decided to give particular priority to the prevention of damage to health through industrial products. For this purpose it set up the

Programme for the prevention of health hazards caused by industrial substances.

In addition to other activities, the BG Chemie has begun to investigate, particularly for long-term effects, chemicals whose possible hazards to health are so far only suspected, so that additional safety measures can promptly be introduced into the factories when they are indicated by the results of these investigations.

The work of the BG Chemie in this field has now been incorporated into the Federal Government's scheme for systematic testing and evaluation of existing chemicals. Its contribution is made avai-

---

[1] Verband der Chemischen Industrie

[2] Chemikaliengesetz

lable in these **Toxicological Evaluations** and in further material to be published.

For evaluating purposes, the existing chemicals have been compiled in a list. The prerequisites for inclusion in this list are as follows:

1. The substances in question should be those used in industry in the manufacture of primary, intermediate, final or auxiliary products.
2. The volume of production and the method of handling the substances are also relevant considerations.
3. Special priority is given to substances that are destined for the consumer sector.
4. There should be evidence of a potential risk to health. This could include, for example, experience gathered in the workplace or by occupational physicians, unconfirmed indications in the literature or a similarity of the chemical structure to other substances that have proved to be hazardous (e.g. alkylating agents, aromatic amines).
5. Basically, the list compiled by the BG Chemie will not include substances for which MAK[3]-values have been fixed or which have proved to be carcinogenic in man or in animal studies (section III A1 and III A2, respectively, in the list of MAK[7]-values). Chemicals proposed for further discussion or investigation in the "yellow-pages" of the list of MAK[3]-values will only be investigated by the BG Chemie after prior consultation of the MAK-Kommission[4].
6. In order to avoid unnecessary duplication of work, BG Chemie will not study substances which are known to be the subject of investigations already being carried out by other national or international groups, provided these studies pursue objectives similar to those of the BG Chemie.

---

[3] Maximum workplace concentration

[4] German Commission for the Investigation of Health Hazards of Chemical Compounds in the Work Area (Senatskommission zur Prüfung gesundheitsschädlicher Arbeitsstoffe)

Substances are proposed by the member companies and by the technical supervision section of the BG Chemie as well as by other persons or organizations, e.g. the Federal Agency for Occupational Safety[5]. BAU[5] is working systematically on substances cited in the above mentioned survey of the VCI[1]. If the chemical is mainly of occupational relevance BAU[5] proposes the inclusion in the list of substances of the BG Chemie. Several substances have been accepted to be evaluated by the BG Chemie resulting from BAU's proposals.

The work of the BG Chemie is directed on chemicals with possible health endangering effects to employees after exposition at the work place. Numerous of the substances, however, are of environmental relevance, additionally, and might therefore be subject of the endeavours of BUA[6]. To avoid double-work BG Chemie and BUA[6] come to arrangements for preparation of the section "toxicity in warm-blooded animals", which is of relevance for both, the maintenance of occupational and environmental health and safety standards. Furthermore arrangements are made with the MAK-Kommission[4], ECETOC[7], and IPCS[8] for the prevention of double-work.

In assessing individual substances, the BG Chemie is supported by a scientific advisory committee (see Annex 1), which includes experienced toxicologists, occupational physicians and chemists. Representatives of the Federal Institute for Occupational Safety[6] and the Federal Health Office[9] also participate. The decision-making body for all these activities is the Principles and Substances Programme Committee (Annex 2).

After a substance has been included in the list, a painstaking investigation must be undertaken to decide whether that particular substance poses a health hazard to employees (Figure 1).

---

5 Bundesanstalt für Arbeitsschutz (BAU)

6 Advisory Committee on Existing Chemicals of Environmental Relevance (Beratergremium für umweltrelevante Altstoffe)

7 European Chemical Industry Ecology and Toxicology Centre

8 International Programme on Chemical Safety

9 Bundesgesundheitsamt

Figure 1

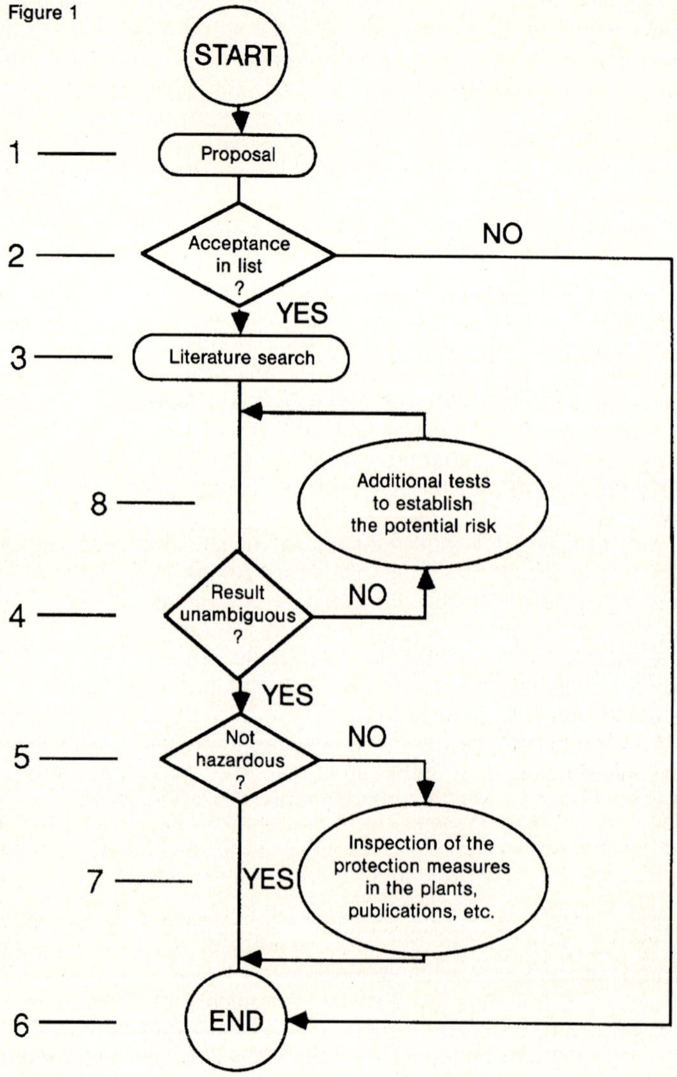
START
1
Proposal
2
Acceptance in list ?
NO
YES
3
Literature search
8
Additional tests to establish the potential risk
4
Result unambiguous ?
NO
YES
5
Not hazardous ?
NO
7
YES
Inspection of the protection measures in the plants, publications, etc.
6
END

The full procedure is as follows:

- Proposal for acceptance in the BG Chemie list of substances (1).
- Decision on whether or not to accept the substance (2).
- After acceptance in the list, a toxicological institute will conduct a search and review of the literature to see if there are any scientific publications or other study findings that report on acute or chronic toxicity, or on teratogenic, genotoxic or carcinogenic properties (3).
- On the basis of the literature search and review, a decision will be made as to whether a conclusive evaluation of the chemical in question is possible (4).
- If this shows that the substance is not hazardous (5), studies on this chemical can be concluded (6).
- If the substance studied has properties hazardous to health, the BG Chemie will check the safety precautions in the organizations where this chemical is used and, if necessary, will ensure that adequate improvements are made. At the same time, these results will be published and made available to interested and affected parties; for example, to the Commission for the Investigation of Health Hazards of Chemical Compounds in the Work Area[4] (7).
- If the literature search does not permit a conclusive evaluation of the substance (4), further studies must be conducted to determine the potential risk (8).
- Once these studies have been completed, a decision must be taken as to whether the available documentation is sufficient for a final evaluation (4).
- If the results are conclusive (4), no further tests are necessary. If on the other hand the chemical does pose risks, appropriate measures must be taken (7).
- However, if the results are inconclusive (4), additional tests will be necessary to assess the potential risk (8). The procedures to be followed will be decided on a case-to-case basis.

So far, the following tasks have been accomplished:

- Some 4000 substances were subjected to preliminary investigations to ascertain whether they fulfilled the above-mentioned prerequisites for inclusion in the list.
- The question of acceptance of 514 of the substances has been discussed intensively by the advisory committee, in some cases repeatedly.
- 304 substances have been placed on the list of substances (see Annex 4).
- In the meantime, literature searches have been conducted and toxicity reviews have been worked out on 210 of these substances.
- For a number of substances the literature searches have produced no clear-cut results. Hence, a decision has been made to pursue the question further by conducting investigations to ascertain the potential risk, especially in terms of teratogenic, embryotoxic, neurotoxic, genotoxic or carcinogenic effects. For 111 substances, tests – in some cases several tests (358 altogether) – have been planned, commissioned or already completed. For one substance, the performance of a long-term study on carcinogenicity has been planned, for further 5 chemicals carcinogenicity studies are in discussion.

On the basis of the work so far completed, evidence exists that the following 10 substances in the list are carcinogenic:

- N-Methyl-bis(2-chloroethyl)amine [CAS-No. 51-75-2]
- Vinylidene fluoride [CAS-No. 75-38-7]
- Diethylcarbamyl chloride [CAS-No. 88-10-8]
- 5-Chloro-2-aminotoluene [CAS-No. 95-69-2]
- Benzotrichloride [CAS-No. 98-07-7]
- 4-Nitro-2-aminotoluene [CAS-No. 99-55-8]
- 1,2-Butylene oxide [CAS-No. 106-88-7]
- Hydrazobenzene [CAS-No. 122-66-7]
- 3,3′-Dimethyl-4,4′–diaminodiphenyl methane [CAS-No. 838-88-0]
- 2-Chloroacrylonitrile [CAS-No. 920-37-6]

In each individual case, the technical supervisory officer of the BG Chemie has investigated the use of these substances on the plant premises and, wherever necessary, has introduced improvements to the occupational safety measures. At the same time these results are reached to the German Commission for the Investigation of Health Hazards of Chemical Compounds in the Work Area.

In order to make our results available to all interested parties, and in particular to specialists, the BG Chemie began in 1987 to publish the **Toxicological Evaluations** in German. In all, 101 such evaluations have now been published. They have been prepared on the basis of collaboration by scientists, toxicological research institutes (see Annex 3) and the secretariat of the advisory committee, which also undertook the work of sub-editing (see Annex 1).

These evaluations are based on documentation found in the scientific literature, on experimental studies commissioned by the BG Chemie and on experience gathered by the staff of the specialised institutes commissioned to draft the toxicological profiles, as well as by the members of the advisory committee. The members of this committee are in agreement with the toxicological evaluations submitted. The BG Chemie's Principles and Substances Programme Committee has also accepted these evaluations.

The increasing international interest in the **Toxicological Evaluátions** has led to the preparation of this publication in English, the forth volume of which is presented now. Therefore for 60 existing chemicals "Toxicological Evaluations" are available in English at the moment, further 30 will be published within the next few months.

With its "Programme for the prevention of health hazards caused by industrial substances", the BG Chemie intends to ensure that the risks for employees in contact with industrial substances of unknown, but potentially adverse effects are recognized as early as possible and, if necessary, reduced by examining the situation at the workplace as well as by introducing improvements. The BG Chemie is grateful to all persons named in this report, without whose active cooperation the research could not have been effectively pursued. We wish to thank also the many persons, who cannot be named individually here, who have contributed their time and energy to the success of these endeavours.

Annex 1

Members of the Advisory Committee

Dr. G. Fleischhauer (Chairman)
Berufsgenossenschaft der chemischen Industrie
(Employment Accident Insurance Fund of the Chemical Industry)
Postfach 101480, 6900 Heidelberg

Dr. K. H. Adlfinger
Initiative umweltrelevante Altstoffe
(Initiative on Existing Chemicals of Environmental Relevance)
Kennedyallee 93, 6000 Frankfurt 70

Dr. L. Dix
Ciba-Geigy AG, Werksärztlicher Dienst (Works Medical Service),
Betriebsstätte Grenzach (Plant site Grenzach)
Postfach 1120, 7889 Grenzach-Wyhlen 1

Professor Dr. Dr. H. P. Gelbke
BASF AG, Abteilung Toxikologie (Department of Toxicology),
ZNT – Z 470
6700 Ludwigshafen

Direktor Dr. H.-J. Henne
BASF AG,
Abteilung Arbeitssicherheit und Umweltschutz
(Department of Occupational Safety and Environmental Protection)
6700 Ludwigshafen

Professor Dr. D. Henschler
Institut für Pharmakologie und Toxikologie der Universität Würzburg
(Institute of Pharmacology and Toxicology
at the University of Würzburg)
Versbacher Strasse 9, 8700 Würzburg

Professor Dr. H. Herrmann
Jürgensallee 44 m, 2000 Hamburg 52

Dr. R. Jung
Hoechst AG, Abteilung Toxikologie (Department of Toxicology)
6230 Frankfurt 80

Dr. H. Jungen
Deutsche Wissenschaftliche Gesellschaft für Erdöl, Erdgas und Kohle e.V. (German Scientific Association of Oil, Gas and Coal)
Steinstrasse 7, 2000 Hamburg 1

Professor Dr. D. Kayser
Bundesgesundheitsamt (Federal Health Office)
Postfach 330013, 1000 Berlin 33

Dr. U. Korallus
Bayer AG, Früher Ärztliche Abteilung
(Former Chief Works Physician)
5090 Leverkusen-Bayerwerk

Dr. E. Löser
Bayer AG, Institut für Toxikologie (Department of Toxicology)
Friedrich-Ebert-Strasse 217, 5600 Wuppertal 1

Professor Dr. A. Manz
Alter Achterkamp 61, 2070 Großhansdorf 2

Professor Dr. H. G. Miltenburger
Laboratorium für Mutagenitätsprüfung (Laboratory for Mutagenicity Testing)
Technische Hochschule Darmstadt
(Technical University of Darmstadt)
Schnittspahnstrasse 3, 6100 Darmstadt

Professor Dr. R. Preussmann
Deutsches Krebsforschungszentrum
(German Cancer Research Center)
Institut für Toxikologie und Chemotherapie
(Institute of Toxicology and Chemotherapy)
Im Neuenheimer Feld 280, 6900 Heidelberg

Dr. N. Rupprich
Bundesanstalt für Arbeitsschutz
(Federal Agency for Occupational Safety)
Postfach 170202, 4600 Dortmund 17

Dr. H. Schnierle
Hoechst AG, Sicherheitsüberwachung (Safety Monitoring)
Bau C 769
6230 Frankfurt 80

Dr. H. Schweinfurth
Schering AG, Industrie-Chemikalien (Industrial Chemicals)
Waldstrasse 14, 4709 Bergkamen

Permanent Guests

Frau Dipl.-Geoökol. A. Geschke
Bayer AG, Institut für Toxikologie
(Department of Toxicology)
Friedrich-Ebert-Straße 217, 5600 Wuppertal 1

Dr. H.-J. Klimisch
BASF AG, Abteilung Toxikologie
(Department of Toxicology)
ZNT – Z 470
6700 Ludwigshafen

Frau Dr. I. Mangelsdorf
GSF-Forschungszentrum für Umwelt und Gesundheit GmbH
(Research Center of Environment and Health)
Institut für Toxikologie (Institute of Toxicology)
Ingolstädter Landstrasse 1, 8042 Neuherberg

Secretariat of the Advisory Committee

Frau Dr. M. Beth
Frau G. Haass
Frau C. Heumann
Dr. H. T. Hofmann
Dr. W. Huber
Frau Dr. G. Martens
Dr. J. Oberhansberg
Dr. H. Zeller

Address: Berufsgenossenschaft der chemischen Industrie
(Employment Accident Insurance Fund of the Chemical Industry)
Postfach 101480, 6900 Heidelberg 1

Annex 2

Members of the Principles and Substances Programme Committee

W. Schultze
Industriegewerkschaft Chemie-Papier-Keramik
(Chemicals-Paper-Ceramics Trade Union)
Postfach 3047, 3000 Hannover

E. Lechelt
Industriegewerkschaft Chemie-Papier-Keramik
(Chemicals-Paper-Ceramics Trade Union)
Postfach 3047, 3000 Hannover

Dr. K. Molitor
Bundesarbeitgeberverband Chemie e.V.
(German Employers' Association)
Postfach 1280, 6200 Wiesbaden

Professor Dr. K. Kleine-Weischede
Bayer AG, 5090 Leverkusen-Bayerwerk

Chairman of the Board
of the Berufsgenossenschaft der chemischen Industrie
(Employment Accident Insurance Fund of the Chemical Industry)
Dr. D. Dibbern
BASF AG, 6700 Ludwigshafen

Vice-Chairman of the Board
of the Berufsgenossenschaft der chemischen Industrie
(Employment Accident Insurance Fund of the Chemical Industry)
B. Oldach
Uhlandstrasse 78, 2105 Seevetal 1

Managing Director
of the Berufsgenossenschaft der chemischen Industrie
(Employment Accident Insurance Fund of the Chemical Industry)
Direktor H. Lauer
Berufsgenossenschaft der chemischen Industrie
Postfach 101480, 6900 Heidelberg 1

Annex 3

In addition to the members of the advisory committee and the secretariat the following persons were involved supporting the publication of the Toxicological Evaluations:

Dr. V.A. Fung
National Toxicology Program
Department of Health and Human Services
Public Health Service, Bethesda, MD 20892, USA

Dr. B. Görlitz
Fraunhofer-Institut für Toxikologie und Aerosolforschung
Institutsteil Hannover
Nikolai-Fuchs-Strasse 1, 3000 Hannover 61

Professor Dr. F. Leuschner
Laboratorium für Pharmakologie und Toxikologie
Redderweg 8, 2104 Hamburg 92

Dr. J. Leuschner
Laboratorium für Pharmakologie und Toxikologie
Redderweg 8, 2104 Hamburg 92

Professor Dr. H. Marquardt
Direktor der Abteilung für allgemeine Toxikologie
Universitätskrankenhaus Eppendorf
Grindelallee 117, 2000 Hamburg 13

Ms. T. Russel
British Industrial Biological Research Association
Woodmansterne Road, Surrey SM5 4DS
Great Britain

Annex 4

List of substances compiled by the Berufsgenossenschaft der chemischen Industrie (including informations about studies and toxicity profiles)

Name of substance	CAS-No.	Tox. Evaluations			Studies
		S	L	E	
N–Methyl–bis(2–chloroethyl)amine	51–75–2				
Acetamide	60–35–5				
Thiourea	62–56–6				
N,N'–Diphenyl–p–phenylene-di-amine	74–31–7		(1992)		
Chloromethane	74–87–3	05/90			
Vinyl fluoride	75–02–5	05/90	09/89	Vol. 2	A 3; MNT 3
Bromoform	75–25–2	05/90	09/89	Vol. 3	
Vinylidene fluoride	75–38–7	03/88			
Methyldichlorosilane	75–54–7	02/92			
Trimethylmonochlorosilane	75–77–4				
Dichloro dimethylsilane	75–78–5				
Trichloro methylsilane	75–79–6				
Acetone cyanohydrin	75–86–5				
Dicyclopentadiene	77–73–6	03/88	03/88	Vol. 1	
Isoprene	78–79–5	05/90	05/90	Vol. 2	
2–Methylpropane–1–ol	78–83–1	03/88	03/88	Vol. 1	D14orlrat 3; D90orlrat 3; TERAihlrat 3; TERAihlrbt 3
Methacroleine	78–85–3				D90ihlrat 1; CTC 2; D14ihlrat 2; IRS 2; TERAihlrat 2

Methylvinylketone	78–94–4				
Trichloroethene	79–01–6				
Chloroacetyl chloride	79–04–9				
Chloroacetamide	79–07–2	03/88	03/88	Vol. 1	
Acrylic acid	79–10–7	05/90	05/90	Vol. 2	
Chloroacetic acid	79–11–8	11/86	11/86	(Vol. 6)	
Chlorocarbonic acid methylester	79–22–1	03/88	03/88		CLTihlrat 1; D05ihlrat 2; D28ihlrat 2;A 3; AP 3; CTC 3; D90ihlrat 1
Dichloroacetyl chloride	79–36–7				D14 1
Methacrylamide	79–39–0				
Methacrylic acid	79–41–4				
Dichlorodiphenylsilane	80–10–4				
Benzenesulphonic acid hydrazide	80–17–1	02/92	02/92	(Vol. 6)	
2–Nitro–1,3–dimethylbenzene	81–20–9				D28orlrat 2; A 3; CTC 3
1,8–Naphthalic anhydride	81–84–5				
1-Aminoanthraquinone	82–45–1				
3–Nitro–1,2–dimethylbenzene	83–41–0				D28orlrat 2; A 3; CTC 3
Anthraquinone	84–65–1			(Vol. 6)	
1–Nitronaphthalene	86–57–7				
7–Amino–4–hydroxy–naphthalene sulfonic acid	87–02–5				
(Z)–2,3–Dichloro–4–oxo–2–butenoic acid	87–56–9				

Name of substance	CAS-No.	Tox. Evaluations			Studies
		S	L	E	
Diethylcarbamyl chloride	88–10–8	05/90	09/89	Vol. 3	
o–Chlorobenzotrifluoride	88–16–4	05/90	05/90	Vol. 3	A 3; CTC 3
o–Nitrotoluene	88–72–2				
o–Chloronitrobenzene	88–73–3	05/90			D05orlmouse 2; D28orlmouse 2; CTC 3; HGPRT 3
o–Nitroaniline	88–74–4	05/90			
2–(1–Methylpropyl)–1–hydroxy–4,6–dinitrobenzene	88–85–7				
Nitro–p–xylene	89–58–7				
2–Nitro–4–methylaniline	89–62–3				D90orlrat 1
4–Chloro–2–nitroaniline	89–63–4	02/89	02/89	Vol. 1	
Thymol	89–83–8				
4–Nitro–1,3–dimethylbenzene	89–87–2				CTV 3; D28orlrat 2; HGPRT 2; A 3
N–Phenyl–1–naphthylamine	90–30–2				
6–Amino–4–hydroxy–2–naphthalene sulfonic acid	90–51–7				
o–Phthalodinitrile	91–15–6	03/88	03/88	Vol. 2	D14NTorlrat 2; D90NTorlrat 2; HGPRT 3; MNT 3

Quinoline	91–22–5				
4–Nitro–4'–aminodiphenylamine–2–sulfonic acid	91–29–2				SENS 1; D14orlrat 2; D28orlrat 2
Diphenyl	92–52–4	03/88			
o–Chlorotoluene	95–49–8				
o–Chloroaniline	95–51–2				
2–Fluorotoluene	95–52–3				D05ihlrat 1; D28ihlrat 1; A 2; D01ihlrat 2; IRE 2 ; IRS 2; MNT 2
2,4–Xylidine	95–68–1	11/86	11/86		CTCF 2; CTC 2; D01ihlrat 3; D28ihlrat 3; IRE 3; IRS 3
5–Chloro–2–aminotoluene	95–69–2	03/88			DNAC 3; MNT 3
Chloro–p–xylene	95–72–7				
2,4–Dichlorotoluene	95–73–8				
3,4–Dichlorotoluene	95–75–0				
3,4–Dichloroaniline	95–76–1	(1992)			A 3; A 3; DNAC 3; MNT 3
4–Chloro–2–aminotoluene	95–79–4				
2,4–Toluylenediamine	95–80–7				
2,5–Dichloroaniline	95–82–9				
2,4,5–Trichlorophenol	95–95–4	11/86	11/86		
2–Butanone oxime	96–29–7				
Chloroacetic acid methylester	96–34–4	05/90	09/89	Vol. 3	D01ihlrat 3; D28ihlrat 3
Ethylenethiourea	96–45–7	02/89	02/89	Vol. 1	D28ihlrat 3; DNAV 3; HGPRT 3

Name of substance	CAS-No.	Tox. Evaluations			Studies
		S	L	E	
gamma–Butyrolactone	96–48–0	02/89	02/89	Vol. 1	D90ihlrat 1; D01ihlrat 2; D14ihlrat 2; TERAihlrbt 2
1–Chloro–2,4–dinitrobenzene	97–00–7	02/92	02/92	(Vol. 5)	CTC 3; DNAV 3
N–(2,4–Dimethylphenyl)–3–oxobutanoic acid amide	97–36–9				
1,3–Di–o–tolylguanidine	97–39–2	02/92	02/92	(Vol. 6)	
2–Methoxy–4–nitroaniline	97–52–9				D14orlrat 1; D90orlrat 1; D01derrat 2; SENS 2
o–Aminoazotoluene	97–56–3	03/88			
Tetramethyl thiuram monosulfide	97–74–5				
Benzotrichloride	98–07–7	05/90	05/90	Vol. 4	
Benzotrifluoride	98–08–8				A 3
Trichlorophenylsilane	98–13–5				
m–Chlorobenzotrifluoride	98–15–7	05/90	05/90	Vol. 3	D90NTihlrat 1; A 3; CTC 3; CTC 3; D01NTihlrat 2; SENS 2
p–t–Butylphenol	98–54–4	03/88			
p–Chlorobenzotrifluoride	98–56–6				
p–t–Butylbenzoic acid	98–73–7	05/90	09/89	(Vol. 5)	D90NTrat 1; FERTorlrat 3; D14NTrat 1

Benzalchloride	98–87–3	05/90	05/90	Vol. 4	D01ihlrat 2; D14ihlrat 2; D90ihlrat 2
Benzoylchloride	98–88–4	05/90	05/90	Vol. 4	AP 3; MNT 3
Nitrobenzene	98–95–3				
m–Nitrotoluene	99–08–1				
m–Nitroaniline	99–09–2	05/90	05/90	Vol. 2	
4–Nitro–1,2–dimethylbenzene	99–51–4				A 3; CTC 3; D28orlrat 2
5–Nitro–2–aminotoluene	99–52–5	05/90	05/90	Vol. 2	A 3; DNAC 3; MNT 3
4–Nitro–2–aminotoluene	99–55–8				DNAC 3; MNT 3
5–Nitro–o–anisidine	99–59–2	02/89	02/89	Vol. 1	CTC 3; DNAC 3
N,N–Dimethyl–p–phenylene-diamine	99–98–9				D01derrat 1; D28orlrat 1; SENS 1
p–Nitrotoluene	99–99–0				
4–Nitrophenol	100–02–7		(1992)		
Terephthalic acid	100–21–0	05/90	05/90	Vol. 3	
Benzylchloride	100–44–7	05/90	05/90	Vol. 4	
Benzonitrile	100–47–0				
p–Aminodiphenylamine	101–54–2	02/92	05/91	(Vol. 5)	
Dioctyldiphenylamine	101–67–7	05/90	05/90	(Vol. 5)	
Dicyclohexylamine	101–83–7				
N,N'–Di–sec–butyl–p–phenylene-diamine	101–96–2	02/89	02/89	Vol. 1	D28gavrat 2; CTC 3; HGPRT 3
N–Phenyl–3–oxobutanoic acid amide	102–01–2				

Name of substance	CAS-No.	Tox. Evaluations			Studies
		S	L	E	
1,3–Diphenylguanidine	102–06–7				
2–Amino–5–methoxytoluene	102–50–1	02/89	02/89	Vol. 1	
Triethanolamine	102–71–6	05/90	05/90	Vol. 4	D05NTihlrat 2; D28NTihlrat 2; SENS 3
2–Ethylhexyl acrylate	103–11–7				
Phenyl isocyanate	103–71–9	02/92	05/91	Vol. 4	D90 1; TERA 1
Dimethylbenzylamine	103–83–3				D28gavrat 3; D28Fgavrat 3; IRS 3; AP 3; MNT 3
4–Chlorophenyl isocyanate	104–12–1	02/92	05/91	Vol. 4	D01ihlrat 2; D14ihlrat 2; D90ihlrat 2
2–Ethylhexanol	104–76–7	02/89	02/89	Vol. 1	D14ihlrat 2; D90ihlrat 2
p–Nitrosophenol	104–91–6	05/90	09/89	Vol. 2	D28orl 1; CBD 3; D01MHBorlcat 3; D28orlrat 3; DNAC 3; META 3; MNT 3; CLT rat 1
Vinyl propionate	105–38–4				
Chloroacetic acid ethyl ester	105–39–5	02/92	02/92	(Vol. 6)	
Carbonic acid diethyl ester	105–58–8				
2,4–Dimethylphenol	105–67–9				D05orlrat 2; D28orlrat 2

Di–2–ethylhexylamine	106–20–7				TERAihl 1; D28PPihlrat 1; D90PPihlrat 1; D01ihlrat 3; ALARihlmouse 2
p–Chlorotoluene	106–43–4				
p–Chloroaniline	106–47–8	11/86	11/86		MNT 3
p–Toluidine	106–49–0				
Diethylene glycol bis–chloroformic acid ester	106–75–2				
1,2–Butylene oxide	106–88–7	11/86	11/86		
Allyl chloride	107–05–1				
Propargylalcohol	107–19–7	05/90	09/89	Vol. 2	D14ihlrat 2; D90ihlrat 2; MNT 3
Ethyleneglycol	107–21–1				
Glyoxal	107–22–2				DNAV 2
Vinylmethylether	107–25–5	02/92	02/92	(Vol. 6)	D28ihlrat 3; D28Fihlrat 3; MNT 3
2–Acetoxy propene	108–22–5				
m–Chlorotoluene	108–41–8				
3–Chloroaniline	108–42–9	11/86	11/86	(Vol. 5)	A 3; A 3; MNT 3
3,5–Dimethylphenol	108–68–9				D05orlrat 2; D28orlrat 2
Cyanuric acid chloride	108–77–0				
Cyanuric acid	108–80–5		(1992)		
Toluene	108–88–3				TERAihlrbt 3; TERAFihlrbt 3
Isopropyl ethylene glycolether	109–59–1	05/90	09/89	Vol. 3	D28ihlrat 3; D28Fihlrat 3; TERAihlrat 3; TERAihlrbt 3

Name of substance	CAS-No.	Tox. Evaluations			Studies
		S	L	E	
Chlorocarbonic acid propylester	109–61–5				D28rat 1; AP 3
Ethoxyethene	109–92–2				
Tetrahydrofurane	109–99–9				
Tetrahydrothiophene	110–01–0	03/88			D28ihlrat 2; AP 3; CTC 3
1,4–Butanediol	110–63–4		(1992)	(Vol. 6)	D14ihlrat 1; D90ihlrat 1; D01ihlrat 3
2–Butyne–1,4–diol	110–65–6	02/89	02/89	Vol. 1	D05NTorlrat 2; D28NTorlrat 2; TERAorlrat 2; CTC 3; SENS 3; D01derrat 3
Trioxane	110–88–3				
Piperidine	110–89–4				D05NTihlrat 2; D28NTihlrat 2; TERAihlrat 3; MNT 3
Diisopropanolamine	110–97–4	02/92	05/91	Vol. 4	
Diethylenetriamine	111–40–0				
Diethanolamine	111–42–2	05/90	05/90	Vol. 2	D90NTihlrat 2; D14NTihlrat 2; SENS 3; TERAihlrat 2
Diethyleneglycol	111–46–6	02/89	02/89	Vol. 1	D28orlrat 3; TERAgavrbt 3
1,4–Dicyanobutane	111–69–3	02/89	02/89	Vol. 1	

Diethylene glycol methylether	111–77–3	03/88	03/88		
Diethylene glycol ethylether	111–90–0	02/92	02/92		D05ihlrat 2; D01ihlrat 2; D28ihlrat 2
Triethylenetetramine	112–24–3	02/92	05/91	Vol. 4	
2–Methylpropene	115–11–7	02/89	02/89	Vol. 2	META 3; CBDihl 1
2–Methyl–3–butyn–2–ol	115–19–5	02/92	05/91	(Vol. 5)	
Tris(2–chloroethyl)–phosphate	115–96–8	11/86	11/86		A 3; MNT 3; MNT 2
Isatoic acid anhydride	118–48–9	02/92	02/92		MNT 1
4,4'–Methylene–bis(2,6–di–tert–butylphenol)	118–82–1	05/90	05/90	(Vol. 5)	
o–Chlorobenzoic acid	118–91–2				
3–Amino–4–methoxybenzanilide	120–35–4				
Terephthalic acid dimethylester	120–61–6	02/89	02/89	Vol. 1	CTV 3; TERAorlrat 3
2,4–Dichlorophenol	120–83–2	11/86	11/86		
Trimethyl phosphite	121–45–9				
4–Aminobenzenesulfonic acid	121–57–3				
m–Chloronitrobenzene	121–73–3				D28gavrat 2; CTC 3; CTV 3; D01derrat 3; HGPRT 3; IRS 3; SENS 3
Triethyl phosphite	122–52–1				D28orlrat 2; MNT 2; SENS 2
Phenylglycidylether	122–60–1	05/90	05/90	Vol. 3	
Hydrazobenzene	122–66–7	05/90	05/90	Vol. 4	
4–Aminoacetanilide	122–80–5				

Name of substance	CAS-No.	Tox. Evaluations			Studies
		S	L	E	
2–Ethylhexanal	123–05–7	05/90	09/89	Vol. 2	ALARihlmouse 2; D01ihlrat 2; D28PPihlrat 2
Propionaldehyde	123–38–6	02/92	05/91	(Vol. 5)	
3–Methylbutane–1–ol	123–51–3	03/88	03/88	Vol. 1	D14orlrat 3; D90orlrat 3; TERAihlrat 3; TERAihlrbt 3
Acetylacetone	123–54–6				
Diazene dicarboxamide	123–77–3	02/92	05/91	(Vol. 5)	
Dioxane	123–91–1				
Isobornylacetate	125–12–2				
Triisobutylphosphate	126–71–6				D90orlrat 1; A 2; IRSrbt 3; TERAorlrat 3; D01ihlrat 3; SENS 3
Tributyl phosphate	126–73–8	02/89	02/89	Vol. 1	
Dimethylacetamide	127–19–5				TERAihlrbt 3
1,4–Diaminoanthraquinone	128–95–0	02/92	05/91	Vol. 4	
1,4–Naphthoquinone	130–15–4	03/88	03/88		CTC 3; CTV 3; HGPRT 3; ALARihlmouse 2; D01ihlrat 2
1–Naphthylamine	134–32–7				
2–Naphthol	135–19–3				D28orlrat 1; SENS 2
Thiram	137–26–8	05/90	05/90	Vol. 3	

Trimethylphenylammonium chloride	138–24–9	02/89	02/89	Vol. 1	A 3; D01ihlrat 3; D01CHEorldog 3; HGPRT 3; MNT 3
3–Oxobutanoic acid ethyl ester	141–97–9				
n–Heptane	142–82–5				
2–Mercaptobenzothiazole	149–30–4	05/90	05/90	Vol. 4	
Triethylenediamine	280–57–9				D28ihlrat 2; AP 3; IRE 3; MNT 3; SENS 3; SENSF 3
Imidazole	288–32–4				A 2; MNT 2
4–Bromofluorobenzene	460–00–4				TERA 1; A 2; CTC 2; IRE 2; IRS 2; SENS 2; D05ihlrat 1; D28ihlrat 1; D01orlrat 2
Fluorobenzene	462–06–6				IRS 2; MNT 3; SENS 2; D05ihlrat 1; D28ihlrat 1
Dicyclohexylcarbodiimide	538–75–0	11/86	11/86		A 3; CTC 3
Chlorocarbonic acid ethylester	541–41–3	02/89	02/89	Vol. 1	D28rat 1; AP 3
β–Methallyl chloride	563–47–3				
2,6–Dimethylphenol	576–26–1				D05orlrat 2; D28orlrat 2
Mercaptobenzimidazole	583–39–1				
Chlorocarbonic acid butylester	592–34–7				CTC 2; D05ihlrat 2; D28ihlrat 2; AP 3
Carbamic acid butylester	529–35–8				
α–Chloropropionic acid	598–78–7				
1,2–Dichlorobutane	616–21–7				

Name of substance	CAS-No.	Tox. Evaluations			Studies
		S	L	E	
Maleic acid dimethylester	624–48–6	05/90	09/89	Vol. 2	A 3; D01derrat 3; D28derrat 3; IRS 3; MNT 3; SENS 3
Propargylchloride	624–65–7				ALARihlmouse 2; A 3; MNT 2
3–Chloropropanoic acid chloride	625–36–5				D90ihlrat 1; SENS 1; TERA 1; A 3; ALARihlmouse 2; D01ihlrat 2; D05ihlrat 2; D28ihlrat 2; CTC 2
Methoxy acetic acid	625–45–6	05/90	09/89	Vol. 3	D05ihlrat 2; D28ihlrat 2
Manganese (II) acetate	638–38–0				
2,3,5–Trimethylhydroquinone	700–13–0	02/92	02/92	(Vol. 6)	D14gavrat 2; D28gavrat 1
3,4–Dichlorobutene–1	760–23–6				
Diethyl phosphite	762–04–9				D28orlrat 2; MNT 2; SENS 2
1,4–Dichlorobutene–2	764–41–0	11/86	11/86		
4–Nitrodiphenylamine	836–30–6				
3,3'–Dimethyl–4,4'–diaminodi-phenylmethane	838–88–0	11/86	11/86		
Dimethylhydrogen phosphite	868–85–9				
2–Chloroacrylonitrile	920–37–6	11/86	11/86		A 3
N–Methylolmethacrylamide	923–02–4				
Trimethylquinone	935–92–2	05/90	05/90	Vol. 2	CTVorl 2; D28rat 1

Diphenyl–2–ethylhexyl phosphate	1241–94–7				D28PPorlrat 2; TERArbt 2
Manganese dioxide	1313–13–9	02/89	02/89	Vol. 1	D14ihlrat 1; D90 Ihlrat 1
Sodium sulfide (anhydrous)	1313–82–2				
Sodium sulfide (nonahydrate)	1313–84–4				
Antimony (V) oxide	1314–60–9				
Antimony (V) sulfide	1315–04–4				
Iron oxide (Magnetite)	1317–61–9				
Phthalocyanine Green	1328–53–6				
Tricresyl phosphate (mixed isomers)	1330–78–5				
Antimony (III) sulfide	1345–04–6				
tert–Butylacrylate	1663–39–4				
Dimethylaminopropionitrile	1738–25–6				D14ihlrat 3
2–Amino–6–methoxybenzthiazole	1747–60–0				D01derrat 2; SENS 2
1,2–Diaminoanthraquinone	1758–68–5				
4,4'–Diaminodicyclohexylmethane	1761–71–3	11/86	11/86		A 3; MNT 3
p–Nitrocumene	1817–47–6				D28orlrat 2; HGPRT 2; MNT 2; SENS 2
Dimethyloldihydroxyethylene urea	1854–26–8				A 1
2,4–Dinitro–N–methylaniline	2044–88–4	05/90	09/89	Vol. 2	A 3; CTC 3; D01orlrat 3; D01MHBcat 3; IRE 3; IRS 3; D28orlrat 2
o–Chlorobenzotrichloride	2136–89–2	05/90	05/90	Vol. 3	D01derrat 2; HGPRT 2; MNT 2; SENS 3

Name of substance	CAS-No.	Tox. Evaluations			Studies
		S	L	E	
Diglycidylether	2238–07–5	05/90	09/89		
1,5–Naphthalenediamine	2243–62–1	05/90	05/90	Vol. 2	CBD 3; CTC 3; HGPRT 3
2,3,4–Trichlorobutene–1	2431–50–7	11/86	11/86		
Dimethoxy thiophosphonyl chloride	2524–03–0				
Aminoguanidinebicarbonate	2582–30–1	03/88			AP 3; D28gavrat 3; MNT 3; DNAV 2; HGPRT 2
Ethylene glycol mono propyl ether	2807–30–9				
Glycidyl trimethyl ammonium chloride	3033–77–0				
Ethene sulfonic acid, sodium salt	3039–83–6				
(3–Chloro–2–hydroxypropyl)trimethyl ammoniumchloride	3327–22–8				
1–(2,4–Dinitrophenylazo)–2–naphthol	3468–63–1				
2,4–Dichloro–6–methoxy–1,3,5–triazine	3638–04–8	05/90			
2–Methoxy–2,3–dihydro–4H–pyran	4454–05–1				
4–Chlorobutanoic acid chloride	4635–59–0				SENS 1; ALARihlmouse 2; D01ihlrat 2; D05ihlrat 2; D28ihlrat 2; CTC 2

N,N–Dicyclohexyl–2–benzo-thiazole sulfenamide	4979–32–2				
p–Chlorobenzotrichloride	5216–25–1	05/90	05/90	Vol. 3	
Hydroxylamine hydrochloride	5470–11–1	02/92	05/91	(Vol. 5)	
Isobutylidenediurea	6104–30–9	02/92	05/91	(Vol. 5)	MNT 1; TERAorlrbt 2
Manganese (II) acetate (tetrahydrate)	6156–78–1				
2,5–Dimethoxy–4–chloroaniline	6358–64–1				D14orlrat 2; D90orlrat 2
o–Nitrocumene	6526–72–3				
Gallium	7440–55–3				
Aluminium chloride	7446–70–0				
Antimony (V) chloride	7647–18–9				
Thioglycolic acid 2–ethylhexylester	7659–86–1				D07orlrat 2; A 2; CTC 2; D07Forlrat 2; D28PPrat 2
Sodium hypochlorite	7681–52–9	02/92	05/91	Vol. 4	
Hydrogen peroxide	7722–84–1				
Ammoniumperoxidisulfate	7727–54–0	03/88	03/88		
Sodium chlorite	7758–19–2				
Manganese (II) chloride	7773–01–5				
Hydrogen sulfide	7783–06–4				
Antimony (III) fluoride	7783–56–4				
Antimony (V) fluoride	7783–70–2				
Aluminium chloride hexahydrate	7784–13–6				
Aluminium fluoride	7784–18–1				

Name of substance	CAS-No.	Tox. Evaluations			Studies
		S	L	E	
Aluminium nitrate nonahydrate	7784–27–2				
Aluminium sulfate octadecahydrate	7784–31–8				
Manganese (II) sulfate	7785–87–7				
Ammoniumbichromate	7789–09–5				
Antimony (III) bromide	7789–61–9				
Chloro sulfonic acid	7790–94–5				
Sulfuryl chloride	7791–25–5	02/92	05/91	(Vol. 5)	A 1
Hydroxylamine	7803–49–8	02/92	05/91	(Vol. 5)	
Antimony (III) chloride	10025–91–9				
Manganese (II) sulfate (monohydrate)	10034–96–5				
Hydroxylamine sulfate	10039–54–0	02/92	05/91	(Vol. 5)	MNT 2; TERAorlrat 2
Aluminium sulfate	10043–01–3				
Hydroxylamine hydrogene sulfate	10046–00–1	02/92	05/91	(Vol. 5)	
Manganese (II) sulfate (tetrahydrate)	10101–68–5				
Manganese (II) nitrate	10377–66–9				
Sodium bichromate	10588–01–9				
Dimethylaminosulfochloride	13360–57–1	11/86	11/86		

Manganese (II) chloride (tetrahydrate)	13446–34–9				
Aluminium nitrate	13473–90–0				
Sodium tetrafluoroborate	13755–29–8				
Ammonium tetrafluoroborate	13826–83–0				
Potassium tetrafluoroborate	14075–53–7				D05gavrat 1; D28gavrat 1
Zinc diethyl dithiocarbamate	14324–55–1				
Zinc ethylphenyl dithiocarbamate	14634–93–6	02/92	05/91	(Vol. 5)	MNT 1
p–(2,4–Dichlorophenoxy)aniline	14861–17–7				
Sodium hexafluoroaluminate	15096–52–3	02/92	02/92	(Vol. 6)	D14ihl 1; D28ihl 1; D01ihl 1; CTV 1
Sodium bisulfide	16721–80–5				
Tetrafluoro boric acid	16872–11–0				
Di-t-butyl tin chloride	19429–30–2	11/86	11/86		A 3; MNT 3
Manganese (II) chloride (dihydrate)	20603–88–7				
Manganese (II) nitrate (tetrahydrate)	20694–39–7				
Ethylene glycol mono propyl ether acetate	20706–25–6				
Tellurium diethyl dithiocarbamate	20941–65–5				
Dinonyldiphenylamine	24925–59–5				
Diphenyl cresyl phosphate	26444–49–5	02/92	02/92	(Vol. 6)	TERAorlrat 1; MNT 1; D05orlrat 1; D28orlrat 1
4–Isopropyl phenyl isocyanate	31027–31–3				
Styrenated diphenylamine	68442–68–2				D28orlrat 1; MNT 1

Abbreviations

Study type

A	Ames test
AP	Ames test with preincubation
ALAR	Alarie test
CBD	Covalent binding DNA
CLT	Combined long term carcinogenicity study
CTC	Cytogenetic test in vitro (cultures)
CTV	Cytogenetic test in vivo
D01	Acute toxicity study (LD_{50}, LC_{50})
Dnn	Toxicity study after repeated application/exposure (nn=05–90 days)
DnnCHE	Cholinesterase inhibition
DnnMHB	Methemoglobin formation
DnnNT	Neurotoxicity study (+ Irwin screen)
DnnPP	Peroxisome proliferation
DNAC	DNA-repair test in vitro (cultures)
DNAV	DNA-repair test in vivo
F	Follow-up study
FERT	Fertility study
HGPRT	Hypoxanthine-guanine phosphoribosyl transferase test
IRE	Eye irritation study
IRS	Skin irritation study
META	Metabolism/kinetic study
MNT	Micronucleus test
SENS	Sensitization study
TERA	Embryotoxicity/teratogenicity study

Species

rat	Rat
mouse	Mouse
rbt	Rabbit
hamst	Hamster
gpig	Guinea pig
cat	Cat
dog	Dog

Application route

orl	Oral
gav	Gavage
ihl	Inhalation
der	Dermal
ip	Intraperitoneal
iv	Intravenous

Status

1	Planned
2	Contracted
3	Finalized

Toxicological Evaluations

S	Short version (German)
L	Long version (German)
E	English version
( )	Planned for publication

Benzotrichloride

1. Summary and assessment

On repeated inhalation of benzotrichloride by rats, a rise in the excretion of hippuric acid is observed.

Benzotrichloride is toxic on acute inhalation exposure (LC_{50}, rat, 4 hours, 0.5–0.6 mg/l); orally it is of low acute toxicity (LD_{50}, rat, oral, 700–6000 mg/kg).

Repeated oral administration to rats (28 days at 0.5, 5, 50 or 500 mg benzotrichloride/kg feed) leads to slight, dose-dependent, histopathological changes in the liver, kidneys and thyroid gland. There are no effects at 0.5 mg benzotrichloride/kg feed.

On inhalation, benzotrichloride is acutely irritating to the respiratory tract in animal studies. On repeated exposure to rats (28 days – 2 months), in addition to the marked local damage to the upper respiratory tract, the exposed animals develop bronchitis, pneumonia with haemorrhages, weight loss and leukopenia. Degenerative damage to the parenchymal organs and damage to the nuclei in the cortical cells of the central nervous system also occurs. Exposure to a concentration of 5.1 µg/l for 6 hours per day for 28 days can be tolerated without damage.

Locally, the chemical exerts a strong irritant effect on the skin, eyes and respiratory system of rabbits, which can increase to ulcers and necroses on repeated application. Systemically, damage to the testes and proliferation of the bile duct have been described on repeated dermal application to rabbits of doses of 100 mg/kg or more. No systemic effects occur at 50 mg/kg.

After metabolic activation, benzotrichloride is mutagenic in strains TA 1535, TA 98 and TA 100 in the Salmonella/microsome test and in the *Escherichia coli* strain WP2 hcr; it is also mutagenic in *Bacillus subtilis*.

After inhalation exposure at 1 ppm (8.1 mg/m^3) for 6 hours daily, 5 times per week for 1, 3 or 6 months, chromosome aberrations are seen in the bone marrow cells of male Sprague-Dawley rats in all three exposure groups, as well as sister chromatid exchange and chromosome aberrations in the peripheral blood lymphocytes.

Benzotrichloride is carcinogenic to mice treated orally and dermally. In long-term studies involving dermal application of down to 2.3 µl (3.16 mg)/mouse, not only local tumours develop, but lung adenomas and carcinomas are also observed. Also, on oral administration of benzotrichloride in relatively low doses (threshold dose 0.04 mg/mouse, roughly 1 mg/kg) carcinomas are found in the lungs as well as epithelial carcinomas in the stomach. In two carcinogenicity studies in mice, inhalation of the vapours produced at 50 °C and at room temperature (no information on concentration) leads to skin and lung tumours, malignant lymphomas, and a dose-related increase in tumours of the nasal cavities, larynx and lungs.

In an inhalation study in rats and mice over 107 weeks (exposure for 6 hours per day, 5 times per week) at concentrations of 2, 1, 0.4 or 0.1 ppm (16.2, 8.1, 3.2, 0.8 mg/m^3) tumours of the respiratory tract (nasal cavities, larynx, lungs) developed in rats (concentration-dependent) and in mice. A no-effect level was not reported (individual data and data from control animals missing).

Inhalation exposure at 1 ppm (8.1 mg/m^3) for 6 hours daily, 5 times per week for 1, 3 or 6 months leads to metaplasia and hyperplasia of the epithelial cells in the respiratory tract and to papillomas in the nasal cavities in male rats after 6 months exposure; after an observation period of 5 months, malignant and benign tumours of the respiratory tract, skin and external ear canal were found.

Studies on reproductive toxicity are not available, but after repeated dermal application to rabbits, multinuclear giant cells in the testes and degeneration of the seminiferous tubules are seen, as well as local skin damage.

No increase in microsomal enzyme induction is seen in the liver of rats given five intraperitoneal injections of benzotrichloride.

In man, marked irritation of the skin, eyes and respiratory tract have been described after single exposure to the chemical or its vapour. Skin sensitization effects have not been reported.

There are no epidemiological studies on the carcinogenic effect of benzotrichloride alone. Tumours of the respiratory organs have been observed in workers involved in the chlorination of toluene. These individuals had been exposed to benzoyl chloride, and to its precursor benzotrichloride as well as benzal chloride. As these chemicals occur together in the manufacturing process, it is not possible to comment on the carcinogenicity of the individual chemicals involved.

In two epidemiological studies on workers engaged in the manufacture of chlorinated toluenes, there were indications of an elevated mortality from cancer of the respiratory tract and, in one of the studies, cancer of the gastrointestinal tract.

From the available results of carcinogenicity studies on mice and rats and from the established mutagenic activity of benzotrichloride, it can be concluded that the chemical is carcinogenic to animals under conditions which correspond to the possible exposure of humans in the workplace.

The main acute effect of benzotrichloride is its local irritant activity on the skin, eyes and respiratory tract. Benzotrichloride is mutagenic, and carcinogenic to rats and mice treated dermally, orally and by inhalation exposure.

2. Name of substance

2.1	Usual name	Benzotrichloride
2.2	IUPAC-name	α,α,α-Trichlorotoluene
2.3	CAS-No.	98-07-7

3. Synonyms, common and trade names

Benzenyl chloride
Benzenyl trichloride
Benzylidyne chloride
Benzyl trichloride
Phenylchloroform
Phenyltrichloromethane
Toluene trichloride
1-(Trichloromethyl)benzene
Trichlorophenylmethane
Trichlormethylbenzene
Benzotrichlorid

4. Structural and molecular formulae

4.1 Structural formula

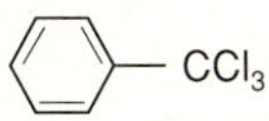

4.2 Molecular formula $C_7H_5Cl_3$

5. Physical and chemical properties

5.1	Molecular mass, g/mol	195.48
5.2	Melting point, °C	-4.8 (Lipper, 1975)
5.3	Boiling point, °C	220.7 (Lipper, 1975)
5.4	Vapour pressure, hPa	0.2 (at 20 °C) 0.49 (at 30 °C) 1.33 (at 40 °C) 1.8 (at 50 °C) (Bayer, 1988)
5.5	Density, g/cm^3	1.3723 (at 20 °C) (Lipper, 1975)
5.6	Solubility in water	Slightly soluble, hydrolyses in water (Lipper, 1975)
5.7	Solubility in organic solvents	Alcohol, ether, chloroform carbon tetrachloride, benzene (Windholz, 1976; CRC, 1981)
5.8	Solubility in fat	No information available
5.9	pH-value	–
5.10	Conversion factor	1 ppm $\hat{=}$ 8.11 mg/m^3 1 mg/m^3 $\hat{=}$ 0.12 ppm (at 25 °C and 1013 hPa)

6. Uses

Manufacture of benzoyl chloride. Intermediate for dyestuffs and pesticides (Lipper, 1975).

7. Experimental results

7.1 Toxicokinetics and metabolism

In 10 rats (strain not specified) which inhaled benzotrichloride vapour (30 mg/m^3) for 2 hours daily for 20 days, the urinary excretion of hippuric acid increased from 14–20 mg before exposure, up to 47 mg after 20 exposures (no information on volumes). The authors suggested that sodium benzoate is one of the initial breakdown products produced from benzotrichloride, and this is metabolized to hippuric acid; however, it was assumed that other metabolites were also formed (Archipova et al., 1963).

7.2 Acute and subacute toxicity

Data on the acute toxicity of benzotrichloride are presented in Table 1:

Table 1. Acute toxicity of benzotrichloride

Species	Sex	Route	LD_{50}/LC_{50} or effect	Reference
Rat		Oral	6 g/kg (14 days[a])	Smyth et al., 1951
Rat	♂	Oral	770 (614–966) mg/kg (14 days[a])	Dean, 1979
Rat	♀	Oral	702 (524–941) mg/kg (14 days[a])	Dean, 1979
Rat	♂	Oral	2188 mg/kg	Bayer, 1978
Rat	♀	Oral	1590 mg/kg	Bayer, 1978
Mouse	♂	Oral	845 (674–1060) mg/kg (14 days[a])	Dean, 1978
Mouse	♀	Oral	770 (614–966) mg/kg (14 days[a])	Dean, 1978
Rat	♂, ♀	Dermal	>5000 mg/kg	Bayer, 1978
Rabbit	♂, ♀	Dermal	4 (2–8) g/kg	Dean, 1979
Rat		Inhalation	LC_{50} (1 hour) 8.39 (7.81–8.97) mg/l	Dean, 1979
Rat		Inhalation	30 minutes was the maximum exposure period during which no deaths occurred on inhalation of a saturated atmosphere	Smyth et al., 1951
Rat		Inhalation	123 ppm (1 mg/l) for 4 hours 5/6 rats died	Smyth et al., 1951
Rat Mouse		Inhalation	1 mg/l (123 ppm) lethal after 2 hours 0.1 mg/l (12.3 ppm) irritation of the mucous membranes 0.03 mg/l (3.6 ppm) no effect	Archipova, 1963
Rat	♂	Inhalation	LC_{50} (4 hours) >0.6 mg/l (73.6 ppm)	Bayer, 1978
Rat	♀	Inhalation	LC_{50} (4 hours) ca. 0.5 mg/l (61.5 ppm)	Bayer, 1978
Rat	♂	Inhalation	LC_{50} (2 hours) 0.15 mg/l at 0.1 mg/l 3/10 rats died	Archipova, 1963
Mouse		Inhalation	LC_{50} (2 hours) 0.06 mg/l	Archipova, 1963

[a] observation period

Groups of 5 male and 5 female Charles River CD rats inhaled benzotrichloride aerosols at concentrations of 2, 4.01, 4.82, 6.01, 10.86 and 20.03 mg/l for 1 hour. The rats showed the following dose-related signs of toxicity: salivation, dyspnoea, reduced activity, gasping for breath, weight loss, marked congestion of the lungs with localized bleeding and, at the highest dose level, dark areas in the gastric mucosa (Cavender, 1979).

The LC_{16}, LC_{50} and LC_{84} values (2-hour exposure) for male rats were reported to be 90, 150 and 240 mg/m^3 respectively, and for mice were 30, 60 and 120 mg/m^3 respectively (strains not specified). The observation periods were 4 weeks for rats and 2 weeks for mice. Symptoms of toxicity seen in rats and mice included excitation, irritation of the conjunctiva and the mucous membranes of the respiratory tract, and hyperaemia of the ears, paws and tail. Histopathological examination revealed inflammation of the respiratory tract with secondary bacterial infection, fatty dystrophy of the liver cells, necrosis of the epithelia of the kidney tubules, dystrophic effects in the myocardium, and swelling of the cortical cells of the central nervous system (Mikailova, 1964).

In another study, 10 male rats were exposed for 2 hours to 100 mg benzotrichloride/m^3 (0.1 mg/l), and were observed for 4 weeks. Three of the 10 animals died (cause of death not specified); after exposure, the remaining 7 showed weight loss (the initial weight was reached again after 4 weeks), leukopenia and a reduction in the daily volume of urine (Mikailova, 1964).

Groups of 10 male and 10 female Sprague-Dawley rats (average weight 60 g) received benzotrichloride at concentrations of 0, 0.5, 5.0, 50.0 or 500.0 mg/kg in their feed for 28 days. Weight gain and feed consumption were not affected, and no deaths occurred. In male rats, an increase in sorbitol dehydrogenase activity was found at dose levels of 5 mg/kg feed and above, and an increase in lactate dehydrogenase activity occurred at 500 mg/kg feed. Haematological parameters were unaffected. Histological examination of the liver, kidneys and thyroid gland revealed slight, dose-dependent effects (liver: pyknosis, vacuoles in the nuclei, necrotic hepatocytes; kidneys: eosinophilic inclusions in the tubule cells; thyroid gland: reduction in follicle size, decrease in colloid density). No pathological changes were evident at 0.5 mg/kg feed. No benzotrichloride was detectable in the liver or the fat of any of the treated rats (limit of detection <0.1 ppm; Chu et al., 1984).

Exposure of 10 male and 10 female rats to benzotrichloride at a concentration of 460 µg/l for 6 hours each working day for 4 weeks resulted in dyspnoea and gasping for breath; all of the exposed rats had died by the end of the first week of treatment. A concentration of 48 µg/l caused dyspnoea and weight loss in 10 male and 10 female rats. In both treatment groups histopathological changes were seen in the nasal conchae and the trachea (inflammation, metaplasia of the epithelium); in the lungs, epithelial degeneration, ulceration of the mucous membranes and general inflammation were seen. A concentration of 5.1 µg/l had no adverse effects (Levin, 1981).

After dermal application of 1 ml (ca. 1.4 g) benzotrichloride to rabbits 3 times a week (duration of treatment not known) erosions developed which were slow to heal, and which were sloughed off after 1 month. Absorption resulted in a fall in the number of leukocytes, from an average of 14,000 to 8000/mm^3 (no further details; Archipova et al., 1963).

The application of 100 or 200 mg/kg/day (on working days only) to the shaved skin of New Zealand rabbits (4 males and 4 females at each dose) for 3 weeks led to an increased incidence of multinucleated giant cells and degeneration of the seminiferous tubules in the testes. Doses of 50, 100 and 200 mg/kg/day caused concentration-dependent skin reddening, scab formation, skin necrosis and swelling of the lymph nodes; histological examination revealed cell infiltration in the dermis, hyperkeratosis and proliferation of the bile duct (Nair, 1980).

7.3 Skin and mucous membrane effects

In a range-finding test, severe eye irritation (grade 10) and moderate skin irritation (grade 5) were found (Smyth et al., 1951).

In a further study, there was a marked irritant effect on the conjunctiva (after instillation of 0.1 ml into the conjunctival sac), but no skin irritation was seen (4-hour patch test with 0.5 ml, 3 male and 3 female New Zealand rabbits, examination after 24, 48 and 72 hours; Dean, 1979).

The intact and abraded skin of white New Zealand rabbits (males and females, weight 3–4 kg, 6 animals in total) was treated with benzotrichloride (dose not specified) for 24 hours, according to the ETAD method (Code of Federal Regulations, Title 16, Section 1500.41). Examination for primary skin irritation took place 24 and 72 hours and 7 days after application. Benzotrichloride caused slight skin irritation (primary irritation index 2.8), which was not reversible after 7 days (Bayer, 1978).

The eye irritancy of benzotrichloride (dose not specified) was tested in male and female white New Zealand rabbits (weight 3–4 kg, 6 animals in total), according to the ETAD method (Code of Federal Regulations, Title 16, Section 1500.42). The eyes were examined 1, 24, 48 and 72 hours and 7 days after instillation. Benzotrichloride caused slight irritation of the conjunctiva and slight, transient clouding of a limited area of the cornea (Bayer, 1978).

7.4 Sensitization

No information available.

7.5 Subchronic and chronic toxicity

Thirty rats (170–200 g, sex and strain not specified) were repeatedly exposed (2 hours daily for up to 2 months) to benzotrichloride vapour [30 and 100 mg/m^3 (0.03 and 0.1 mg/l)]. Ten rats served as controls. The rats in both test groups showed weight loss of 35–76 g/rat after 1 week. Continued exposure led to leukopenia, with an average reduction in the leukocyte count from 14,000 to 8000/mm^3 (down to 5200/mm^3 in a few animals) and then a slight increase to 9000/mm^3, and a fall in blood pressure from 90 mm Hg to 60 mm Hg (method of measurement not specified). Histopathological examination revealed purulent bronchitis, pneumonia, fatty degeneration of the liver cells and karyolysis of the cortical cells of the CNS. A no-effect-level was not recorded. The report of the findings is inadequate (Archipova et al., 1963).

When 25 μl (34.3 mg) or 10 μl (13.7 mg) benzotrichloride was applied to the shaved dorsal skin of female ICR mice (SPF-maintenance), either neat or as a 50% solution in benzene, 2–3 times a week for up to 9.8 months, the mice showed motor disturbances and clear irritation and swelling of the skin, with subsequent hair loss and induration. In a few cases, keratinization, ulceration and necroses were observed at the application site. In addition, irritation of the mucous membranes of the eyes and the respiratory tract occurred (Fukuda et al., 1981).

7.6 Genotoxicity

7.6.1 In vitro

Benzotrichloride (purity and contaminants not specified) was mutagenic in the Salmonella/microsome test in strains TA 1535, TA 98 and TA 100 and in *Escherichia coli* strain WP2 hcr at doses of 0.5 to 2.0 μmol/plate, after metabolic activation by S9-mix from

Aroclor-induced rat liver. Without the addition of S9-mix, the mutagenic effect on TA 100 and E. coli WP2 hcr was less pronounced (data to support this were not provided; Yasuo et al., 1978).

Benzotrichloride (purity not specified) was also shown to be mutagenic in another Salmonella/microsome test in strains TA 98, TA 100 and TA 1538 with metabolic activation (Khudoley et al., 1987).

In the *Salmonella typhimurium* strains TA 100 and TA 98, benzotrichloride had a dose-dependent mutagenic effect at concentrations from 1000 to 100,000 μg/plate, both in the presence and absence of S9-mix from Aroclor-induced rat and hamster livers (Zeiger et al., 1988).

The substance was also mutagenic in a Rec assay (without S9-mix) in *Bacillus subtilis* strains H 17-rec$^+$ and M 45-rec$^-$, at concentrations of 1.5, 2.6 and 3.6 μmol/plate (Yasuo et al., 1978).

DNA strand breaks were detected (by alkaline elution) in human epithelial bronchial cells incubated for 1 hour with 0.1 or 1 μg benzotrichloride/ml. Dose-dependent strand breaks occurred. Benzotrichloride was 3 to 4 times more effective than benzo(a)pyrene in this study (Ming You et al., 1986).

7.6.2 In vivo

Chromosomal aberrations (mainly gaps) were found in the bone marrow of male Sprague-Dawley rats exposed to 1 ppm benzotrichloride (8.11 mg/kg) for 6 hours/day, 5 times a week for 1, 3 or 6 months. Sister chromatid exchange in the peripheral blood lymphocytes was increased in all of the test groups compared with the controls. Chromosomal aberrations in these lymphocytes were no higher than in the controls after 1 month, but were significantly higher after 6 months (Koshi and Fukuda, 1986).

7.7 Carcinogenicity

In a carcinogenicity study, groups of 40 female ICR mice (9 weeks old) were given benzotrichloride by stomach tube at doses of 0, 0.043, 0.17, 0.7 and 2.7 mg/mouse, twice weekly for 25 weeks. All of the surviving mice were killed 18 months after the beginning of treatment. The total numbers of malignant tumours were 0/35 in the control group and 2/37, 11/38, 28/40 and 27/35 in the respective dose groups. The incidence of squamous cell carcinomas of the stomach was 0/35 in the control group and 0/37, 2/38, 22/40 and 24/35 in the treated groups; the incidence of adenocarcinomas of the lungs was 0/35 in the control group and 1/37, 9/38, 16/40 and 10/35 in the treated groups (IARC, 1982; Fukuda et al., 1978).

Fukuda et al. (1981) carried out three dermal carcinogenicity studies in mice (see Table 2).

In the first study, groups of 19–22 female ICR mice (14 weeks old, body weight not specified, SPF-maintenance) received skin applications of 25 µl (34.4 mg) neat benzotrichloride (purity not specified; ca. 860–1380 mg/kg at an assumed body weight of 25–40 g) or 12.5 µl (17.2 mg) benzotrichloride as a 50% solution in benzene (ca. 430–690 mg/kg). The control group was treated with 25 µl (22 mg) benzene. The applications were made twice weekly for 3 weeks and then once a week until the mice were killed in the 32nd week. The total doses of benzotrichloride were 1170 and 585 mg/mouse. At the end of the study, none of the mice in the control group had died, 10% had died in the low-dose group and 46% in the high-dose group. In the high-dose group, 21 out of 22 mice had developed tumours: 12 mice had skin carcinomas, 4 had skin papillomas, 8 had adenomas and 1 a carcinoma of the lungs, and six mice had lymphomas. Of the 19 mice in the low-dose group, 17 had developed tumours: 6 carcinomas and 5 papillomas of the skin, 8 adenomas and 2 carcinomas of the lungs and 1 lymphoma. No tumours occurred in the benzene-treated controls (Fukuda et al., 1981).

In the second study, groups of 10 female ICR mice (3 weeks old, body weight not specified) received skin applications of 10 µl (13.7 mg) benzotrichloride (ca. 340–920 mg/kg at an assumed body weight of 15–40 g) or 10 µl (6.9 mg) of a 50% solution of benzotrichloride in benzene (ca. 170–460 mg/kg). The control mice were treated with 10 µl (8.8 mg) benzene. The applications were made 3 times a week for 4 weeks and then twice weekly until the mice were killed in the 43rd week (controls and low-dose group) or the 24th week (high-dose group). The total doses of benzotrichloride were 580 mg/mouse in the low-dose group and 685 mg/mouse in the high-dose group. At the end of the study, no animals had died in the control group, 60% had died in the low-dose group and 80% in the high-dose group. With the exception of 1 mouse in the high-dose group, all of the animals in the two treatment groups developed tumours. The tumours seen were 3 papillomas and 11 carcinomas of the skin, 11 adenomas and 2 carcinomas of the lungs, 8 lymphomas, 2 lip carcinomas and 1 stomach carcinoma. There were no tumours in the benzene-treated controls (Fukuda et al., 1981).

Table 2. Tumours in female ICR mice after dermal application of benzotrichloride (Fukuda et al., 1981)

	Dose µl/mouse (mg/mouse)	Mortality (%)	1st papilloma after x days	Number of mice with tumours (%)	Number of mice with tumours[a] Skin Ca	Skin Sa	Skin Pa	Lungs Ca	Lungs Ad[b]	Lymphomas	Others
1st study											
Neat benzotrichloride	25 (34.4)	46	70	21/22 (95)	12	0	4	1	8(6)	6	0
Benzotrichloride 50% in benzene	12.5 (17.2)	10	153	17/19 (39)	6	0	5	2	8(0)	1	0
Benzene control	25 (22)	0	–	0/20 (0)	0	0	0	0	0(0)	0	0
2nd study											
Neat benzotrichloride	10 (13.7)	80	58	8/9 (89)	4	0	2	0	3(1)	5	0
Benzotrichloride 50% in benzene	5 (6.8)	60	131	10/10 (100)	7	0	1	2	8(2)	3	3[c]
Benzene control	10 (8.8)	0	–	0/10 (0)	0	0	0	0	0(0)	0	0
3rd study											
Benzotrichloride 9.2% in benzene	2.3 (3.2)	35	210	13/19 (95)	13	0	5	2	9(9)	0	19[d]
Benzene control	25 (22)	20	–	2/20 (10)	0	0	0	0	2(0)	0	0

[a] Ca=carcinoma, Sa=sarcoma, Pa=papilloma, Ad=adenoma
[b] ( )=Mice with multiple adenomas
[c] 2 Squamous cell carcinomas of the lips and 1 cell carcinoma of the fore-stomach
[d] 8 Squamous cell carcinomas and 3 papillomas of the lips, 2 squamous cell carcinomas of the tongue, 2 squamous cell carcinomas of the oesophagus, 2 squamous cell carcinomas and 1 papilloma of the fore-stomach, 1 adenocarcinoma of the stomach

In the third study, groups of 20 female ICR mice (7 weeks old, weight not specified) were treated with 25 µl 9.2% benzotrichloride in benzene [2.3 µl (3.2 mg) benzotrichloride/mouse, ca. 80–160 mg/kg at an assumed body weight of 20–40 g]. The control mice were treated with 25 µl (22 mg) benzene. The applications were made twice weekly for 50 weeks (total dose 316 mg/mouse). The treated animals were killed in the 57th week, the controls in the 82nd week. The mortality at the end of the study was 20% in the control group and 35% in the treated group. In the treated group there were 13 mice with carcinomas and 5 with papillomas of the skin and 2 mice with carcinomas and 9 with adenomas of the lungs. Furthermore, 19 other tumours of different types were observed in various locations (8 squamous cell carcinomas and 3 papillomas of the lips, 2 squamous cell carcinomas of the tongue, 2 squamous cell carcinomas of the oesophagus, 2 squamous cell carcinomas and 1 papilloma of the fore-stomach and 1 adenocarcinoma of the stomach). Only 2 lung adenomas were found in the benzene-treated controls (Fukuda et al., 1981).

Mice (sex distribution, strain, weight etc. not specified) were exposed to benzotrichloride vapour produced at 50 °C (no details of concentration) for 30 minutes/day, twice weekly for 5 months. Lung tumours were found in 17/32 mice (53.1%, $p < 0.001$), skin tumours in 8/32 mice (25%, $p < 0.02$) and malignant lymphomas in 8/32 mice (25%, $p < 0.02$) 10 months after exposure. Only lung tumours occurred in 3/30 (10%) of the control mice. Under the same experimental conditions, benzotrichloride vapour produced at room temperature (no details of concentration) caused lung tumours in 30/37 mice (81.1%), skin tumours in 10/37 mice (27%) and malignant lymphomas in 4/37 mice (10.8%). This study was evaluated 15 months after the end of exposure (Yoshimura et al., 1986).

Female Sprague-Dawley rats and female ICR mice (all 7 weeks old, 50 animals/group) were exposed to benzotrichloride concentrations of 2, 1 (rats only), 0.4 and 0.1 ppm for 104 weeks (6 hours/day, 5 days/week), and killed after 107 weeks. The initial concentration of 2 ppm was reduced in stages during the study because of the increasing number of deaths (no further details). With the exception of the animals in the low-dose group (0.1 ppm), the mortality rate was significantly higher than in the controls. At 2 ppm all of the rats and mice died after 39 and 45 weeks respectively. Tumours of the respiratory tract were seen in 12–92% of the rats (concentration-dependent), and more than half were malignant. Tumours of the nasal cavities occurred in 28–64% of the rats; at 2 ppm they were predominantly squamous cell carcinomas, while at the lower concentrations more than 60% were adenocarcinomas. Tumours of the larynx and trachea were found in 18–24% and 6–12% of the rats respectively. These were predominantly squamous cell carcinomas. Lung tumours were found in 10–35% of the rats (no data on individual incidences, comparison with controls not made). In the mice, 40–46% of the animals had tumours of the respiratory tract, mainly pulmonary adenocarcinomas; dose-dependency was not seen in this species (Fukuda and Takemoto, 1980).

Groups of 30 strain A/J mice (15 male and 15 female) received intraperitoneal injections of 12, 30 or 60 mg benzotrichloride/kg in tricaprylin, 3 times a week for 8 weeks. The total doses were 287, 719 and 1440 mg/kg. The number of lung tumours was determined 24 weeks after the beginning of the study. The mean numbers of lung adenomas per mouse were 18, 43 and 127 respectively, compared with 0.46 in the controls. The carcinogenic potency of benzotrichloride measured in the A/J mouse strain was half that of benzo(a)pyrene (You et al., 1986; Stoner et al., 1986).

Male Sprague-Dawley rats (number not specified) were exposed to benzotrichloride vapour at a concentration of 1 ppm (8.11 mg/m^3) for 6 hours a day, 5 days a week for 1, 3 or 6 months. No neoplastic changes were seen in the groups exposed for 1 or 3 months. Exposure for 6 months induced metaplasia and hyperplasia of the epithelial cells in the upper respiratory tract, as well as papillomas in the nasal cavities. In the rats that were exposed for 6 months and then observed for 5 months, benign and malignant tumours were seen in the respiratory tract, on the skin and in the external ear canal (no further details; Koshi and Fukuda, 1986).

7.8 Reproductive toxicity

When doses of 100 or 200 mg/kg/day were applied dermally to groups of 4 male and 4 female New Zealand rabbits for 3 weeks, there was an increased incidence of multinucleated giant cells in the testes and degeneration of the seminiferous tubules (Nair, 1980).

7.9 Effects on the immune system

No information available.

7.10 Neurotoxicity

No information available.

7.11 Other effects

In order to study the effect of benzotrichloride on microsomal enzyme induction in the rat liver, adult male Holtzman rats (250–300 g) were given daily intraperitoneal injections of 50 mg benzotrichloride/kg for 5 days. The animals were killed 24 hours after the last dose and the activities of O-demethylase (substrate p-nitroanisole), N-demethylase (substrate aminopyrine) and a phosphorothioate detoxification system [substrate EPN = O-ethyl-O-(p-nitrophenyl)-phenylthiophosphonate] were measured. The enzyme systems studied were not affected by benzotrichloride (Ehrich and Carlson, 1979).

The alkylating activity of benzotrichloride was tested in a study of the relationship between depigmentation, carcinogenic activity and tumour promotion. C57-black mice were given benzotrichloride intradermally 4 times at a dose of 5 mg/mouse. In the course of the next 6 months, depigmentation of the hair occurred (Aw and Boyland, 1981).

In an in vitro study, the threshold dose and the no-effect dose were determined for benzotrichloride in cultures of NER-2 cells (no further details) and in human embryo fibroblasts. The cells were incubated for 3 days at 37 °C. The cytotoxic effect was graded microscopically at low magnification according to 4 degrees of severity. A grade 2 effect was viewed as the threshold dose and was detected in both cell cultures at 2 mg/l. Benzotrichloride had no effect at 0.2 mg/l (Grigor'eva et al., 1974).

8. Experience in humans

Benzotrichloride and its vapours are severely irritating to the skin, eyes and mucous membranes of the respiratory tract of humans on acute exposure (IARC, 1982; Windholz, 1976). Another source reports that benzotrichloride vapour appears to be minimally irritating to the mucous membranes, although it has a narcotic effect (Lipper, 1975).

There are no data available on the carcinogenic effect of benzotrichloride alone in humans. However, 6 cases of cancer of the respiratory tract have been observed in workers who had contact with, or were involved in the manufacture of, benzoyl chloride, during which exposure to benzotrichloride also occurred (Sakabe et al., 1976, 1977).

The mortality of 163 workers exposed to various chlorinated toluenes was compared with that of 790 unexposed workers. Analysis of the data was carried out with the aid of standardized mortality ratios and regression models in life tables; for comparison, the mortality rates in England and Wales were used. The evaluation revealed indications of increased cancer mortality in the exposed workers. No other causes of death in the exposed group were increased. Tumours were reported in the respiratory tract and the gastrointestinal tract. Although the workers were exposed to a mixture of chemicals, the authors considered benzotrichloride to be the cause of the increased tumour incidence (Sorahan et al., 1983).

In a prospective mortality study of 697 employees at a chlorination plant in the USA who were exposed to benzyl chloride, benzoyl chloride, benzotrichloride and related chemicals, a total of 47 deaths was observed during the period 1943–1982, of which 44 could be evaluated. No statistically significant increase in mortality was found in the total cohort, but there were 7 cases of cancer of the respiratory tract compared with 2.84 expected. Mortality was increased only in white workers who had been employed for more than 15 years. Because of the small number of cases and the absence of precise information on smoking (only 1 of the dead workers was a non-smoker) the value of the study is limited. However, the data do suggest an association between the toluene chlorination process and an increased risk of cancer of the respiratory tract (Wong, 1988).

9. Threshold limit values

Since 1979, benzotrichloride has been included in section IIIB of the list of MAK values (DFG, 1979).

References

Archipova, O.G., Kochetkova, T.A., Shinkarenko, B.N.
Toxic properties and biotransformation of benzotrichloride
Gig. Sanit., 28, 30–34 (1963)

Aw, T.G., Boyland, E.
Depigmentation of hair in mice by chemicals
ICRS Med. Sci., 9, 29–30 (1981)

Bayer AG, Institut für Toxikologie
Benzotrichlorid – akute toxikologische Untersuchungen
Unpublished report no. 7839 (1978)

Bayer AG
DIN-Sicherheitsdatenblatt (1988)

Cavender, F.L.
FYI Submissioin FYI-OTS-1180-0107
Benzotrichloride acute inhalation toxicity study in rats
Washington DC, Office of Toxic Substances, U.S. Environmental Protection Agency (1979)
Cited in Chemical Hazard Information Profile
Draft Report „Benzotrichloride", March 3, 1982

Chu, I., Shen, S.Y., Villeneuve, D.C., Secours, V.E., Valli, V.E.
Toxicity of trichlorotoluene isomers:
A 28-day feeding study in the rat
J. Environ. Sci. Health, B 19 (2), 183–191 (1984)

CRC-Handbook of Chemistry and Physics
62nd ed., C-166
CRC-Press, Boca Raton, Florida, 1981/82

Dean, W.P.
FYI Submission FYI-OTS-1180-0107
Benzotrichloride acute oral toxicity (LD_{50}) study in mice
Washington DC, Office of Toxic Substances, U.S. Environmental Protection Agency (1978)
Cited in Chemical Hazard Information Profile
Draft Report „Benzotrichloride", March 3, 1982

Dean, W.P.
FYI Submission FYI-OTS-1180-0107
Benzotrichloride acute toxicity study in rabbits and rats
Washington DC, Office of Toxic Substances, U.S. Environmental Protection Agency (1979)
Cited in Chemical Hazard Information Profile
Draft Report „Benzotrichloride", March 3, 1982

DFG (Deutsche Forschungsgemeinschaft)
Maximale Arbeitsplatzkonzentrationen (MAK), Mitteilung XV der Senatskommission zur Prüfung gesundheitsschädlicher Arbeitsstoffe
Boldt Verlag, Boppard (1979)

Ehrich, M., Carlson, G.P.
Hepatic microsomal enzyme induction by trifluoromethyl compounds and some halogenated and nonhalogenated analogs
Res. Commun. Chem. Pathol. Pharmacol., 25, 333–342 (1979)

Fukuda, K., Matsushita, H., Takemoto, K.
Carcinogenicity of benzotrichloride by the oral route of administration (J-4774) (1978)
In: Proceedings of the 52nd annual meeting of the Japanese Industrial Health Association, p 516–517, cited in IARC (1982)

Fukuda, K., Takemoto, K.
Species difference and concentration-effect-relationship in cancers induced by inhalation of benzotrichloride (BTC)
The 44th General Meeting of the Japanese Cancer Association (1980)

Fukuda, K., Matsushita, H., Sakabe, H., Takemoto, K.
Carcinogenicity of benzyl chloride, benzal chloride, benzotrichloride and benzoyl chloride in mice by skin application
Gann, 72, 655 (1981)

Grigor'eva, L.V., Korchak, G.I., Kudzima, G.D.
Determination of the toxic action of organochlorine compounds by the cell culture method
Gig. Sanit., 3, 93–95 (1974)
Cited in Chemical Hazard Information Profile
Draft Report „Benzotrichloride", March 3, 1982

IARC (International Agency for Research on Cancer, Lyon)
Monographs on the evaluation of the carcinogenic risk of chemicals to humans
Some industrial chemicals and dyestuffs, Vol. 29 (1982)

Khudoley, V.V., Mizgireuv, I., Pliss, G.B.
The study of mutagenic activity of carcinogens and other chemical agents with Salmonella typhimurium assays: testing of 128 compounds
Arch. Geschwulstforsch., 57, 453–462 (1987)

Koshi, K., Fukuda, K.
Cytogenetic and morphological findings in rats exposed to benzotrichloride
Mutat. Res., 164, 272 (1986)

Levin, A.A.
FYI Submission FYI-OTS-0981-0122
Benzotrichloride subchronic inhalation study
Washington DC, Office of Toxic Substances, U.S. Environmental Protection Agency (1981)
Cited in Chemical Hazard Information Profile
Draft Report „Benzotrichloride“, March 3, 1982

Mikailova, T.V.
Comparative toxicity of chlorous toluene compounds – benzyl chloride, benzal chloride and benzotrichloride
Gig. Tr. Prof. Zabol., 8, 14–19 (1964)

Nair, K.P.C.
FYI Submission FYI-OTS-1180-0107
Benzotrichloride three-week dermal toxicity study in rabbits
Washington DC, Office of Toxic Substances, U.S. Environmental Protection Agency (1980)
Cited in Chemical Hazard Information Profile
Draft Report „Benzotrichloride“, March 3, 1982

Sakabe, H., Matsushita, H., Koshi, S.
Cancer among benzoyl chloride manufacturing workers
Ann. N.Y. Acad. Sci., 271, 67–70 (1976)

Sakabe, H., Fukuda, K.
An updating report on cancer among benzoyl chloride manufacturing workers
Ind. Health, 15, 173–174 (1977)

Smyth, H.F., Carpenter, C.P., Weil, C.S.
Range-finding toxicity data: List IV
Arch. Ind. Hyg. Occup. Med., 4, 119–122 (1951)

Sorahan, T., Waterhouse, J.A.H., Cooke, M.A., Smith, E.M.B., Jackson, J.R., Temkin, L.
A mortality study of workers in a factory manufacturing chlorinated toluenes
Ann. Occup. Hyg., 27, 173–182 (1983)

Stoner, G.D., You, M., Morgan, M.A., Superczynski, M.J.
Lung tumor induction in strain A mice with benzotrichloride
Cancer Lett., 33, 167–173 (1986)

Lipper, K.A.
Chlorkohlenwasserstoffe, aromatische, seitenkettenchlorierte
In: Ullmanns Enzyklopädie der technischen Chemie
4th ed., Vol. 9, p. 526
Verlag Chemie, Weinheim (1975)

Windholz, M. (ed.)
The Merck Index
9th ed., p. 145
Merck & Co., Rahway, N.J. (1976)

Wong, O.
A cohort mortality study of employees exposed to chlorinated chemicals
Am. J. Ind. Med., 14, 417–431 (1988)

Yasuo, K., Fujimoto, S., Katoh, K., Kikuchi, Y., Kada, T.
Mutagenicity of benzotrichloride and related compounds
Mutat. Res., 58, 143–150 (1978)

Yoshimura, H., Takemoto, K., Fukuda, K., Matsushita, H.
Carcinogenicity in mice by inhalation of benzotrichloride and benzoyl chloride
Jpn. J. Ind. Health, 28, 352–359 (1986)

You, M., Hsu, I.C., Morgan, M., Stoner, G.D.
Induction of lung adenomas in strain A mice and DNA strand breaks in human bronchial epithelial cells with benzotrichloride
Proc. AACR (American Association for Cancer Research), 27, 94, Abstract 369 (1986)

Zeiger, E., Anderson, B., Haworth, S., Lawlor, T., Mortelmans, K.
Salmonella mutagenicity tests: IV. Results from the testing of 300 chemicals
Environ. Mol. Mutagen., 11, Suppl. 12, 1–158 (1988)

Benzal chloride

1. Summary and assessment

On acute oral administration, benzal chloride is only slightly toxic (LD_{50}, oral, male rats, 3250 mg/kg).

A single (7-hour) exposure to the vapour formed at 23 °C causes breathing difficulties together with irritation of the eyes and mucosa. A 1-hour exposure period was tolerated without clinical symptoms. The LC_{50} value (2 hours) for rats is 400 mg/m^3. Local irritation of the eyes and respiratory tract is prominent in these animals, as well as weight loss which is reversible during the observation period. Histological examination reveals inflammation of the respiratory tract, with dystrophic changes in the liver, kidneys and myocardium. No deaths are seen in rats and mice exposed for 1 hour at a concentration of 2000 mg/m^3. More recent studies give an LC_{50} value (4 hours) for male rats of 4300 mg/m^3.

When applied dermally for 24 hours to rabbits' ears, benzal chloride causes marked reddening and swelling of the skin with subsequent necrosis.

In the eyes, benzal chloride produces only transient reddening and swelling of the conjunctiva.

Repeated inhalation exposure (from 14 to 32 days) up to 0.74 mg/l of benzal chloride as vapour results especially in irritation symptoms like lachrymation and salivation. Reduced body weight gain, but no differences in organ weights, macroscopic and microscopic pathology between exposed and control rats are observed.

On long-term (approx. 10–12 months) repeated open application to mouse skin, it gives rise to alopecia, skin hardening and keratinization, in addition to acute skin changes; there are no reports concerning symptoms of systemic toxicity.

After metabolic activation, benzal chloride is mutagenic in *Salmonella typhimurium* (strain TA 100) and *Escherichia coli* (strain WP2 hcr). A mutagenic effect is also observed in *Bacillus subtilis* (rec assay).

In a carcinogenicity study involving dermal application to mice, benzal chloride induces skin tumours (carcinomas and sarcomas). Lung adenomas also occur, but these are seen in a few of the control animals too. The number of mice used in the study groups (10 and 19) is relatively low.

No information is available on human exposure to benzal chloride alone, although there are indications that the vapour can lead to irritation of the upper respiratory tract.

Lung tumours have been observed in workers engaged in the production of benzoyl chloride, in which benzal chloride occurs as a by-product. Two further epidemiological studies on workers involved in the chlorination of toluene suggest a relationship between this process and an increased number of lung tumours. However, because the workers are also exposed to benzoyl chloride, benzotrichloride, benzyl chloride and benzal chloride, an assessment of the carcinogenic effects of benzal chloride and the other three chemicals is not possible on the basis of these observations.

Since 1979, benzal chloride has been classified in group III B of the German list of MAK values.

Benzal chloride causes local irritation and is mutagenic. A possible carcinogenic effect has been noted in the handling of this chemical.

2. Name of substance

2.1	Usual name	Benzal chloride
2.2	IUPAC-name	α,α-Dichlorotoluene
2.3	CAS-No.	98-87-3

3. Synonyms, common and trade names

Benzalchlorid
Benzyl dichloride
Benzylene chloride
Benzylidene chloride
Chlorobenzal
Dichlorophenyl methane
α,α-Dichlorotoluol
Dichloromethyl benzene

4. Structural and molecular formulae

4.1 Structural formula

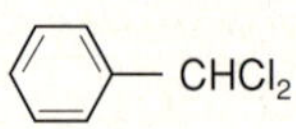

4.2 Molecular formula $C_7H_6Cl_2$

5. Physical and chemical properties

5.1	Molecular mass, g/mol	161.0
5.2	Melting point, °C	–16 (Lipper, 1975)
5.3	Boiling point, °C	205.2 (at 1013 hPa) (Lipper, 1975)
5.4	Vapour pressure, hPa	0.5 (at 20 °C) (Bayer, 1988) 8.0 (at 75 °C) (Lipper, 1975)
5.5	Density, g/cm^3	1.2536 (at 20 °C) (Lipper, 1975)
5.6	Solubility in water	0.2 g/l (at 40 °C; decomposition) (Bayer, 1988)
5.7	Solubility in organic solvents	Soluble in ethanol, ether, chloroform, carbon tetrachloride (Lipper, 1975)
5.8	Solubility in fat	No information available
5.9	pH value	The aqueous solution is acidic (Bayer, 1988)
5.10	Conversion factor	1 ppm $\hat{=}$ 6.6 mg/m^3 1 mg/m^3 $\hat{=}$ 0.15 ppm (at 25 °C and 1013 hPa)

6. Uses

Manufacture of benzaldehyde (Lipper, 1975).

7. Experimental results

7.1 Toxicokinetics and metabolism
No information available.

7.2 Acute and subacute toxicity

The oral LD_{50} value for benzal chloride in male Sprague-Dawley rats following a 14-day observation period was 3250 (2360–4470) mg/kg, and in male CF-1 mice the value was 2460 (1790–3390) mg/kg (no comments were made on symptoms of toxicity; Vernot et al., 1977; Back et al., 1972).

In male Wistar rats, an oral LD_{50} value of 1.80 ml/kg (1.71–1.91 ml/kg; 14-day observation) was obtained following the administration of neat benzal chloride by stomach tube. Signs of toxicity observed included narcosis, lying on the side and general malaise (Bayer, 1978).

Five male and 5 female Wistar rats survived an inhalation-risk test (exposure for 7 hours at 23° C, 14-day observation period). Breathing difficulties, ruffled fur and signs of irritation of the eyes and mucous membranes were observed during the investigation, although these were not seen at the end of the study. Localized emphysematous areas were found in the lungs of the animals dissected at the end of the observation period (Bayer, 1979).

The LC_{16}, LC_{50} and LC_{84} values for male rats (strain not specified) were 0.16, 0.4 and 1.0 mg/l, respectively, and for mice (sex and strain not specified) were 0.08, 0.21 and 0.55 mg/l respectively. The animals were exposed once for 2 hours, and the observation period was 4 weeks for rats and 2 weeks for mice. Symptoms observed in both species were agitation, irritation of the conjunctiva and of the mucous membranes of the respiratory tract, and hyperaemia of the ears, paws and tail. Histological examination of the animals which died revealed inflammation of the airways; during the 12- to 14-day observation period, secondary bacterial infections, fatty degeneration of the liver cells, necrosis of the kidney tubule epithelia, dystrophic changes in the myocardium and swelling of the cortical cells of the central nervous system occurred (IARC, 1982; Mikhailova, 1964).

In other inhalation studies, rats and mice survived 1-hour exposures to 0.5 and 2.0 mg benzal chloride/l (no further details; Back et al., 1972).

A 4-hour LC_{50} of 4.3 mg/l was determined for male Sprague-Dawley rats (HRC, 1991a).

In a further study 10 male rats (strain not specified) inhaled 0.1 mg benzal chloride/l for 2 hours, and were observed for 4 weeks. One of the 10 rats died (cause of death not given). The remaining 9 showed a temporary weight loss after exposure, an effect which was reversed after 21 days (IARC, 1982; Mikhailova, 1964).

In a preliminary 14-day inhalation study male and female Sprague-Dawley rats (5 animals/group; body weights 170–250 g) were exposed to 0.314, 0.742 and 1.496 mg/l benzal chloride as vapour 6 hours a day, 5 days a week for 2 consecutive weeks. Control animals were exposed to air. During exposure signs consistent with exposure to an irritant substance were seen in exposed rats including lachrymation, salivation, irregular breathing, hunched posture and closed/half-closed eyes. In the higher dosage groups body weight gain was significantly lower than controls in both sexes, the food consumption was reduced and the water consumption increased. No differences in organ weights were seen, but in 2/5 males of the highest dosage group petechiae in the lungs were observed (HRC, 1991b).

Male and female Sprague-Dawley rats (10 animals/group; body weights 170–250 g) were exposed to benzal chloride as vapour in concentrations of 0.015, 0.102 and 0.738 mg/l 6 hours per day for 5 days per week for 4 consecutive weeks and 4 further days. Control animals were exposed to air. During exposure half-closed eyes and a diminished reactivity compared with controls were observed in the two higher dosage groups. Salivation, damp orange staining of the front part of the body, red staining around the eyes and/or snout were seen in the highest concentration. A statistically significant reduction in body weight gain compared with the controls was noted in both sexes of the highest concentration groups, also reduced food and increased water consumption. Reduced erythrocyte cholinesterase activity was noted in female rats from all exposed groups and in males from the two highest dosage groups. The highest dosage groups produced a lower volume of urine with a lower pH-value. There were no differences in organ weights as well as in macroscopic and microscopic pathology between exposed and control rats. (HRC, 1991b)

7.3 Skin and mucous membrane effects

Benzal chloride (0.5 ml) was applied semi-occlusively to the hairless skin of the ears of 2 New Zealand rabbits for 24 hours (observation period 7 days). Very marked reddening of the skin and moderate oedema were seen, and skin necrosis developed during the observation period (Bayer, 1979).

The instillation of 0.1 ml into the conjunctival sac of the eye of the rabbit caused slight reddening and swelling of the conjunctiva, increased watering of the eyes and temporary clouding of the cornea (Bayer, 1979).

Irritation of the skin, eyes and respiratory tract were seen in female ICR mice treated dermally with benzal chloride (10 µl neat or 2.3 µl diluted with benzene) for 10 or 12 months (see also the sections on subchronic/chronic toxicity and carcinogenicity). Precise details of irritation at the various doses were not provided (Fukuda et al., 1981).

7.4 Sensitization

No information available.

7.5 Subchronic and chronic toxicity

In the course of a carcinogenicity study in female ICR mice (see also the section on carcinogenicity), dermal application (2–3 times per week) of neat benzal chloride (10 μl/mouse, for 10 months) or of a solution of benzal chloride in benzene (2.3 μl/mouse, for 12 months) caused erythema and swelling at the application site, with subsequent alopecia, induration and keratinization. Decreased motor activity was also found. Compared with benzotrichloride, benzoyl chloride and benzyl chloride, which were studied at the same time and produced similar symptoms, the local effects of benzal chloride were less pronounced. There were no indications of systemic toxicity (Fukuda et al., 1981).

7.6 Genotoxicity

7.6.1 In vitro

Benzal chloride (purity not specified) induced dose-dependent mutations in the Salmonella/microsome assay in strain TA 100 with metabolic activation (S9-mix from Aroclor-induced liver from Wistar rats). The doses tested were 0, 0.6 and 1.2 μmol/plate. The number of revertants at the top dose was higher than the controls by a factor of 5.9. Benzal chloride was not toxic at these dose levels. Benzal chloride also induced dose-dependent mutations in *Escherichia coli* (strain WP2 hcr) in the presence of a metabolic activation system. The doses used were 0, 0.6 and 1.2 μmol/plate, and at the top dose the number of revertants was increased by a factor of 23 (Yasuo et al., 1978).

In a Rec-assay with *Bacillus subtilis* (M45 Rec^- and H17 Rec^+), benzal chloride concentrations of 31 and 62 μmol/plate gave positive results (Yasuo et al., 1978).

7.6.2 In vivo

No information available.

7.7 Carcinogenicity

Benzal chloride was tested for carcinogenicity in mice following skin application. The commercial product was used without further purification (impurities not specified). The chemical was applied to the clipped dorsal skin of ICR mice (SPF origin). In the first study, 10 μl neat benzal chloride was applied to each of 10 female mice (3 weeks old), 3 times weekly for 4 weeks and then twice weekly until the mice were killed at the age of 9.8 months. A control group of 10 mice were treated with 10 µl benzene. In the second study, 19 female mice (7 weeks old) were treated with 2.3 µl benzal chloride (diluted to 25 µl with benzene) twice weekly for 11.7 months. As control twenty mice were treated with 25 µl benzene. All of the mice in the 10 µl group survived. After application of 2.3 µl, 26% of the animals survived the 11.7-months treatment period. At the end of the study, all of the surviving mice were killed, and the organs and tumours histologically examined. Following treatment with 10 µl neat benzal chloride, all 10 mice survived the 9.8-months period, and 4 of them had developed tumours (2 mice had skin papillomas and 3 had lung adenomas). The first tumour occurred after 187 days. No tumours were observed in the controls (10 µl benzene). After treatment with 2.3 µl benzal chloride dissolved in benzene, only 5 of the 19 mice survived to the end of the 11.7-months period. Even so, 16 out of 19 mice had tumours (9 skin carcinomas, 2 skin sarcomas and 1 lymphoma), and 5 had lung adenomas. In the 20 control mice treated with benzene alone, 2 had lung adenomas, but no skin tumours were seen (Fukuda et al., 1981).

7.8 Reproductive toxicity

No information available.

7.9 Effects on the immune system

No information available.

7.10 Neurotoxicity

No information available.

7.11 Other effects

No information available.

8. Experience in humans

No data are available on human exposure to benzal chloride alone.

Benzal chloride (together with benzyl chloride) has been identified as a contaminant in technical grade butyl benzyl phthalate, which is used a plasticizer in the manufacture of PVC floor tiles.

Workers using technical grade butyl benzyl phthalate (contaminated with 0.03% benzyl chloride and 0.3% benzal chloride) in the manufacture of PVC tiles have reported irritation of the upper airways. Concentrations of 0.15 mg benzal chloride/m^3 (PVC tile factory), 0.2 mg benzal chloride/m^3 (manufacture of the coating of the PVC tiles) and 0.03 mg/m^3 benzyl chloride were measured in the air in the workplace. In addition to benzyl chloride, benzal chloride was also detected in the air above a 10-day-old PVC floor covering. The emission rate of benzal chloride at room temperature was estimated to be about 0.01 mg/hour/m^2 (Rittfeldt et al., 1983).

Lung tumours have been observed in workers engaged in the manufacture of benzoyl chloride. In these cases, however, those affected were exposed to toluene, benzotrichloride and to a lesser extent benzal chloride and benzyl chloride (concentrations not specified; Sakabe and Fukuda, 1976, 1977).

In a mortality study of 163 workers exposed to various chlorinated toluenes and 790 unexposed workers, there were indications of increased cancer mortality in the exposed workers (evaluated by means of standardized mortality ratios and regression models in life tables). No other causes of death in the exposed group were increased. The tumours occurred in the respiratory tract and gastro-intestinal tract. The report gave no indications of a carcinogenic effect for benzal chloride alone, and the authors favoured benzotrichloride as the probable cause of the increased number of tumours in the exposed subjects (Sorahan et al., 1983).

In a further mortality study of 697 employees at a chlorination plant, who were exposed to benzyl chloride, benzoyl chloride, benzotrichloride and other chemicals (e.g. benzal chloride), a total of 47 deaths was observed in the period from 1943–1982, of which 44 could be evaluated. No statistically significant increase in mortality was found for the total cohort, but there were 7 cases of cancer of the respiratory tract compared with 2.8 expected. Mortality was increased only in white workers who had been employed for more than 15 years. Because of the small number of cases and the absence of precise information on smoking (only one of the dead workers was a non-smoker), the study is limited in value. However, the data do suggest an association between the toluene chlorination process and an increased risk of cancer of the respiratory tract (Wong, 1988).

9. Threshold limit values

Since 1979, benzal chloride has been included in section IIIB of the list of MAK values (DFG, 1979).

References

Back, K.C., Thomas, A.A., MacEwen, J.D.
Reclassification of materials listed as transportation health hazards
6570th Aerospace Medical Research Laboratory
Wright-Patterson Air Force Base, Ohio (1972)
NTIS-PB 214-270

Bayer AG, Institut für Toxikologie
Unpublished report of 3. 11. 1978

Bayer AG, Institut für Toxikologie
Benzalchlorid, Gewebetoxikologische Untersuchungen
Unpublished study, report no. 8420 (1979)

Bayer AG
Safety data sheet (1988)

DFG (Deutsche Forschungsgemeinschaft)
Maximale Arbeitsplatzkonzentrationen (MAK), Mitteilung XV der Senatskommission zur Prüfung gesundheitsschädlicher Arbeitsstoffe
Boldt Verlag, Boppard (1979)

Fukuda, K., Matsushita, H., Sakabe, H., Takemoto, K.
Carcinogenicity of benzyl chloride, benzal chloride, benzotrichloride and benzoyl chloride in mice by skin application
Gann, 72, 655–664 (1981)

HRC (Huntingdon Research Centre Ltd)
Benzalchloride (No. 58) acute inhalation toxicity in rats, 4-hour exposure (1991a)
Commissioned by BG Chemie

HRC (Huntingdon Research Centre Ltd)
Benzalchloride, 32-day inhalation study in the rat (1991b)
Commissioned by BG Chemie

IARC (International Agency for Research on Cancer)
IARC Monographs on the evaluation of the carcinogenic risk of chemicals to humans
Vol. 29, May 1982 and Suppl. 4, October 1982

Mikhailova, T.V.
The relative toxicity of chlorinated toluenes: benzyl chloride, benzal chloride and benzotrichloride
Gig. Tr. Prof. Zabol., 8, 14–19 (1964)

Rittfeldt, L., Ahlberg, M.S., Zingmark, P.A., Santesson, J.
Occupational exposure to benzylchloride and benzalchloride due to contaminated butyl benzyl phthalate
Scand. J. Work Environ. Health, 9, 367–368 (1983)

Sakabe, H., Matsushita, H., Koshi, S.
Cancer among benzoyl chloride manufacturing workers
Ann. N.Y. Acad. Sci., 271, 67–70 (1976)

Sakabe, H., Fukuda, K.
An updating report on cancer among benzoyl chloride manufacturing workers
Ind. Health, 15, 173–174 (1977)

Sorahan, T., Waterhouse, J.A.H., Cook, M.A., Smith, E.M.B., Jackson, J.R., Temkin, L.
A mortality study of workers in a factory manufacturing chlorinated toluenes
Ann. Occup. Hyg., 27, 173–182 (1983)

Lipper, K.A.
Chlorkohlenwasserstoffe, aromatische, seitenkettenchlorierte
In: Ullmanns Enzyklopädie der technischen Chemie
4th edition, Vol. 9, p. 525
Verlag Chemie, Weinheim (1975)

Vernot, E.H., MacEwen, J.D., Haun, C.C., Kinkead, E.R.
Acute toxicity and skin corrosion data for some organic and inorganic compounds and aqueous solutions
Toxicol. Appl. Pharmacol., 42, 417–423 (1977)

Wong, O.
A cohort mortality study of employees exposed to chlorinated chemicals
Am. J. Ind. Med., 14, 417–431 (1988)

Yasuo, K., Fujimoto, S., Katoh, M., Kikuchi, Y., Kada, T.
Mutagenicity of benzotrichloride and related compounds
Mutat. Res., 58, 143–150 (1978)

Benzoyl chloride

1. Summary and assessment

On intramuscular application, ^{14}C-labeled benzoyl chloride remains predominantly at the site of injection, with only small quantities found in the urine and the faeces after 5 days.

On acute oral administration, benzoyl chloride is only slightly toxic (LD_{50} rat, oral, 2529 mg/kg). The dermal LD_{50} in rabbits is 790 mg/kg.

On inhalation at room temperature of an atmosphere enriched with benzoyl chloride vapour, five out of ten rats die after 7 hours of exposure. Exposure times of 3 and 1 hour are not fatal. The LC_{50} (4 hours) for rats lies between 1450 mg/m^3 (230 ppm) in males and more than 1980 mg/m^3 (314 ppm) in females. All animals show breathing difficulties and irritation of the eyes and nose. Autopsy reveals emphysema, dark-red spotted lungs and lung oedema.

When applied dermally for 24 hours to rabbits' ears (semiocclusive), benzoyl chloride causes marked reddening and oedema with subsequent necrosis.

Benzoyl chloride is severely irritating to corrosive when instilled into rabbits' eyes.

On long-term, repeated, dermal application (uncovered) of undiluted benzoyl chloride, skin hardening, alopecia, ulceration and necroses develop in addition to the local inflammation. Signs of systemic toxicity have not been observed.

Genotoxicity tests carried out with benzoyl chloride in vivo and in vitro give no indication of mutagenic activity.

In two carcinogenicity studies on mouse skin (test period in the first study, 43 weeks; in the second study application for 50 weeks with observation up to 82 weeks) no increase in the incidence of local or systemic tumours was found.

In an inhalation study in mice (30-minute exposures to the vapours formed at 50 °C, twice a week for 5 months, with an observation period of ten months, vapour concentration not specified) there was no increase in the number of tumours of the lungs and skin in comparison with the controls.

In an inhalation study which was not described in detail (estimated concentration 6.8 ppm, exposure twice a week for 30 minutes over 5 months) no lung tumours were seen, and in a second similarly inadequately-reported inhalation study (1.6 ppm, twice a week for 30 minutes) three lung tumours were observed after 14 months. The results of these investigations are of little value as the control levels are not given.

Tumours of the respiratory tract have been observed in workers engaged in the manufacture of benzoyl chloride; however, it is not possible to attribute these tumours specifically to benzoyl chloride, as other products such as benzyl chloride, benzotrichloride and benzal chloride occur in the process of toluene chlorination. Two epidemiological studies on workers in chlorination plants suggest a relationship between the process of toluene chlorination and an increased risk of cancer of the respiratory tract. However, as there is mixed exposure to benzotrichloride, benzyl chloride, benzal chloride and benzoyl chloride in the above process, an assessment of the carcinogenic effect in man based on these observations is not possible either for benzoyl chloride or for the other three chemicals.

Benzoyl chloride is a local irritant; there are no indications that it is mutagenic; the appropriate findings for a carcinogenic effect are absent.

2. Name of substance

2.1	Usual name	Benzoyl chloride
2.2	IUPAC-name	Benzoyl chloride
2.3	CAS-No.	98-88-4

3. Synonyms, common and trade names

Benzoic acid chloride
Benzene carbonyl chloride
α-Chlorobenzaldehyde
Benzoylchlorid
Benzoesäurechlorid

4. Structural and molecular formulae

4.1 Structural formula

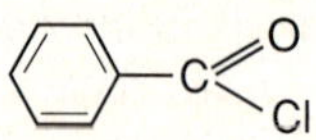

4.2 Molecular formula C_7H_5ClO

5. Physical and chemical properties

5.1	Molecular mass, g/mol	140.57
5.2	Melting point, °C	-0.6 (Wilhelm, 1979)
5.3	Boiling point, °C	198.3 (Wilhelm, 1979)
5.4	Vapour pressure, hPa	0.5 (at 20 °C) 1.33 (at 32.1 °C) 13.3 (at 73.8 °C) 133.0 (at 128 °C) (Wilhelm, 1979; Verschueren, 1977)
5.5	Density, g/cm^3	1.21 (at 20 °C) (Wilhelm, 1979)
5.6	Solubility in water	Insoluble, hydrolyses (Wilhelm, 1979)
5.7	Solubility in organic solvents	Miscible with benzene, carbon tetrachloride, ether, carbon disulphide (IARC, 1982; Kirk-Othmer, 1978)
5.8	Solubility in fat	No information available
5.9	pH-value	No information available
5.10	Conversion factor	1 ppm $\hat{=}$ 5.83 mg/m^3 1 mg/m^3 $\hat{=}$ 0.17 ppm (at 25 °C and 1013 hPa)

6. Uses

Intermediate product; manufacture of pharmaceuticals and dyestuffs; used for benzoylation (Neumüller, 1979).

7. Experimental results

7.1 Toxicokinetics and metabolism

When 10 µl ^{14}C-benzoyl chloride was applied to 3 cm of the dorsal musculature of male Wistar rats, through an incision, only small amounts were found in the urine and faeces after 5 days (3 and 20×10^{-2} cpm, respectively). The equivalent figures for benzoic acid, studied at the same time, were 10^2 and 10^4 cpm, respectively. In 2 further analogous studies it was found that, 3 days after application, the highest radioactivity from benzoyl chloride was present at the application site (27×10^4 cpm), whilst for benzoic acid the equivalent value was only 2116 cpm (Wang and Evans, 1977).

7.2 Acute and subacute toxicity

The oral LD_{50} value for benzoyl chloride in male rats (Wistar TNO/W 74) following a 14-day observation period was 2.09 (1.77–2.44) ml/kg. The symptoms of toxicity were sedation and prolonged convulsions (Bayer, 1979).

In addition, an oral LD_{50} for rats of 2460 mg/kg has been reported (CHIP, 1982).

A single oral dose of 1750 mg/kg given to NMRI/SPFHan mice was fatal to 1 of the 10 mice; signs of toxicity observed were apathy, spasms and shortness of breath (Bayer, 1988).

In an inhalation hazard test, groups of 5 male and 5 female rats were exposed for 1, 3 or 7 hours to an atmosphere enriched with benzoyl chloride vapour at room temperature. After exposures of 1 and 3 hours, all of the rats survived the 14-day observation period. After exposure for 7 hours, 2/5 males and 3/5 females died. Rats in all of the groups had breathing difficulties and irritation of the eyes and nose. Autopsy revealed emphysema, dark red spots on the lungs and pulmonary oedema (Bayer, 1979).

After a single 1-hour nose-only exposure of 10 male and 10 female rats (Wistar TNO/W 74) to 2343 mg/m^3 (398 ppm), all of the males survived but 2 of the females died during the 21-day observation period. For up to 19 days after exposure the rats showed inactivity, ruffled fur and breathing difficulties. Autopsy at the end of the observation period revealed emphysematous changes in the lungs of some animals. After a 4-hour nose-only exposure followed by a 21-day observation period, an LC_{50} of ca. 1450 mg/m^3 (247 ppm) was determined for male Wistar rats and >1980 mg/m^3 (>337 ppm) for females. The rats became inactive and showed dirty, ruffled fur and breathing difficulties, symptoms which lasted for up to 19 days. The visible mucous membranes showed marked irritation. Post-mortems on the dead animals revealed dark red spots on the lungs, emphysema and pulmonary oedema in places (Bayer, 1979).

A dermal LD_{50} of 790 mg/kg was reported for rabbits (CHIP, 1982).

7.3 Skin and mucous membrane effects

Benzoyl chloride (0.5 ml on a 2.5×2.5 cm piece of cellulose) was applied semi-occlusively to the hairless skin of the ears of rabbits for 24 hours. Very marked reddening and marked swelling of the skin were observed at the application site after 24 hours. After 7 days, skin necrosis was evident (Bayer, 1979).

The instillation of 100 µl neat benzoyl chloride into the conjunctival sac of rabbits' eyes caused marked reddening and moderate to severe swelling of the conjunctiva, effects that were present for the entire 7-day observation period. In addition, marked eye-watering occurred, the iris was swollen and reddened and the cornea showed slight, diffuse cloudiness (Bayer, 1979).

7.4 Sensitization

No information available.

7.5 Subchronic and chronic toxicity

In the course of a carcinogenicity study (see also Sect. 7.7) in female ICR mice (SPF-maintenance), 10 µl neat benzoyl chloride or a 50% solution in benzene were applied to the shaved dorsal skin, 2–3 times a week for up to 9.8 months. Marked redness and swelling of the skin occurred, with subsequent hair loss and induration. In a few cases, keratinization, ulceration and necrosis were also seen at the application site. In addition to the local effect on the skin, irritation of the eyes and the mucous membranes of the respiratory tract also occurred. The mice showed no systemic effects apart from over-excitement (Fukuda et al., 1981).

7.6 Genotoxicity

7.6.1 In vitro

Benzoyl chloride was not mutagenic in a Salmonella/microsome test in strains G 46 (his^-), TA 1535, TA 100, C 3076 (his^-), TA 1536, TA 1538, D 3052 or TA 98 (at concentrations of 0.1–1000 µg/plate) or in the *E. coli* strain WP2 (2.1–3.6 µmol/plate) with or without metabolic activation (S9-mix from Aroclor-induced rat liver; McMahon et al., 1979; Yasuo et al., 1978). There was no indication of the purity of the samples tested or the identity of any contaminants, and no mention of bacteriotoxic activity. The authors suggested that the lack of mutagenicity of benzoyl chloride was connected with its rapid hydrolysis (Yasuo et al., 1978).

In another publication, benzoyl chloride was reported to be weakly mutagenic in strain TA 98 at a dose of 10 µmol/plate without metabolic activation (Chiu et al., 1978). However, the precise details are unclear, so that an evaluation is not possible.

Benzoyl chloride was studied in a pre-incubation test (30 minutes at 30 °C) in the *Salmonella typhimurium* strains TA 1535, TA 100, TA 1537 and TA 98 at concentrations of up to 3600 µg/tube.

No bacteriotoxic effect was seen at up to 900 µg/tube, but benzoyl chloride was toxic at higher levels (1200 to 3000 µg/tube). Precipitation of the substance occurred from 450 µg/tube. There was no evidence of mutagenic activity (Bayer, 1989).

In a Rec-assay in *Bacillus subtilis* (strains M45-Rec$^-$ and H17-Rec$^+$) benzoyl chloride was not genotoxic at concentrations of 0.4 and 0.7 µmol/plate (Yasuo et al., 1978).

7.6.2 In vivo

In a micronucleus test, a single oral dose of 1750 mg benzoyl chloride/kg was given by stomach tube to groups of 5 male and 5 female mice, and their bone marrow was studied 24, 48 and 72 hours later. In a preliminary study, this dose was lethal to 1/10 mice and caused clear toxic effects (apathy, spasms, shortness of breath) in all of the animals. No evidence of a clastogenic effect was seen in the micronucleus test (Bayer, 1988).

7.7 Carcinogenicity

Benzoyl chloride was tested for carcinogenic activity in female ICR mice following dermal application. Three groups of 10 mice (3 weeks old, body weight not specified) were treated with 10 µl of the neat commercial product (equivalent to 12.1 mg; ca. 300–800 mg/kg with an assumed body weight of 15–40 g) or 10 µl of a 50% solution of benzoyl chloride in benzene (equivalent to 6.1 mg; ca. 150–400 mg/kg). This was applied to the clipped dorsal skin 3 times a week for 4 weeks and then twice weekly until week 43. The controls were treated with 10 µl benzene. The mice were killed after 43 weeks (all had survived up to this time); the benzoyl chloride-treated mice had each received total doses of 1065 or 533 mg. No information was given on body weight gain. Two mice in the low-dose group had skin tumours (1 papilloma, 1 squamous epithelial carcinoma), and within 3 mice in the high-dose group 3 lung adenomas were found. No tumours occurred in the control group (which suggests that the study duration was inadequate).

In a second study, 2 groups of 20 female ICR mice were used (7 weeks old, body weight not specified). One group was treated with 25 µl of a 9.2% solution of benzoyl chloride in benzene (2.3 µl equivalent to 2.8 mg benzoyl chloride, corresponding to ca. 70–140 mg/kg with an assumed body weight of 20–40 g), the control group received 25 µl benzene. The solutions were applied to the shaved dorsal skin of the mice twice weekly for 50 weeks, with a total dose per mouse of 278 mg. The mice were killed in the 82nd week. At this time, 5% of the animals in the test group were either dead or moribund, while the corresponding figure for the control group was 20%. Two out of 20 mice in the test group had squamous epithelial carcinomas of the skin; no skin tumours were found in the controls. Lung adenomas were found in 5 of the treated mice and 2 of the controls. There was no significant difference between the incidence of skin tumours in the test groups and that in the controls in either study (Fukuda et al., 1981).

Twenty female ICR mice (5 weeks old) were exposed to an estimated average benzoyl chloride concentration of 6.8 ppm for 30 minute periods, twice weekly for 5 months (no further details of the protocol are available). There was no increase in the incidence of lung tumours. On histological examination, slight adenoid proliferation was found in the trachea and bronchi of 2 mice (Takemoto et al., 1978).

Female ICR-ICL mice (5 weeks old, exact number not specified) were exposed to an estimated average concentration of 1.6 ppm benzoyl chloride for 30 minutes, twice weekly for 5 months. The mice were then observed for a further 14 months. No lesions or tumours were found after 6 months. After 10 months, examination of 13 mice revealed skin papillomas and tracheal epithelial proliferation in 2 animals. After 14 months, adenocarcinomas of the lungs were found in 2 of a further 7 mice, and 1 other animal had a lung adenoma. Details of controls were not given (Yoshimura et al., 1979).

In an inhalation study, white mice (number, sex, strain, age etc. not specified) were exposed to a benzoyl chloride-containing atmosphere at 50 °C (no details on vapour generation or concentration measurements) for 30 minutes daily, twice weekly for 5 months and were then observed for 10 months. Lung tumours were found in 3/28 mice (10.7%) and skin tumours in 2/28 (7.1%; no details of histological examination given). According to the authors, this was not significantly different from the controls. Only an English summary of this Japanese study is currently available (Yoshimura et al., 1986).

7.8 Reproductive toxicity

No information available.

7.9 Effects on the immune system

No information available.

7.10 Neurotoxicity

No information available.

7.11 Other effects

No information available.

8. Experience in humans

Benzoyl chloride is classified as being a strong lacrimatory irritant and irritating to the skin, eyes and mucous membranes, although original work to support this statement is not available (Kirk-Othmer, 1978; Windholz, 1976).

Three cases of lung cancer have been reported amongst workers at a factory which manufactured benzoyl chloride from 1954–1972. Of the 147 people employed during this period, 41 were involved in benzoyl chloride production, and 4 of these 41 developed malignant tumours after 6–15 years of employment. A 44-year-old non-smoker had a squamous cell carcinoma in the left hilum of the lung. Two 44-year-old smokers developed lung tumours which were not histologically classified. The fourth case was diagnosed as a maxillary malignant lymphoma in a 49-year-old worker. The time between the start of exposure and diagnosis ranged from 6 to 18 years (Sakabe et al., 1976).

The same authors reported 2 more cases of lung cancer in a factory where benzoyl chloride was produced. One was a 40-year-old smoker involved in benzoyl peroxide production for 17 years, who was also exposed to benzoyl chloride for 7 years during this period; the latent period was 13 years. The second was a 35-year-old non-smoker involved in benzoyl peroxide production for 4 years, who was then employed in the manufacture of benzoyl chloride for about 2 years. He subsequently worked in an office for 7 years. From the age of 25 he had been treated for obstructive lung disease with chronic bronchitis, emphysema and bronchial ectasia, before lung cancer (squamous epithelial carcinoma) was diagnosed (Sakabe and Fukuda, 1977).

In all these cases, the people affected were exposed not only to benzoyl chloride but also to the precursors (toluene, benzotrichloride and, in smaller quantities, benzal chloride and benzyl chloride) involved in its production (Sakabe et al., 1976; Sakabe and Fukuda, 1977).

In a mortality study of 163 workers exposed to various chlorinated toluenes and 790 unexposed workers, there were indications of increased cancer mortality in the exposed workers (evaluated by means of standardized mortality ratios and regression models in life tables). No other causes of death in the exposed group were increased. The tumours occurred in the respiratory tract and gastro-intestinal tract. The authors favoured benzotrichloride as the probable cause of the increased number of tumours in the exposed subjects (Sorahan et al., 1983).

In a further mortality study of 697 employees at a chlorination plant, who were exposed to benzyl chloride, benzoyl chloride, benzotrichloride and other chemicals, a total of 47 deaths was observed in the period from 1943–1982, of which 44 could be evaluated. No statistically significant increase in mortality was found for the total cohort, but there were 7 cases of cancer of the respiratory tract compared with 2.84 expected. Mortality was increased only in white workers who had been employed for more than 15 years. Because of the small number of cases and the absence of precise information on smoking (only one of the dead workers was a non-smoker), the study is limited in value. However, the data do suggest an association between the toluene chlorination process and an increased risk of cancer of the respiratory tract (Wong, 1988).

9. Threshold limit values

No information available.

References

Bayer AG, Institut für Toxikologie
Benzoylchlorid, Gewerbetoxikologische Untersuchung
Unpublished report No. 8418 (1979)

Bayer AG, Fachbereich Toxikologie
Benzoylchloride, Micronucleus test on the mouse to evaluate for clastogenic effects
Unpublished report No. 17383 (1988)
commissioned by BG Chemie, Heidelberg

Bayer AG, Fachbereich Toxikologie
Benzoylchloride, Salmonella/microsome test to evaluate for point mutagenic effects. Preincubation method
Unpublished report No. 17635 (1989)
commissioned by BG Chemie, Heidelberg

CHIP (Chemical Hazard Information Profile)
Draft Report Benzoylchloride
June 30 (1982)

Chiu, C.W., Lee, L.H., Wang, C.Y., Bryan, G.T.
Mutagenicity of some commercially available nitro compounds for *Salmonella typhimurium*
Mutat. Res., 58, 11 (1978)

Fukuda, K., Matsushita, H., Sakabe, H., Takemoto, K.
Carcinogenicity of benzyl chloride, benzal chloride, benzotrichloride and benzoyl chloride in mice by skin application
Gann, 72, 655 (1981)

IARC (International Agency for Research on Cancer)
IARC Monographs on the evaluation of the carcinogenic risk of chemicals to humans
Vol. 29, p. 83–91
IARC, Lyon, France (1982)

Kirk-Othmer (eds.)
Encyclopedia of chemical technology
3rd ed., Vol. 3, p. 786
John Wiley and Sons, New York (1978)

McMahon, R.E., Cline, J.C., Thompson, C.Z.
Assay of 855 test chemicals in ten tester strains using a new modification of the Ames Test for bacterial mutagens
Cancer Res., 39, 682 (1979)

Neumüller, O.A. (ed.)
Römpps Chemie-Lexikon
8th ed., p. 408
Franckh'sche Verlagsbuchhandlung, Stuttgart (1979)

Sakabe, H., Matsushita, H., Koshi, S.
Cancer among benzoyl chloride manufacturing workers
Ann. N.Y. Acad. Sci., 271, 67–70 (1976)

Sakabe, H., Fukuda, K.
An updating report on cancer among benzoylchloride manufacturing workers
Ind. Health, 15, 173 (1977)

Sorahan, T., Waterhouse, J.A.H., Cooke, M.A., Smith, E.M.B., Jackson, J.R., Temkin, L.
A mortality study of workers in a factory manufacturing chlorinated toluenes
Ann. Occ. Hyg., 27, 173–182 (1983)

Takemoto, K., Yoshimura, H., Matsushita, S.
Experiment of pulmonary tumorigenicity of benzotrichloride
Proc. of 51st Annual Meeting of Japan. Assoc. of Ind. Health, p. 514–515 (1978)
cited in: CHIP (1982)

Wilhelm, W.
Benzoesäure
in: Ullmann's Encyclopedia of chemical technology
4th ed., Vol. 8, p. 372
Verlag Chemie, Weinheim (1979)

Verschueren, K.
Handbook of environmental data on organic chemicals, p. 124
Van Nostrand Reinhold, New York (1977)

Wang, P.Y., Evans, D.W.
Adhesion of synthetic organic polymer to soft tissue
IV. Evaluation of a silicon adhesive system
Biomat. Med. Dev. Art. Org., 5 (3), 277–291 (1977)

Windholz, M. (ed.)
The Merck Index
9th ed., p. 146
Merck and Co., Rahway, N.J. (1976)

Wong, O.
A cohort mortality study of employees exposed to chlorinated chemicals
Am. J. Ind. Med., 14, 417–431 (1988)

Yasuo, K., Fujimoto, S., Katoh, M., Kikuchi, Y., Kada, T.
Mutagenicity of benzotrichloride and related compounds
Mutat. Res., 58, 143 (1978)

Yoshimura, H., Takemoto, K., Fukuda, K., Matsushita, S.
Carcinogenicity in mice by inhalation of benzotrichloride and benzoyl chloride
Sangyo Igaku, 28, 352–359 (1986)

Yoshimura, H., Katayama, H., Takemoto, K., Matsushita, S.
Experimental lung tumors induced by exposure to benzotrichloride
Proc. Japan Assoc. Ind. Health, p. 332–333 (1979)
Cited in: CHIP (1982)

Benzyl chloride

1. Summary and assessment

On oral administration, benzyl chloride is rapidly absorbed, distributed and excreted in the urine (65–75%) and the faeces (14–16%) within 24 hours. The concentration of ^{14}C in the forestomach after 24 hours is approximately four times higher than that in the stomach. Following inhalation exposure, the level of radioactivity is roughly the same in the urine and the faeces, whereas after oral administration excretion is predominantly in the urine.

In vivo studies have shown that in the liver, under conditions where glutathione is depleted, benzyl chloride is metabolised to mercapturic acid and to benzoic acid in the rabbit and hippuric acid in the rat, and is largely excreted in the urine. It is also quickly eliminated after subcutaneous and intravenous administration. On intravenous injection after 1 hour there is a high rate of alkylation of DNA in the central nervous system, liver and testes, but this falls rapidly.

Local irritation of the mucous membranes, eyes and skin is prominent among the acute effects of benzyl chloride. On repeated dermal application, erythema, swelling, skin hardening and keratinization occur.

The LD_{50} value (rat, oral) is 1230 mg/kg, the animals showing inflammation and ulceration of the gastric mucosa, oedema of the heart, lungs and liver, as well as myocardial necrosis. An LC_{50} value (rats, 4 hours) of approximately 4 mg/l (760 ppm) has been reported, with inflammation of the airways and damage to the liver, kidneys and heart muscle. Reversible disturbances of liver function are observed on single exposure by the oral, parenteral and inhalation routes.

Sensitization studies indicate a possible skin sensitization potential, although the designs of these studies do not meet current standards.

Repeated oral administration (15, 30 or 62 mg/kg by stomach tube for 6 months) gives rise to hyperkeratosis and hyperplasia in the forestomach and to necroses in the heart muscle. A basalcell carcinoma was found in the fore-stomach of one female rat after repeated administration of 62 mg/kg for 6 months. The no effect level is 15 mg/kg in females, and <15 mg/kg in males. Similar changes were seen in rats in a further 6-months study involving oral administration three times a week; hyperplasia of the epithelium of the fore-stomach and myocardial necrosis occured at 30 mg/kg in rats. In B6C3F1 mice, liver damage was observed at 50 mg/kg.

In a 4-week inhalation study in rats, guinea-pigs and hamsters, the no effect level in rats and hamsters was 35 ppm (180 mg/m^3) and in male guinea-pigs was 12 ppm (60 mg/m^3). Higher concentrations caused irritatioin of the eyes and mucous membranes, together with breathing difficulties and weight loss. In a 27-week inhalation study in Sprague-Dawley rats and guinea-pigs, the no effect levels after daily 6-hr exposures were 62 mg/m^3 (about 12 ppm) in rats and 5 mg/m^3 (about 1 ppm) in guinea-pigs.

Benzyl chloride causes alkylation in vitro and in vivo. On intravenous administration to mice, alkylation of the DNA occurs in the brain and testes, and also in the liver, lungs and spleen. Alkylation of the haemoglobin is also seen. The alkylating activity in vitro parallels the direct mutagenic activity of benzyl chloride in *Salmonella typhimurium* strains TA 98 and TA 100 (base-pair mutations without S9 mix); with S9 mix the mutagenic effect is diminished in most cases. Benzyl chloride is mutagenic to animal cells and yeasts tested in vitro. Benzyl chloride causes DNA-damage in bacteria, mouse lymphoma cells and human cells in culture. It also induces unscheduled DNA synthesis in animal cells in vitro. Chromosome aberrations and sister chromatid exchange are observed in rodent cells tested in vitro, but in human lymphocytes only sister chromatid exchange has been seen. In *Drosophila melanogaster* there are no conclusive results to support a mutagenic effect. Negative results have been obtained with benzyl chloride in the micronucleus test in mice, in tests for chromosome aberrations in rats and in the host-mediated assay. Benzyl chloride causes cell transformation in embryonic Syrian hamster/BHK cells.

No anomalies are seen in the sperm of mice given benzyl chloride.

In a 2-year gavage study in rats and mice, an increased incidence of C-cell carcinomas and papillomas of the thyroid gland is observed in female rats in the high-dose group (30 mg/kg) and an increased number of forestomach tumours is seen in male and female mice in the high-dose group (100 mg/kg). Subcutaneous injection of benzyl chloride to rats gives rise to local sarcomas and lung metastases. In skin-painting studies on mice, a few skin tumours are formed, but the increased incidence is not significant. Interim reports are available from two studies involving skin application of benzyl chloride to mice, either alone or after prior application of a promoter, croton oil. No tumours have yet been observed after 7 and 10 months, respectively. No significant increase in lung adenomas is found in mice after intraperitoneal administration of benzyl chloride for 24 weeks.

In man, irritation of the eyes and respiratory tract is observed on inhalation exposure to benzyl chloride. More marked eye-watering occurs at 50 mg/m^3 (10 ppm), and 80 mg/m^3 (16 ppm) leads to severe irritation. In people exposed to 10 mg/m^3 (about 2 ppm) general systemic effects such as fatigue, headache and disturbance of liver functions were reported in addition to the irritant effects. According to a further communication, 25 mg/m^3 (5 ppm) should be considered unacceptable in the working environment. Pustule-formation on the skin has been reported as a local effect of benzyl chloride. Lung tumours have been observed in workers engaged in the production of benzoyl chloride. As benzyl chloride also appears in the manufacturing process, a carcinogenic risk from the latter cannot be excluded. A similar judgement was reached in two further epidemiological studies of workers involved in the chlorination of toluene.

Since 1979, benzyl chloride has been classified in category III B in the German list of MAK values.

Benzyl chloride causes local irritation, alkylation and mutation. It has been shown to have carcinogenic potential.

2. Name of substance

2.1	Usual name	Benzyl chloride
2.2	IUPAC-name	α-Chlorotoluene
2.3	CAS-No.	100-44-7

3. Synonyms, common and trade names

Benzylchlorid
Chloromethylbenzene
Chlorophenylmethane
α-Tolyl chloride

4. Structural and molecular formulae

4.1 Structural formula

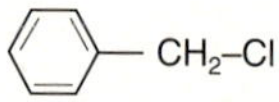

4.2 Molecular formula C_7H_7Cl

5. Physical and chemical properties

5.1	Molecular mass, g/mol	126.59
5.2	Melting point, °C	–39.2 (Lipper, 1975)
5.3	Boiling point, °C	179.4 (Lipper, 1975)
5.4	Vapour pressure, hPa	0.51 (at 10 °C) (Lipper, 1975) 1.3 (at 22 °C) 13.3 (at 60.8 °C) 79.6 (at 100 °C)
5.5	Density, g/cm^3)	1.1002 (at 20 °C) (Lipper, 1975)
5.6	Solubility in water	Slight (0.46 g/l at 30 °C) (Lipper, 1975)
5.7	Solubility in organic solvents	Slightly soluble in alcohol, ether, chloroform, carbon tetrachloride (Lipper, 1975)
5.8	Solubility in fat	No information available
5.9	pH-value	–
5.10	Conversion factor	1 ppm $\hat{=}$ 5.25 mg/m^3 1 mg/m^3 $\hat{=}$ 0.19 ppm (at 25 °C and 1013 hPa)

6. Uses

Manufacture of benzyl alcohol and butylbenzyl phthalate (70–80%), production of synthetic penicillin, disinfectants, dyestuffs, aromatic oils, antioxidants and emulsifiers (Lipper, 1975).

7. Experimental results

7.1 Toxicokinetics and metabolism

Benzyl chloride was rapidly absorbed following oral administration and was mainly excreted in the urine. ^{14}C-benzyl chloride in corn oil was administered to male and female rats (Fischer 344/N) at a dose of 25 mg/kg, and 4 animals were killed 3, 6 and 24 hours after administration. The radioactivity was measured in the blood, heart, stomach, gut, lungs, liver, kidneys, muscle tissue, fat, urine and faeces. In the urine, 15, 41 and 65% of the administered radioactivity was found after 3, 6 and 24 hours respectively in the males, while in females the corresponding figures were 23, 54 and 74%. After 24 hours, 14% and 16% of the activity was found in the faeces of males and females respectively. After 3 hours, ca. 6–8% of the activity was present in the gastro-intestinal tract, while 0.6–0.8% was detectable after 24 hours; 3.5–3.6% of the activity was found in the muscle tissue after 3 hours, and 1.5–1.7% after 24 hours. In the liver, ca. 1% was found after 3 hours and 0.6–0.7% after 24 hours. The corresponding figures for the blood were 1.3–1.7% after 3 hours and 0.9–1.3% after 24 hours. Based on the distribution of ^{14}C (expressed as microgram equivalents of ^{14}C-benzyl chloride) the highest levels of radioactivity were found in the gastro-intestinal tract. However, it was noticed that after 24 hours the concentration of ^{14}C in the fore-stomach (14 μg × eq/g in females, 22 μg × eq/g in males) was about 4 times higher than that in the stomach (4 μg × eq/g in females, 5 μg × eq/g in males). The liver and kidneys had constantly higher isotope concentrations than the blood (at 3 hours, 10–12 and 12–70 μg × eq/g, respectively in the liver and kidneys compared with 5–6.6 μg × eq/g in the blood). The isotope concentration in the heart, muscle and fat was at no time higher than that in the blood (Bunner and Creasia, 1982).

According to Rao (1985) the half-life for elimination from the blood was 1.12 hours (no further details).

Groups of 10 male B6C3F1 mice were given ^{14}C-benzyl chloride either once orally by stomach tube at doses of 100 or 10 mg/kg body weight or once by inhalation (6 hours) at concentrations of 15 or 5 mg/m^3 (uptake by the mice 10 and ca. 3 mg/kg body weight respectively). Some of the animals were killed 1 day after oral administration or inhalation exposure, and the rest 5 days after treatment. The radioactivity in the various tissues of the mice was determined. Whole body autoradiography was carried out as well as studies of the covalent binding in the various organs. After oral administration of the high dose the radioactivity was eliminated mainly in the urine (about 62% in the urine and 0.32% in the faeces, measured at 24 hours), while after administration of the low dose similar levels of activity were found in the urine and faeces (about 34 and 45% respectively). After oral administration of 100 mg/kg, a significantly higher level of activity was found in the fore-stomach (5.29 µg/g tissue) than in the stomach (0.8 µg/g tissue), liver (0.6 µg/g tissue, kidneys (0.65 µg/g tissue) and blood (0.19 µg/g blood). This difference was still detectable after 5 days (fore-stomach 0.78 µg/g tissue, maximum 0.1 µg/g tissue in all other tissues analysed). On administration of 10 mg/kg the tissue levels were distinctly lower. The activity in the fore-stomach after 24 hours was still 0.61 µg/g tissue, while in the other tissues a maximum of 0.15 µg/g tissue was measured. After 5 days, this difference could no longer be detected. The results of these measurements were confirmed by whole body radiography. For the most part, the radioactivity in the tissues analysed was bound covalently to cellular macromolecules (measured in pmol/mg protein). The degree of covalent binding was higher in the fore-stomach than in the stomach, and covalent binding to the haemoglobin was greater than that in the liver. The levels were clearly dose-dependent for the haemoglobin, stomach and liver, but not for the fore-stomach. After inhalation exposure, the radioactivity was excreted in equal amounts in the urine and faeces. In general the covalent binding (pmol/mg protein) and the radioactivity (µg/g tissue) in the tissues examined were lower than they were after oral administration. The following values were recorded based on approximately equivalent absorbed doses:

Table 1. Covalent binding (pmol/mg protein)

	10 mg/kg body weight oral	15 mg/m^3, inhalation (≈10 mg/kg body weight)
Liver	2.00	0.09
Haemoglobin	0.29	0.10
Stomach	6.71	0.87
Fore-stomach	52.38	1.96

Specific radioactivity after 24 hours (µg /g tissue)

	10 mg/kg body weight oral	15 mg/m^3, inhalation (≈10mg/kg body weight)
Kidneys	0.044	0.008
Liver	0.052	0.015
Stomach	0.112	0.052
Fore-stomach	0.611	0.066
Lungs	0.014	0.065
Erythrocytes	0.006	0.004

The results of whole body autoradiography confirmed the low radioactivity in the tissues. Only low levels were found in the nasal mucous membranes and in the lungs after exposure to the two different concentrations (Monsanto, 1987 b).

Male NMRI mice (25 g) received a single intravenous injection of ^{14}C-benzyl chloride at doses of 57–384 µg/mouse (5–30 µCi), and were killed 1, 6 and 24 hours later. The blood, liver, spleen, lungs, testes and brain were removed, and haemoglobin was isolated from the erythrocytes, DNA from the tissues. The degree of alkylation of the DNA (nmol/g DNA) reached a maximum after 1 hour in the brain, testes and liver, and was about 3 times higher in the testes and brain than in the other organs studied; it then declined again within 24 hours. In contrast, the degree of alkylation of the haemoglobin and of the DNA in the lungs and spleen increased over 24 hours, the value for haemoglobin at this time exceeding the highest (1-hour) level for the testes and brain by a factor of about 3 (Walles, 1981 a).

After a single intramuscular injection of 200 mg benzyl chloride/kg into Sprague-Dawley rats, 62% of the substance was found at the site of application (time of measurement not specified). The highest plasma level was found 15 minutes after administration, and after 2 hours, rapid elimination from the plasma began (α-phase half-life 20 minutes, β-phase half-life 30 hours). 4% of the administered dose was excreted in the urine as benzylmercapturic acid, and 1% was eliminated unchanged in the exhaled air (Gerges et al., 1985).

Following intravenous injection of 0.063 µl (57 µg, 5 µCi) of ^{14}C-benzyl chloride into mice, elimination of the radioactivity from the liver and blood occurred within 6 hours and conformed to a non-linear two-compartment model [liver 200 dpm/mg wet weight (1 hour), ca. 150 dpm/mg wet weight (6 hours); blood 30 dpm/mg wet weight (1 hour), ca. 20 dpm/mg wet weight (6 hours)]. In contrast, the radioactivity in the testes and brain dropped linearly within 6 hours from about 40 (1 hour) to about 8 dpm/mg wet weight and from 12 (1 hour) to 3 dpm/mg wet weight, respectively (Walles, 1981 b).

Benzyl chloride reacted with protein in the tissues after subcutaneous injection into rats and rabbits (no further details) or after oral administration to dogs; following conjugation with glutathione it was metabolized to benzylmercapturic acid (Von Oettingen, 1955).

After oral administration of benzyl chloride to 2 dogs (weight ca. 8 kg) at a dose of 1 g/dog, mercapturic acid was excreted in the urine (no further details; Stekol, 1938).

No acid-labile precursors of benzylmercapturic acid were found in the urine of rats given benzyl chloride, from which it was deduced that benzyl chloride is converted directly to mercapturic acid in the body (Knight and Young, 1958).

In rats and rabbits, benzyl chloride is partly excreted as mercapturic acid in the urine. Following oral administration of 158 µmol/100 g to female rats, 27% (20–32%) of the administered dose was excreted as mercapturic acid within 10 hours. At the same time, there was a clear reduction in glutathione in the liver (Barnes et al., 1959).

A similar reaction was also seen in rats after inhalation exposure to benzyl chloride (220 ppm) for 6 hours, with a drop in the glutathione levels in the liver and kidneys to 13.5 and 46% of the control values, respectively (Rao, 1985).

A 45% reduction in glutathione was also seen in vitro within 15 minutes of incubation of liver homogenate with 1 mM benzyl chloride (Gerges et al., 1985).

When benzyl chloride was administered orally to rats at a dose of 44 mg/kg/day for 7 days, 30% of the substance was eliminated in the urine as hippuric acid (Maitrya and Vyas, 1970).

After administration of 200 mg/kg orally to rabbits, 49 (37–67%) of the dose was eliminated as mercapturic acid within 24 hours; in addition, 37% of the administered dose was excreted as benzoic acid, 17% as the free acid and 20% as the glycine conjugate (Bray et al., 1958).

7.2 Acute and subacute toxicity

In male Wistar rats, the oral LD_{50} value for benzyl chloride (neat, 14-day observation period) was 0.40 ml/kg (0.34–0.46 ml/kg). The signs of toxicity included sedation and general malaise (Bayer, 1978).

An oral LD_{50} value of 1230 mg/kg (1150–1660 mg/kg) was determined in male Sprague-Dawley rats, and in male CF-1 mice a value of 1620 mg/kg (1150–2185 mg/kg) was obtained (14-day observation period; Vernot et al., 1977).

In another paper, oral LD_{50} values of 780 mg/kg and 625 mg/kg were reported for the white mouse and for the rat, respectively (Rudnev et al., 1979).

The LD_{50} for benzyl chloride on subcutaneous injection into rats (strain BD, 100 days old, sex unspecified) was determined as 1000 mg/kg. The rats showed apathy, dyspnoea, pulmonary oedema and bloody diarrhoea. Death occurred 1–4 days after treatment (Druckrey et al., 1970).

Oral administration of 250 mg/kg (single dose) or of 125 mg/kg (4 doses) to female Fischer-344/N rats caused 100% mortality. Male Fischer-344/N rats died after up to 5 doses of 250 mg/kg or 6–9 doses of 125 mg/kg (number of animals and time interval between doses not specified). Histological examination of the dead animals that had received 250 mg/kg revealed congestion and oedema in the heart, liver and lungs of the females and acute myocardial necrosis in the males. Rats that had received 125 mg/kg showed acute gastritis and ulceration of the fore-stomach (Bunner and Creasia, 1982).

In an inhalation study, rats and mice survived benzyl chloride concentrations of 0.5 and 2 mg/l for 1 hour (no further details; Back et al., 1972).

Exposure to 170 ppm benzyl chloride for 8 hours caused severe irritation and inflammation, and some deaths in cats. A concentration of 400 pm inhaled for 7 hours caused immediately irritation with subsequent coughing, clouding of the cornea and, after 2–3 days, inflammation and oedema of the lungs and death. Cats exposed to 1000 ppm for 2 hours developed severe irritation of the airways and signs of paralysis. Higher concentrations of 7–18 mg/l (1400–3500 ppm) for 8 hours were lethal due to pulmonary oedema (Oettel, 1975; Flury and Zernik, 1931).

In dogs, exposure to 370 ppm for 8 hours caused death during the following night (Oettel, 1975; Flury and Zernick, 1931).

In Wistar rats, 4-hour LC_{50} values of about 3500 and 4085 mg/m^3 were obtained in males and females, respectively. The rats had breathing difficulties (which could be observed during the 21-day observation period) as well as signs of irritation of the eyes and mucous membranes (Bayer, 1979).

Groups of 5 male and 5 female Sprague-Dawley rats were exposed for 4 hours to benzyl chloride (purity 99.3%), at average concentrations (hourly measurement by gas chromatography) of 340, 350, 380 or 400 ppm (whole body exposure, observation period 14 days). The 4-hour LC_{50} for male and female rats was calculated as 344 ppm (4.41 mg/l). The rats showed signs of irritation of the respiratory tract and general irritant effects at 540 ppm; apart from congestion of the lungs and clouding of the cornea, no pathological changes were found at post-mortem (Monsanto, 1987 a).

Respective LC_{16}, LC_{50} and LC_{84} values of 0.44, 0.74 and 1.2 mg/l (89, 148 and 240 ppm) have been reported for male rats (strain not specified) and of 0.23, 0.39 and 0.62 mg/l for mice (sex and strain not specified). The animals were exposed once for 2 hours, and the observation period was 4 weeks for rats and 2 weeks for mice. Symptoms observed in both species included excitation, irritation of the conjunctiva and the mucous membranes of the respiratory tract, and hyperaemia of the ears, paws and tail. Histological examination of the dead animals revealed marked inflammation of the airways with secondary bacterial infection, fatty dystrophy of the liver cells, necrosis of the kidney tubule epithelium, dystrophic changes of the myocardium and swelling of the cortical cells of the central nervous system (Mikhailova, 1964).

In another study, 10 male rats (strain not specified) inhaled 0.1 mg benzyl chloride/l for 2 hours and were observed for 4 weeks. Over a period of 14 days after exposure the rats showed reversible weight loss compared with the controls. Effects on blood composition and kidney function (daily urine quantity, protein concentration) were not seen (no exact details). Likewise there was no significant difference in the threshold of excitation (nerve and muscle excitation) compared with controls (Mikhailova, 1964).

Sensory irritation by inhalation of benzyl chloride was studied in male Swiss OF-1 mice. The reflex decrease in respiratory rate was taken as a measure of sensory irritation. Measurement took place over 5 minutes by means of whole body plethysmography. At least 4 doses of the substance were tested, and the results were used to determine the concentration which would cause a 50% reduction in the respiratory rate. This was found to be 17 ppm for benzyl chloride (de Ceaurriz et al., 1981).

In a further investigation of sensory irritation, groups of 4 male Swiss-Webster mice were exposed for 10 minutes to concentrations of 13.6, 22.8, 26.1 or 31.0 ppm (nose-only exposure, whole body plethysmography). The RD_{50} value for benzyl chloride (the concentration which caused a 50% reduction in the respiratory rate compared with the initial value) was 26.6 ppm ($\hat{=}$ 0.140 mg/l; Monsanto, 1988).

Exposure of cats to a concentration of 48 mg/l (about 93 ppm) for 8 hours daily over 6 days caused increasing signs of inflammation of the mucous membranes of the eyes and respiratory tract. Some deaths occurred. Under the same study conditions rabbits showed only very slight signs of irritation (Flury and Zernick, 1931).

In a 4-week inhalation study, four groups of 10 male and 10 female Sprague-Dawley rats, 10 male Duncan-Hartley guinea-pigs and 10 male Syrian golden hamsters were exposed to benzyl chloride in 10 m^3 Rochester inhalation chambers for 6 hours daily on every week day (24 exposures in total). The concentrations in the chambers (determined 4 times daily) were 0, 12, 35 and 102 ppm ($\hat{=}$ 0, 0.06, 0.18 and 0.53 mg/l). Male and female rats exposed to the highest concentration (102 ppm) showed reduced weight gain, difficult and accelerated breathing, irritation of the nasal mucous membranes and excitation. Likewise the guinea-pigs had breathing difficulties, eye irritation and watering eyes; in addition, their fur was stuck together with saliva and they showed hair loss. In hamsters, decreased weight gain was seen together with irritation of the eyes and upper airways. None of the 3 species showed signs of local irritation in the 35 and 12 ppm dose groups. Histological examination of guinea-pigs in the two higher dose groups (102 and 35 ppm) revealed swelling of the alveoli and lung emphysema. There were no treatment-related histological or pathological findings in rats or hamsters. Based on these experiments (0.06 mg/l daily for 6 hours, 24 exposures), the no-effect-level was assumed to be 35 ppm (0.18 mg/l) for rats and hamsters and 12 ppm (0.06 mg/l) for guinea-pigs (Monsanto, 1983).

7.3 Skin and mucous membrane effects

The hairless skin of the ears of rabbits (White New Zealand) was exposed to 0.5 ml benzyl chloride covered with a dressing for 24 hours. Severe redness and swelling developed with subsequent necrotic skin changes (Bayer, 1979).

Instillation of 0.1 ml neat benzyl chloride into the conjunctival sac of the rabbit caused slight reddening and swelling of the conjunctiva as well as temporary clouding of the cornea (Bayer, 1979).

In the course of a carcinogenicity study in female ICR mice (see also Sect. 7.7), irritation of the eyes, skin and airways was observed after skin application of 10 μl neat benzyl chloride or 2.3 μl benzyl chloride in 25 μl benzene. The mice immediately started to scratch themselves at the site of application. Erythema and swelling were observed at the application site, followed by alopecia, induration and keratinization (the duration of treatment prior to the occurrence of these effects was not specified). Benzyl chloride caused less pronounced effects than benzotrichloride and benzoyl chloride, which were studied at the same time (Fukuda et al., 1981).

7.4 Sensitization

Landsteiner et al. injected guinea-pigs (number and sex not specified) with 0.01 mg benzyl chloride intracutaneously twice weekly for 12 weeks. A challenge was made 2 weeks later when 1 drop of test solution in olive oil was applied to the shaved skin of the flank. A positive effect was observed (no further details; Landsteiner et al., 1936).

A positive sensitization effect was also reported in another guinea-pig study (no further details; von Oettingen, 1955).

7.5 Subchronic and chronic toxicity

When benzyl chloride was administered intradermally to C57 black mice 4 times at a dose of 0.05 ml/mouse, depigmentation of the hair at the site of injection occurred over the course of 6 months (Aw and Boyland, 1981).

After administration by stomach tube of 15, 30 or 62 mg benzyl chloride/kg in corn oil (volume administered 2.5 ml/kg) to male and female Fischer-344/N rats, 3 times a week for 6 months, histological changes occurred mainly in the fore-stomach (hyperkeratosis, hyperplasia) and in the heart (hyperplasia, focal necrosis). At 30 or 62 mg/kg, 50% of the female rats had hyperkeratosis and 50% hyperplasia (62 mg/kg only) of the fore-stomach. One female from the 62 mg/kg group had a basal cell carcinoma of the fore-stomach. No changes of this type were seen in the females given 15 mg/kg. Amongst the males, 80% of the 62 mg/kg group had hyperkeratosis and/or hyperplasia of the fore-stomach, none of the 30 mg/kg group were affected, but 20% of the low-dose males had hyperkeratosis (Bunner and Creasia, 1982).

In a range-finding experiment for a chronic toxicity study, 10 male and 10 female F344 rats (average initial weights 250 g and 128 g, respectively) and 10 male and 10 female B6C3F1 mice (average initial weights 21 and 14 g, respectively) received benzyl chloride in corn oil, 3 times a week for 26 weeks, by stomach tube. The doses used were 0, 15, 30, 62, 125 and 250 mg/kg in rats and 0, 6.3, 12.5, 25.0, 50.0 and 100.0 mg/kg in mice. All of the male and female rats given 250 and 125 mg/kg had died within 2–3 weeks; in these rats, severe acute and chronic gastritis of the fore-stomach and ulcers were seen; in many cases myocardial necrosis and oedema of the heart muscle were found. Only 4 female rats in the 62 mg/kg group survived for the entire duration of the study (26 weeks). In addition to acute myocardial necrosis, hyperplasia of the fore-stomach was seen. Hyperkeratosis of the fore-stomach was seen in a few of the females in the 30 mg/kg group. No observations were made regarding effects in the males. A significant reduction in weight gain was seen in the male rats given 62 mg/kg, an effect which was less marked in the females. The maximum tolerated dose (MTD) for male and female rats (based on the histological and pathological effects seen in this study and the observed reduction in body weight gain) was 30 mg/kg given 3 times a week. No reduction in body weight gain was seen in male and female mice given 100 mg/kg twice a week by stomach tube; histopathological examination of these mice frequently revealed marked hyperplasia of the liver (no further details); occasionally this type of liver damage was also seen dose-dependently at 50 mg/kg and at lower doses. All the male and female mice given 50 mg/kg survived for 26 weeks. The MTD chosen for the chronic study was 100 mg/kg (Lijinski, 1986).

When rats were given 0.6 mg benzyl chloride/kg/day for 6 months, the blood levels of inorganic phosphate, alkaline phosphatase, cholinesterase and succinate dehydrogenase were increased; these effects were not seen at 0.06 or 0.006 mg/kg/day for 6 months (Rudnev et al., 1979).

In a 27-week study on the inhalation toxicity of benzyl chloride, 4 groups consisting of 30 male and 30 female Sprague-Dawley rats together with 30 male Hartley guinea-pigs were exposed to concentrations of 0, 0.005, 0.062 or 0.148 mg/l (≙ 0, 1, 12 or 30 ppm) in 10 m^3 chambers, for 6 hours/day (weekdays only; total 129 exposures). Signs of toxicity observed in both rats and guinea-pigs included alopecia, shedding of bloody tears (chromodacryorrhoea) and diarrhoea, but these effects did not differ within the dose groups or compared with the controls. There were no significant differences in body weight gain between the study and control groups. In guinea-pigs, the highest concentration (0.148 mg/l) caused a reduction in the mean corpuscular volume (MCV) and a significant ($p<0.01$) lowering of the bilirubin level in the blood after 27 weeks. The other haematological and clinical parameters, and the urine analysis, were unremarkable. The relative liver weights in the two higher dose groups (0.148 and 0.062 mg/l) and the relative kidney weight in the high-dose group were increased in guinea-pigs, without any histological or pathological effects being detected in these organs. No pathological changes were seen in the 0.005 mg/l dose group. In the rats, the relative spleen weight was increased in the females only at the highest dose (0.148 mg/l); no pathological or histological effects were seen. All other parameters appeared normal. Based on the available experimental results, a no-effect-level of 0.062 mg/l (≙ 12 ppm) was established for rats, and 0.005 mg/l (≙ 1 ppm) for guinea-pigs (Monsanto, 1984).

In the course of a carcinogenicity study in female ICR mice (see also Sect. 7.7), repeated dermal application of 10 µl neat benzyl chloride or 2.3 µl benzyl chloride in 25 µl benzene resulted in a reduction in motor activity (Fukuda et al., 1981).

7.6 Genotoxicity

Benzyl chloride showed a high alkylating activity [2.925 in the nitrobenzyl pyridine test (NBP-test) Δ E 560 nm], which paralleled a clear, direct mutagenic effect in TA 100 without S9-mix; the mutagenic effect decreased on addition of S9-mix (Neudecker et al., 1980).

Other authors have also described a similar correlation between the strong alkylating effect (NBP-test and guanosine alkylation), the direct mutagenic effect in *Salmonella typhimurium* TA 100 without S9-mix and the ability to induce sister chromatid exchange (Hemminki et al., 1983).

Both positive and negative results have been obtained in numerous studies with a variety of test systems (see Table 1); they can be summarised as follows: (see Table 2, authors given in the table)

Benzyl chloride is a direct mutagen in the Salmonella/microsome test in strains TA 100, TA 98 and TA 1535. In general, the addition of S9-mix leads to a reduction in mutagenic activity. The sometimes variable results presented in the table might be due to the volatility of the substance. The experiments carried out in a desiccator or in a liquid system (to impede evaporation) mainly gave positive results, and produced a direct mutagenic effect in *Salmonella typhimurium* strains TA 100, TA 98 and TA 1535.

In an intraperitoneal host-mediated assay with strains TA 1530, TA 1535 and TA 1538 and with *Saccharomyces cerevisiae* D3, benzyl chloride was inactive.

Benzyl chloride was a dose-dependent mutagen in various reversion tests with *Escherichia coli* WP2 strains and, in addition, DNA damage was detected with *Escherichia coli* $polA^-/polA^+$.

In *Saccharomyces cerevisiae* D3, increased mitotic recombination occurred in vitro.

Dose-dependent gene conversion was seen in 2 strains of *Saccharomyces cerevisiae* (JD1, D7) with and without metabolic activation.

Mitotic crossing-over was found in *Saccharomyces cerevisiae* D6 and *Aspergillus nidulans* P.

Benzyl chloride was a dose-dependent mutagen in the HGPRT test in V79 cells. Two studies showed benzyl chloride to be mutagenic in mouse lymphoma cells, while in another study the results were negative. It gave positive results in a CHO test.

Benzyl chloride was mainly positive in SCE tests in various cell systems in vitro; assays for chromosomal aberrations in vitro have produced some positive and some negative results. In the UDS test, benzyl chloride was active in one study, but inactive in another.

In cultured human cells, benzyl chloride caused DNA damage, which could be partially reversed (breaks in single strands).

Table 2. Mutagenicity tests with benzyl chloride

Test system	Dose Solvent	Metabolic activation	Toxicity	Results	Reference
Salmonella/microsome test TA 1535, TA 1537, TA 1538, TA 98, TA 100 Plate incorporation test	1, 10, 100, 500, 1000, 5000 µg/plate in DMSO	S9-mix from Aroclor-induced rat liver (Wistar)	Toxic at 5000 µg/plate	Dose-dependent mutagen in strain TA 100 from 100 µg/plate with S9-mix	Parry, 1982 p. 65
Salmonella/microsome test TA 1535, TA 1537, TA 1538, TA 98 Plate incorporation test	4, 20, 100, 500, 2500 µg/plate in DMSO	not studied	not toxic	Not mutagenic in the strains tested without S9-mix	Parry, 1982 p. 55
Salmonella/microsome test TA 1535, TA 1537, TA 1538, TA 98, TA 100 Plate incorporation test	7.81, 15.63, 31.25, 62.5, 125, 250 µg/plate in DMSO	not specified	toxic at 250 µg/plate in TA 1538	Not mutagenic in the strains tested at the concentrations used	Parry, 1982 p. 49
Salmonella/microsome test TA 1535, TA 1537, TA 1538, TA 98, TA 100 with urine from mice given benzyl chloride i.p. in a micronucleus test (total dose 1100 mg/kg)	–	–	–	Not mutagenic in the strains tested	Parry, 1982 p. 49

Salmonella/microsome test TA 1535, TA 1537, TA 1538, TA 98, TA 100 Plate incorporation test	31.2, 62.5, 125, 250, 500, 1000 µg/plate in DMSO	S9-mix from Aroclor-induced rat liver (Wistar)	Bacteriotoxic at 1000 µg/plate	Weak mutagenic activity in TA 100 (factor of 2.1) at 500 µg/plate with S9-mix	Parry, 1982 p.45
Salmonella/microsome test TA 1535, TA 1537, TA 1538, TA 98, TA 100 Plate incorporation test	0–10,000 µg/plate in DMSO	S9-mix from rat liver	Toxic from > 250 µg/plate	Weak mutagenic activity in TA 100 with and without S9-mix at 225 µg/plate (factor 1.7–2.0)	Parry, 1982 p.35
Salmonella/microsome test TA 1535, TA 1537, TA 1538, TA 98, TA 100 Plate incorporation test	50, 100, 200, 300, 400 µg/plate in DMSO	S9-mix from phenobarbital and 5,6-benzoflavone induced rat liver (male CRCD rats)	Toxic from 400 µg/plate	No clear increase in the number of revertants	Parry, 1982 p.27
Salmonella/microsome test TA 1535, TA 1537, TA 1538, TA 98, TA 100 Spot test	10, 1000, 10,000, 100,000 µg/ml in DMSO	Not specified	–	Increase in the number of revertants only at 100,000 µg/ml in TA 100, questionable mutagenic effect	Parry, 1982 p.17
Salmonella/microsome test TA 1535, TA 1537, TA 1538, TA 98, TA 100 Plate incorporation test	1, 10, 50, 100, 500, 1000 µg/plate in DMSO	Only tested without metabolic activation	Toxic from 500 µg/plate in TA 100	Mutagenic effect in TA 100 from 50 µg/plate	Parry, 1982 p.21

Table 2 (continued)

Test system	Dose Solvent	Metabolic activation	Toxicity	Results	Reference
Salmonella/microsome test TA 98, TA 100 Plate incorporation test	10, 50, 100, 250, 500, 1000, 2500 µg/plate in DMSO	S9-mix from Aroclor-induced rat liver	Toxic from 500 µg/plate	Mutagenic effect in TA 100 with and without S9-mix	Parry, 1982 p. 39
Salmonella/microsome test TA 1535, TA 1537, TA 1538, TA 98, TA 100 Plate incorporation test	31.25–4000 µg/plate in DMSO	S9-mix from Aroclor-induced rat liver	–	Dose-dependent mutagenic effect in TA 100 with and without S9-mix	Parry, 1982 p. 61
Salmonella/microsome test TA 1535, TA 1538	5–10 µg/plate	S9-mix from non-induced rat liver	–	Dose-dependent mutagen in TA 1535 without S9-mix	Rosenkranz and Poirier, 1979
Salmonella/microsome test TA 98, TA 100 Fluctuation test	1–500 µg/ml in DMSO	None	Toxic in TA 98 from 375 µg/ml	Weakly positive effect in TA 100 at 35 µg/ml and 150 µg/ml, not dose-dependent, mutagenic effect questionable	Parry, 1982 p. 81

Salmonella/microsome test TA 98, TA 100 Fluctuation test	0.1, 1.0, 10, 50, 100, 250 µg/ml in DMSO	S9-mix from Aroclor-induced rat liver	–	Not-mutagenic in either strain	Parry, 1982 p.87
Salmonella/microsome test TA 98, automated fluctuation test	5, 10, 50, 100, 150 µg/ml in DMSO	Not specified	–	Dose-dependent mutagen in TA 98 with and without metabolic activation	Parry, 1982 p.71
Salmonella/microsome test TA 100 "modified liquid test system", see: Rannug, U., Chem. Biol. Interact., 12, 251 (1976)	0–2 µM/plate	No further details	Not toxic	Dose-dependent mutagen without S9-mix, mutagenic activity reduced by S9-mix	Neudecker et al., 1980
Salmonella/microsome test TA 1535, TA 1536, TA 1537, TA 1538, TA 98, TA 100 Plate incorporation test	4.0, 7.9 µmol/plate in DMSO	S9-mix from Aroclor-induced rat liver (male Wistar)	Not toxic at dose levels tested	Dose-dependent mutagen in TA 100 without metabolic activation	Yasuo et al., 1978
Salmonella/microsome test TA 1535, TA 1537, TA 1538, TA 98, TA 100	1000, 2000, 4000 µg/plate in DMSO	S9-mix from Aroclor-induced rat liver	–	Dose-dependent mutagen in TA 100 with and without S9-mix, more effective with S9-mix	Brooks and Gonzales, 1982

Table 2 (continued)

Test system	Dose Solvent	Metabolic activation	Toxicity	Results	Reference
Salmonella/microsome test TA 1535, TA 1536, TA 1537, TA 1538, TA 98, TA 100 Plate incorporation test Tested in the gas phase in a desiccator (7 hours, 37 °C)	250 µg/plate or 0–50 µl in desiccator	S9-mix from Aroclor-induced rat liver (Sprague-Dawley)	Not specified	Not mutagenic up to 250 µg/plate in the plate incorporation test, dose-dependent mutagen in strain TA 100 with and without S9-mix in the desiccator study	Simmon, 1979b
Salmonella/microsome test TA 1530, TA 1535, TA 1538 *Sacch. cerevisiae* D3 Host-mediated assay, mouse, Swiss-Webster, male, test organism administered i.p.	4400 mg/kg i.m. or 450 mg/kg oral	In vivo metabolism	–	Not mutagenic	Simmon et al., 1979
Recombination test with *Bacillus subtilis* M45 (Rec^-), H17 (Rec^+)	79.2 and 118.5 µmol/disc in DMSO	None	–	Questionable	Yasuo et al., 1978
Reversion test with *E. coli* WP2 hcr	0, 3.2, 6.3 µmol/plate in DMSO	S9-mix from Aroclor-induced rat liver	–	Mutagenic without S9-mix	Yasuo et al., 1978

Reversion test with *E. coli* WP2 uvrA	10, 50, 100, 250, 500, 1000 µg/plate in DMSO	S9 -mix from Aroclor-induced rat liver	Toxic from 500 µg/plate	Dose-dependent mutagen with and without S9-mix	Parry, 1982 p.39
Reversion test with *E. coli* WP2 uvrA and WP2	1, 10, 50, 100, 500, 1000 µg/plate in DMSO	None	Toxic in WP2 from 500 µg/plate	Dose-dependent mutagen in *E. coli* strain WP2 uvrA	Parry, 1982 p.21
E. coli polA$^-$/polA$^+$	10 µg/ml	S9-mix from non-induced rat liver	–	Mutagenic with and without S9-mix	Rosenkranz and Poirier, 1979
E. coli polA$^-$/polA$^+$	25 µg/plate	S9-mix from non-induced rat liver	–	Mutagenic with and without S9-mix	Fluck et al., 1976
Sacch. cerevisiae D3 mitotic recombination	concentration of 0.04% in the medium	S9-mix from Aroclor-induced rat liver	–	Increased mitotic recombination with and without S9-mix	Simmon, 1979a
Gene conversion in *Sacch. cerevisiae* JD1	31.3, 62.5, 125, 250, 500 µg/ml in DMSO	S9-mix from Aroclor-induced rat liver	Toxic from 250 µg/ml	Dose-dependent mutagen from 31.3 µg/ml with and without S9-mix	Parry, 1982 p.163
Gene conversion in *Sacch. cerevisiae* JD1	15.6–500 µg/ml in DMSO	Not specified	Survival rate reduced from 125 µg/ml	Dose-dependent mutagen with and without metabolic activation	Parry, 1982 p.157

Table 2 (continued)

Test system	Dose Solvent	Metabolic activation	Toxicity	Results	Reference
Gene conversion in *Sacch. cerevisiae* D7	7.8–500 μg/ml in DMSO	None	Survival rate reduced from 125 μg/ml	Mutagenic from 125 μg/ml	Parry, 1982 p.153
Gene conversion in *Sacch. cerevisiae* JD1	0.5–100 μg/ml in DMSO	Not specified	–	Mutagenic from 1 μg/ml with and without metabolic activation	Parry, 1982 p. 145
Sacch. cerevisiae D7 Inhibition of meiotic cell division	0–100 μg/ml	None	–	No increase in mutation frequency at the ilv-1 locus, inhibition of the sporulation rate	Parry, 1982 p.173
Sacch. cerevisiae D6 mitotic crossing-over	0–200 μg/ml in DMSO	Not specified	–	Increase in mitotic crossing-over in the right arm of chromosome VII, no chromosomal aneuploidy	Parry, 1982 p.139

Aspergillus nidulans P mitotic crossing-over	100, 1000, 5000 μg/plate in DMSO	S9-mix from Aroclor-induced rat liver (Wistar)	–	Slight induction of crossing-over after a 5–6 hour incubation independent of S9-mix, no induction of aneuploidy	Parry, 1982 p.133
Sacch. cerevisiae D6 Detection cf DNA-damage by alkaline sucrose sedimentation	50, 100, 250 μg/ml	None	–	Induction of DNA damage, repair of 70% of damaged cells within 4 hours of the damage arising	Parry, 1982 p.119
Cell transformation test mouse embryo fibroblasts CH 3/10, T 1/2	5, 10, 20 μg/ml in DMSO (1%)	S9-mix from Aroclor-induced rat liver	–	No cell transformation after 24 hr incubation with or without S9-mix	Parry, 1982 p.219
Cell transformation test baby hamster kidney cells (BHK)	16 μg/ml in DMSO	S9-mix from Aroclor-induced rat liver	–	Slight, questionable cell-transforming effect with S9-mix	Parry, 1982 p.215
Azaguanine-resistance in V79 cells	10.3–25.1 μg/ml in DMSO	S9-mix from Aroclor-induced rat liver	–	Dose-dependent mutagen	Parry, 1982 p.245
HGPRT test in V79 cells	100–300 μM in DMSO	None	–	Dose-dependent mutagen after 1 hour incubation	Parry, 1982 p.239
Cell transformation test with BHK 21 C13 cells	25–464 μg/ml	S9-mix from rat liver	–	Indications of cell-transforming activity	Parry, 1982 p.223

Table 2 (continued)

Test system	Dose Solvent	Metabolic activation	Toxicity	Results	Reference
Cell transformation test with BHK cells	0.025–250 µg/ml in DMSO	None	–	No cell-transforming activity	Parry, 1982 p.227
Mouse lymphoma cells L5178Y (tk^+/tk^-)	0–10 µg/ml in DMSO	Not specified	–	No increase in the frequency of mutation	Parry, 1982 p.249
Cell transformation test Golden hamster embryo cells	0.1 µg/ml lowest transforming dose	None	–	Transforming activity	Pienta, 1980
Mouse lymphoma cells L5178Y	No details	No details	–	Positiv	NTP, 1985
Mouse lymphoma cells L5178Y (tk^+/tk^-)	1–32 µg/ml	S9-mix from Aroclor 1254 induced rat liver	Toxic at 32 µg/ml	Positive with and without S9-mix	McGregor et al., 1988
Mouse lymphoma cells L5178Y/(tk^+/tk^-)	1.18×10^{-4} mmol/l 3.93×10^{-4} mmol/l 11.8×10^{-4} mmol/l	–	–	Dose-dependent DNA strand breaks	Garberg et al., 1988

Hamster ovary cells (CHO-K1-BH_4) Chromosomal aberration, SCE, thioguanine resistance mutation	10–50 µg/ml	None	–	Dose-dependent increase in the rate of SCE and chromosomal aberrations, slight increase in thioguanine resistance mutations at 1 dose (18 µg/ml)	Parry, 1982 p. 263; Ishidate et al., 1988
Rat liver epithelial cells RD_4	7.5–30 µg/ml in DMSO	None	–	Dose-dependent increase in chromosomal aberrations	Parry, 1982 p. 279
UDS-test HeLa cell line S3	10^{-7}–10^{-3}M in DMSO	S9-mix from Aroclor-induced rat liver (Wistar)	–	No increase in ^{3}H-thymidine incorporation	Parry, 1982 p. 207
UDS-test HeLa cell line S3	10^{-5}–10^{-3}M	–	toxic from 10^{-3}M	Increased ^{3}H-thymidine uptake, there was a positive correlation between the results in the UDS-test, the Ames test and the NBP-test	Schiffmann et al., 1983

Table 2 (continued)

Test system	Dose Solvent	Metabolic activation	Toxicity	Results	Reference
SCE in hamster ovary cells (CHO)	0–100 µM	None	–	Slight, dose-dependent increase in the rate of SCE, in parallel with slight alkylation of NBP and guanosine and an increase in revertants in TA 100	Hemminki et al., 1983
Human lymphocytes, SCE-test, chromosomal aberrations	1, 5, 10, 25 µg/ml in DMSO	None	Toxic at 25 µg/ml	No increase in the rate of SCE or chromosomal aberrations	Parry, 1982 p. 295
Human lymphocytes, chromosomal aberrations	2.5, 5.0, 7.5, 10.0 µg/ml in DMSO	None	Inhibition of mitosis at >10 µg/ml	No chromosomal aberrations detectable	Parry, 1982 p.297
Human lymphocytes, SCE	2.5, 5.0, 7.5, 10.0 µg/ml in DMSO	None	–	Induction of SCE at 5.0, 7.5 and 10.0 µg/ml	Parry, 1982 p. 301
Human lung tumour cells in culture	125, 250, 500 µg/ml	None	–	Induction of repairable DNA damage	Parry, 1982 p. 203

Lung tumour cells (A549) and XP4LO fibroblasts (Xeroderma pigmentosa) in vitro	2–4 mM	–	–	Induction of repairable DNA damage	Mirzayans and Waters, 1985
Drosophila recessive lethal test	Feeding of larvae (10 mg in 1 ml DMSO (5%) added to 20 ml feed)	–	Dose range not toxic	No increase in sex-linked recessive lethal mutations	Parry, 1982 p. 335
Drosophila, determination of eye colour mutations	0.5, 1.0, 2.0 mM, feeding of larvae	–	Dose range not toxic	Induction of somatic changes on gene expression	Parry, 1982 p. 339
Micronucleus test, mouse, COBS-CD1	1100 mg/kg in Tween 80 in 2 equal doses i.p.	–	Not specified	No increase in micronuclei was detectable in 1000 polychromatic erythrocytes 6 and 24 hours after administration	Parry, 1982 p. 375
Micronucleus test, mouse, Tuck To	75, 150, 300, 600 mg/kg (in Tween 80) i.p. twice at intervals of 24 hours	–	3/4 mice died after 2 doses of 600 mg/kg	No increase in micronuclei was detectable 6 hours after the last dose	Parry, 1982 p. 353

Table 2 (continued)

Test system	Dose Solvent	Metabolic activation	Toxicity	Results	Reference
Micronucleus test, mouse, ♂, CD1	876 mg/kg oral in corn oil	–	LD_{50} oral 1095 mg/kg	No increase in micronuclei was found in 5000 polychromatic erythrocytes after 48, 72 and 96 hours	Parry, 1982 p. 357
Micronucleus test, mouse, ♂ (CBA×Balb/C) F_1	125, 250, 500, 1000, 2000 mg/kg in Tween 80, single s.c., animals killed after 24 and 48 hours 250, 500, 1000 mg/kg in Tween 80, s.c. at intervals of 24 hours, animals killed 6 hours after the 2nd dose	–	Not specified	No increase in the number of micronuclei detectable	Parry, 1982 p. 365

Micronucleus test, mouse, ♀, NMRI	25, 50, 100, 200, 400 mg/kg in methocel orally, twice at 24-hour intervals	–	Not specified	No increase in micronuclei in 500 polychromatic erythrocytes 6 hours after the 2nd dose	Parry, 1982 p.373
Study of sperm head anomalies, mouse, ♂ (CBA×Balb/C) F_1	125, 250, 500 mg/kg in Tween 80, s.c. once daily on 5 consecutive days 50, 100, 200, 400 mg/kg i.p. once daily on 5 consecutive days	–	250 mg/kg s.c. 100 mg/kg i.p. tolerated with no deaths 500 mg/kg s.c. 200 mg/kg i.p. occurrence of deaths	No increased incidence of sperm head anomalies on subcutaneous or intraperitoneal administration	Parry, 1982 p.345
Rat (strain unspecified) chromosomal aberrations in the bone marrow	31.0, 0.006, 0.0006 mg/kg orally once daily for 6 months	–	Dose range not toxic	No increase in chromosomal aberrations	Rudnev et al., 1979

– = not indicated

Strand-breaks were detected in the DNA of mouse lymphoma cells treated with benzyl chloride.

In all micronucleus tests and in chromosomal aberration assays in rat bone marrow, benzyl chloride gave negative results.

No mutagenic activity was found in a test for recessive lethal mutations in *Drosophila*. In contrast, the determination of eye-colour mutations showed that benzyl chloride induced somatic changes.

The studies carried out in various in vitro test systems with different end-points have shown that benzyl chloride has definite mutagenic activity. On the other hand, mutagenic activity could not be detected in in vivo studies (micronucleus test, chromosomal aberration assay in the bone marrow, host-mediated assay).

7.7 Carcinogenicity

Benzyl chloride transformed hamster embryo cells and baby hamster kidney cells. However, both positive and negative results have been found (see Table 2).

A relationship between the direct alkylating effect of benzyl chloride [tested with 4-(nitrobenzyl)pyridine] and its carcinogenic activity following subcutaneous injection into BD rats (9/22 local sarcomas) has been demonstrated (no further details; Preussmann, 1968).

In a 2-year carcinogenicity study groups of 52 male and 52 female F344 rats and B6C3F1 mice were given benzyl chloride (purity 97.5–98%) in corn oil 3 times a week by stomach tube at the following doses: male and female rats 30 and 15 mg/kg, male and female mice 100 and 50 mg/kg. The doses were determined in a subchronic study (see Sect. 7.5). No significant weight loss was seen in any of the test animals compared with the controls, and there was no significant difference in the survival rate of the treated and control animals. All of the animals underwent histopathological examinations. The results are presented in Tables 3 and 4. In this study, a statistically significant increase in C-cell tumours of the thyroid gland was found in the female rats. In 3 male rats in the 30 mg/kg dose group there were 2 carcinomas and 1 papilloma of the fore-stomach, and in 1 female from the same dose group there was a mammary epithelial papilloma (these findings are not presented in Table 3). It was suggested that the MTD of 30 mg/kg established for rats was too low. In the 100 mg/kg dose group there was a significant ($p<0.001$) increase in the number of fore-stomach tumours in male and female mice, an effect which was not observed in the 50 mg/kg

Table 3. Tumours in F-344 rats after oral administration of benzyl chloride in corn oil for 2 years (3 times weekly)

Type of tumour	Dose (mg/kg)					
	♂			♀		
	0	15	30	0	15	30
Mononuclear leukaemias	15/52	19/52	23/51	12/52	11/52	6/52
Liver, neoplastic nodes	3/52	4/52	2/51	2/52	5/52	3/52
C-cell adenoma or carcinoma of the thyroid gland	12/52	7/52	6/51	4/52	8/51	14/52[a]
Pancreatic islet adenoma or carcinoma	14/52	22/52	21/51	3/52	8/52	3/52

[a] p=0.009

group. Other carcinogenic effects were marginal, such as the increased number of adenomas or sarcomas of the lungs only in female mice and the hepatocellular tumours in male mice only in the mid-dose group (Lijinsky, 1986).

Benzyl chloride was tested for carcinogenic activity in mice by skin application. The commercial product was used without further purification (contaminants not specified), and was applied to the clipped dorsal skin of 3-week-old female ICR mice (SPF-maintenance). In the first study, 11 female mice (3 weeks old) were treated with 10 µl neat benzyl chloride 3 times weekly for 4 weeks, and then twice weekly until they were killed at the age of 9.8 months. A control group of 10 mice was treated with 10 µl benzene. None of the animals in the control or test groups died or developed tumours. In the second study, 20 female mice (7 weeks old) were treated with 2.3 µl benzyl chloride diluted to 25 µl with benzene, twice weekly for 11.7 months. A control group of 20 mice was treated with 25 µl benzene. All of the surviving animals were killed at the end of the study, and the organs and tumours from all of the animals (including those that died during the study) were histologically examined. The mortality during the study was 50% in the test group and 20% in the

Table 4. Tumours in B6C3F1 mice after oral administration of benzyl chlori
in corn oil for 2 years (3 times weekly)

Type of tumour	Dose (mg/kg)					
	♂			♀		
	0	50	100	0	50	100
Alveolar/bronchial adenomas or carcinomas	11/52	15/52	11/52	1/52	2/51	6/51 (p=0.05
Haemangiomas or haemangiosarcomas	0/52	0/52	5/52 (p=0.028)	2/52	1/52	3/51
Carcinomas or adenomas of the liver	17/52	28/52 (p=0.024)	20/51	7/52	5/51	3/51
Fore-stomach carcinomas	0/51	2/52	8/52 (p=0.003)	0/52	2/50	3/51
Carcinomas and papillomas of the fore-stomach	0/51	4/52	32/52 (p<0.001)	0/52	5/50	19/51 (p<0.00

control group. Five out of 20 of the treated mice had tumours, of which 3 were carcinomas at the site of application, 2 were lung adenomas and 1 was a leiomyosarcoma of the uterus. Two lung adenomas occurred in the control group. No skin tumours were observed in 120 other control mice in the same laboratory that had also been treated locally with benzene. The increased incidence of skin tumours was not significant (Fukuda et al., 1981).

In another carcinogenicity study, 20 male mice (Alderley-Park Swiss Albino, 4–5 weeks old) were treated with 100 μl benzyl chloride dissolved in 5 μl toluene, which was applied to the clipped dorsal skin twice weekly. Positive and negative controls received benzo(a)pyrene and toluene respectively. According to a preliminary report of the study, no tumours had occurred in the test group or in the negative control group after 7 months. In the positive control group 12 of the 14 surviving mice had developed skin tumours by this time (Ashby et al., 1982).

In a 2-stage carcinogenicity study, 1 mg benzyl chloride dissolved in toluene was applied once to the clipped dorsal skin of 40 T.O. mice (male and female, 3 months old). One week later, 10 μl of a promotor (a 1% solution of croton oil in toluene) was applied to the same area. This was repeated twice weekly. The positive control was a group of 20 mice that had received benzo(a)pyrene as an initiator; a negative control (20 mice) received only croton oil. The only report of this study is a preliminary one after 10 months. No tumours had developed in the 37 surviving mice in the test group, or in the 19 mice in the negative control group. In the positive control group, 8/19 mice had tumours (Coombs, 1982).

Eight rats (BD strain, 100 days old, sex not specified) were given 80 mg/kg purified benzyl chloride in peanut oil once a week for 51 weeks. The total dose was 3.9 g/kg. After an average induction time of 500 days, 6 of the 8 rats had sarcomas at the injection site, and most had lung metastases. Out of 14 rats that received 40 mg/kg once a week for 51 weeks (total dose 2.1 g/kg), 3 developed sarcomas at the injection site after an average induction time of 500 days. Histologically, out of the total of 9 tumours, there were 6 fibrosarcomas, 2 spindle cell sarcomas and 1 myosarcoma. Peanut oil alone did not induce tumours in the control group (no further details; Druckrey, 1970).

Three groups of 20 mice (strain A/He, male and female, 6–8 weeks old) received 8–12 intraperitoneal injections of benzyl chloride in tricaprylin. The mice were injected 3 times a week, and the total doses were 4.7, 11.8 and 15.8 mM/kg (equivalent to 0.6, 1.5 and 2 g/kg). In these groups, 15/20, 16/20 and 8/20 mice survived, respectively. All surviving animals were killed 24 weeks after the first injection. Lung tumours were found in 4/15, 7/16 and 2/8 surviving mice (equivalent to 0.26, 0.50 and 0.25 tumours/mouse). In the control groups, there were 0.22 lung tumours/mouse in the tricaprylin group and 0.21 lung tumours/mouse in the untreated group. The differences were not statistically significant (Student's t-Test; Poirier et al., 1975).

7.8 Reproductive toxicity

Twenty Wistar rats were given oily solution of benzyl chloride orally from day 1 to day 19 of pregnancy. A high embryo mortality rate was seen in the rats given 208 mg/kg; similarly 0.006 and 0.0006 mg/kg led to increased embryo lethality, while 0.00006 mg/kg had no effect. Malformations were not observed. The remaining offspring of the rats that had received 208 mg benzyl chloride/kg showed retarded development, an effect which was not detectable in the 0.00006 mg/kg group (no further details, particularly on choice of doses; Rudnev et al., 1979; Leonskaja, 1980).

Groups of 8 pregnant rats received 0, 50 or 100 mg benzyl chloride/kg in corn oil by stomach tube from day 6 to day 15 of pregnancy. There was no sign of maternal toxicity. The 100 mg/kg dose was foetotoxic, the length of the foetuses being significantly lower than in the controls. The number of skeletal and visceral malformations and variations was not significantly increased (Skowronski and Abdel-Rahman, 1986).

7.9 Effects on the immune system

Benzyl chloride was given orally to groups of 10 rats for 30 days at doses of 31.0, 0.006, 0.0006 and 0.00006 mg/kg, and the rats were assessed for the complement-binding reaction, basophil degranulation and plaque formation (by the Jerne method); an aqueous salt extract of liver tissue from the animals treated with the highest dose was used as the antigen. All of the tests were positive (no further details; Rudnev et al., 1979). By the same method, the lowest effective dose of benzyl chloride in rats was determined as 0.0006 mg/kg (Vinogradov, 1979).

7.10 Neurotoxicity

Changes in the behaviour of mice (male, Swiss OF-1) after inhalation of benzyl chloride were studied by de Ceaurriz using the method of Porsolt et al. [Nature, 226, 730–732 (1977); Arch. Int. Pharmacodyn. Ther., 299, 327–336 (1977)]. Groups of 10 animals were exposed to 12, 17, 18 or 22 ppm benzyl chloride or to pure air for 4 hours. After exposure, the mice were placed in a cylinder filled with water (21 –23°C). Initially the mice exhibited "flight" behaviour, then a calm phase occurred, in which they only moved in order to keep their heads above water ("immobile phase"). The length of the immobile phase was measured, and any changes in its duration were taken as a measure of the effect of the test substance on CNS-controlled behaviour. Benzyl chloride caused a dose-dependent increase in the immobile phase by 32, 52, 71 and 84%. The authors interpreted this as an indication of the neurotoxicity of the chemical (de Ceaurriz et al., 1983).

7.11 Other effects

A single intramuscular injection of 50 mg/kg in corn oil caused an increase in SGOT and SGPT (Skowronski and Abdel-Rahman, 1984).

After a single intravenous injection of 25 or 250 μg/kg (controls received 0.2 ml 10% propylene glycol, which was the vehicle for the benzyl chloride) a significant, dose-dependent increase in SGPT and LDH was seen after 10 minutes. The levels returned to normal within 1 hour. Ornithine-carbamoyl transferase activity reached a peak after 30 minutes and 1 hour, respectively and returned to control levels after 24 hours. The bromsulphthalein value was clearly below control levels at both 30 minutes and 24 hours. The glutathione level in the liver (mg/g tissue) and blood (mg%; assayed after 30 minutes and 4 hours) was significantly reduced compared with controls (Dahab et al., 1986).

Reduced glutathione levels were also seen in the liver and kidneys after oral administration and inhalation exposure (Barnes et al., 1959; Rao, 1985).

Female CD-1 mice exposed to benzyl chloride at a concentration of 1 ppm (TLV-value) for 3 hours, either once or 5 times, did not show an increased sensitivity to aerogenic streptococcal infections nor an increase in bactericidal activity in the lungs (Aranyi et al., 1986).

Isolated rat hepatocytes were incubated for 10, 30, 60 and 120 minutes at 37 °C in benzyl chloride at concentrations of 1.8 and 3.6 mM. The viability of the cells was lowered in a concentration- and time-dependent manner. The parameters used were the exclusion of trypan blue and leakage of lactate dehydrogenase, aspartate transaminase and alanine transaminase. From the observed membrane damage, the authors concluded that benzyl chloride was hepatotoxic (Abdel-Rahman and Saxena, 1988).

8. Experience in humans

A concentration of 16 ppm benzyl chloride (80 mg/m^3) was tolerated by humans for a maximum of 1 minute. A concentration of 10 ppm (50 mg/m^3) caused severe watering of the eyes (Oettel, 1975; Flury and Zernik, 1931).

Concentrations of 32 ppm (160 mg/m^3) caused considerable irritant effects on the eyes and the mucous membrane of the respiratory tract and produced intolerable eye irritation (von Oettingen, 1955; Flury and Zernik, 1931).

A level of 190 ppm (ca. 1000 mg/m^3) was viewed as dangerous to the respiratory tract (Flury and Zernik, 1931).

Exposure to 20 ppm (100 mg/m^3) for 1 minute caused toxic effects, and short exposures to 10 ppm (50 mg/m^3) led to signs of illness. A concentration of 5 ppm (25 mg/m^3) in the workplace air was classified as unsatisfactory (Goldblatt, 1955).

In a small group of workers exposed intermittently to benzyl chloride vapours (up to 500 ppm), conjunctivitis and irritation of the upper airways were observed. After local contact with liquid benzyl chloride, blisters developed on the skin (no further details; Watrous, 1947).

In people exposed to a concentration of 2 ppm (10 mg/m^3), reported effects included fatigue, irritant effects, persistent headaches, disturbances in liver function and slight leukopenia (Mikhailova, 1983).

The odour threshold for benzyl chloride was determined by 4 subjects to be 0.047 ppm (0.24 mg/m^3; Leonardos, 1969).

Tumours of the respiratory tract have been observed in workers involved in benzoyl chloride production. In these cases, the subjects were also exposed to toluene, benzotrichloride and to a lesser extent benzyl chloride and benzal chloride (no details of concentrations; Sakabe et al., 1976; Sakabe and Fukuda, 1977).

The mortality of 163 exposed workers involved in the production of chlorinated toluenes was compared with that of 790 unexposed workers. Analysis of the data was carried out with the aid of standardized mortality ratios and regression models in life tables; for comparison, the mortality rates in England and Wales were used. The evaluation revealed indications of increased cancer mortality in the exposed workers. No other causes of death in the exposed group were increased. Tumours were reported in the respiratory tract and the gastro-intestinal tract. The report gave no indications of a carcinogenic effect for benzyl chloride alone. Benzotrichloride was suggested as the cause of the increased number of tumours in the exposed workers (Sorahan et al., 1983).

In a prospective mortality study of 697 employees at a chlorination plant in the USA who were exposed to benzyl chloride, benzoyl chloride, benzotrichloride and related chemicals, a total of 47 deaths was observed during the period 1943–1982, of which 44 could be evaluated. No statistically significant increase in mortality was found in the total cohort, but there were 7 cases of cancer of the respiratory tract compared with 2.84 expected. Mortality was increased only in white workers who had been employed for more than 15 years. Because of the small number of cases and the absence of precise information on smoking (only 1 of the dead workers was a non-smoker) the value of the study is limited. However, the data do suggest an association between the toluene chlorination process and an increased risk of cancer of the respiratory tract (Wong, 1988).

Workers using butyl benzyl phthalate contaminated with 0.03% benzyl chloride and 0.3% benzal chloride in the manufacture of PVC tiles have reported irritation of the upper airways. Air concentrations of 0.03 mg/m^3 benzyl chloride and 0.2 mg/m^3 benzal chloride were measured in the workplace (no further details; Rittfeldt et al., 1983).

9. Threshold limit values

Since 1979, benzyl chloride has been included in section IIIB of the list of MAK values (DFG, 1979).

References

Abdel-Rahman, M.S., Saxena, S.
Effect of benzyl chloride on rat hepatocytes
J. Toxicol. Environ. Health, 25, 452–459 (1988)

Aranyi, G., O'Shea, W.I., Graham, H.A., Miller, F.I.
The effects of inhalation of organic chemical air contaminants on murine lung host defenses
Fund. Appl. Toxicol., 6, 713–720 (1986)

Ashby, J., Gauni, C., Robinson, M.
Carcinogenicity bioassay of 4 CMB, 4 HMB and benzyl chloride on mouse skin: interim (7 month) report
Mutat. Res., 100, 399–401 (1982)

Aw, T.C., Boyland, E.
Depigmentation of hair in mice by chemicals
IRCS Med. Sci. Libr. Compend., 9, 29–30 (1981)

Back, K.C., Thomas, A.A., MacEwen, J.D.
Reclassification of materials listed as transportation health hazards
Aerospace Medical Research Laboratory
Wright-Patterson Air Force Base, Ohio
NTIS-PB 214 270 (1972)

Barnes, M.M., James, S.P., Wood, P.B.
The formation of mercapturic acids
Biochem. J., 71, 680–690 (1959)

Bayer AG, Institut für Toxikologie
Benzylchlorid: Akute orale Toxizität (männliche Wistar Ratten)
Unpublished report of 6. 12. 1978

Bayer AG, Institut für Toxikologie
Benzylchlorid, Gewerbetoxikologische Untersuchungen
Unpublished report No. 8419 (1979)

Bray, H.G., James, S.P., Thorpe, W.V.
Metabolism of some halogenoalkylbenzenes and related alcohols in the rabbit
Biochem. J., 70, 570–579 (1958)

Brooks, T.M., Gonzales, L.P.
The mutagenic activity of 4-chloromethyl biphenyl (4 CMB) and benzylchloride (BC) in the bacterial microsome assay
Mutat. Res., 100, 61–64 (1982)

Bunner, B.L., Creasia, D.A.
Toxicity, tissue distribution and excretion of benzyl chloride in the rat
J. Toxicol. Environ. Health, 10, 837–846 (1982)

Coombs, M.M.
Attempts to initiate skin tumours in mice in the 2-stage system using 4 CMB, 4 HMB and benzyl chloride. Report of the experiment at 10 months
Mutat. Res., 100, 403–405 (1982)

Dahab, G.M., Gerges, S.E., Abdel-Rahman, M.S.
Effect of benzyl chloride in rat liver functions
J. Toxicol. Environ. Health, 18, 431–439 (1986)

de Ceaurriz, J., Micillino, J.C., Bonnet, P., Guenier, J.P.
Sensory irritation caused by various industrial airbone chemicals
Toxicol. Lett., 9, 137–143 (1981)

de Ceaurriz, J., Desiles, J.P., Bonnet, P., Marignac, B., Muller, J., Guenier, J.P.
Concentration-dependent behavioral changes in mice following short-term inhalation exposure to various industrial solvents
Toxicol. Appl. Pharmacol., 67, 383–389 (1983)

DFG (Deutsche Forschungsgemeinschaft)
Maximale Arbeitsplatzkonzentrationen und biologische Arbeitsstoff-toleranzwerte (1979), Mitteilung XV der Senatskommission zur Prüfung gesundheitsschädlicher Arbeitsstoffe
Verlag Chemie, Weinheim

Druckrey, H., Kruse, H., Preussmann, R., Ivankovic, S., Landschütz, C.
Cancerogene alkylierende Substanzen
Z. Krebsforsch., 74, 241–270 (1970)

Fluck, E.R., Poirier, L.A., Ruelius, H.W.
Evaluation of a DNA polymerase-deficient mutant of *E. coli* for the rapid detection of carcinogens
Chem. Biol. Interact., 15, 219–231 (1976)

Flury, F., Zernik, G. (eds.)
Schädliche Gase
J. Springer, Berlin, p. 339 (1931)

Fukuda, K., Matsushita, H., Sakabe, H., Takemoto, K.
Carcinogenicity of benzyl chloride, benzal chloride, benzotrichloride and benzoylchloride in mice by skin application
Gann, 72, 655–664 (1981)

Garberg, P., Akerblom, E.L., Bolcsfoldi, G.
Evaluation of a genotoxicity test measuring DNA-strand breaks in mouse lymphoma cells by alkaline unwinding and hydroxyapatite elution
Mutat. Res., 203, 155–176 (1988)

Gerges, S.E., Kadrey, A.M., Abu-Hadeed, A.H., Abdel-Rahman, M.S.
Kinetics of benzyl chloride in rats
Soc. Toxicol., 24th annual meeting, San Diego, Calif.
Toxicologist, 5, 204 (1985)

Goldblatt, M.W.
Research in industrial health in the chemical industry
Brit. J. Ind. Med., 12, 1–20 (1955)

Hemminki, K., Falck, K., Linnainmaa, K.
Reactivity, SCE induction and mutagenicity of benzyl chloride derivatives
J. Appl. Toxicol., 3, 203–207 (1983)

IARC (International Agency for Research on Cancer)
IARC Monographs on the evaluation of the carcinogenic risk of chemicals to humans
Vol. 29, 49–63 (1982) and Suppl. 4, 84–86 (1982)

Ishidate, M., jr., Harnois, M.C., Sofuni, T.
A comparative analysis of data on the clastogenicity of 951 chemical substances tested in mammalian cell cultures
Mutat. Res., 195, 151–213 (1988)

Knight, R.H., Young, L.
Biochemical studies of toxic agents
II. The occurrence of premercapturic acids
Biochem. J., 70, 111 (1958)

Landsteiner, K., Jacobs, J.
Studies on the sensitization of animals with simple chemical compounds II
J. Exp. Med., 64, 625–639 (1936)

Leonardos, G., Kendall, D., Barnard, N.
Odor threshold determinations of 53 odorant chemicals
J. Air Pollut. Control Assoc., 19, 91–95 (1969)

Leonskaja, G.I.
Evaluation of the embryotoxic and teratogenic effect of butyl and benzyl chlorides to establish hygienic standards for reservoir water
Gig. Naselen. Mest. (Kiev), 19, 40–43 (1980)
cited in IARC Monographs, Vol. 29

Lijinsky, W.
Chronic bioassay of benzyl chloride in F344 rats and (C57BL/6JxBALB/c) F1 mice
J. Natl. Cancer Inst., 76, 1231–1236 (1986)

Lipper, K.A.
Chlorkohlenwasserstoffe, aromatische, seitenkettenchlorierte
in: Ullmanns Enzyklopädie der technischen Chemie
4th ed., vol. 9, p. 525–537
Verlag Chemie, Weinheim (1975)

Maitrya, B.B., Vyas, C.R.
Studies on conjugation of organic compounds in the rat
Indian J. Biochem., 7, 284–285 (1970)

McGregor, D.B., Brown, A., Cattanach, P., Edwards, J., McBride, D., Casspary, W.I.
Responses of the L5178Y tk^+/tk^- mouse lymphoma cell forward mutation assay II: 18 coded chemicals
Environ. Mol. Mutagen., 11, 91–118 (1988)

Mikhailova, T.V.
Die relative Toxizität von chlorierten Toluolverbindungen: Benzylchlorid, Benzalchlorid und Benzotrichlorid
Gig. Tr. Prof. Zabol., 8, 14–19 (1964)
(German translation from the Russian)

Mikhailova, T.V.
Benzylchloride
Parmeggiani, L. (ed.)
In: Encyclopedia of Occupational Health and Safety
3rd edition, p. 262
International Labor Office (1983)

Mirzayans, R., Waters, R.
Benzyl chloride and 4-chloromethylbiphenyl induced DNA damage and its repair in excision-deficient (XP group A) or -proficient human cells
Mutat. Res., 145, 209–215 (1985)

Monsanto Corporation
Four-week inhalation toxicity study of benzyl chloride to male and female rats, male guinea pigs and male hamsters
Unpublished study, Report MSL-2805 (1983)

Monsanto Corporation
Twenty seven week inhalation toxicity of benzyl chloride vapor to male and female rats and male guinea pigs
Unpublished study, Report MSL-4413 (1984)

Monsanto Corporation
Acute toxicity of benzylchloride administered by inhalation to male and female Sprague-Dawley rats
Unpublished study, Report MSL-6471 (1987 a)

Monsanto Corporation
A study of molecular dosimetry of benzyl chloride following oral administration to mice
Unpublished study, Report MSL-6760 (1987 b)

Monsanto Corporation
Evaluation of the sensory irritation potential of benzyl chloride
Unpublished study, Report MSL-6375 (1988)

Neudecker, T., Lutz, D., Eder, E., Henschler, D.
Structure-activity relationship in halogen and alkyl substituted allyl and allylic compounds: correlation of alkylation and mutagenic properties
Biochem. Pharmacol., 29, 2611–2617 (1980)

NTP (National Toxicology Program)
Annual Plan for Fiscal Year 1985
NTP-85-055, March 1985
Public Health Service, Dept. of Health and Human Services

Oettel, H.
Chlorkohlenwasserstoffe, aromatische seitenkettenhalogenierte
cited in: Ullmanns Enzyklopädie der technischen Chemie
Vol. 9, 536, 4th revised and expanded edition
Verlag Chemie, Weinheim (1975)

Parry, J.M. (ed.)
The UKEMS genotoxicity trial 1981: The results of a collaborative exercise in mutagenicity and carcinogenicity testing
Mutat. Res., 100, 1–433 (1982)

Pienta, R.J.
Transformation of Syrian Hamster embryo cells by diverse chemicals and correlation with their reported carcinogenic and mutagenic activities
In: de Serres, F.J., Hollander, A. (eds.)
Chemical mutagens, principles and methods for their detection, 6, 175–202
Plenum Press, New York (1980)

Poirier, L.A., Stoner, G.D., Shimkin, M.B.
Bioassay of alkyl halides and nucleotide base analogs by pulmonary tumor response in strain A mice
Cancer Res., 35, 1411–1415 (1975)

Preussmann, R.
Direct alkylating agents as carcinogens
Food Cosmetic. Toxicol., 6, 576–577 (1968)

Rao, H.
The kinetics and hepatotoxicity of benzyl chloride vapors in rats
Masters Thesis, New Jersey Institute of Technology
Newark, N.J. (1985)

Rittfeldt, L., Ahlberg, M.S., Zingmark, P.A., Santesson, J.
Occupational exposure to benzyl chloride and benzal chloride due to contaminated butyl benzyl phthalate
Scand. J. Work Environ. Health, 9, 367–368 (1983)

Rosenkranz, H.S., Poirier, L.A.
Evaluation of the mutagenicity and DNA-modifying activity of carcinogens and non-carcinogens in microbial systems
J. Natl. Cancer Inst., 62, 873–891 (1979)

Rudnev, M.I., Tomashevskaya, L.A., Vinogradov, G.I., Kapustin, A.A., Zholdakova, Z.T., Leonskaya, G.I.
Hygienische Begründung des zulässigen Gehalts an Benzylchlorid und 2-Chlorbutan in Wasserreservoiren (German translation from the Russian)
Gig. Sanit., 3, 11–15 (1979)

Sakabe, H., Matsushita, H., Koshi, S.
Cancer among benzoylchloride manufacturing workers
Ann. N.Y. Acad. Sci., 271, 67–70 (1976)

Sakabe, H., Fukuda, K.
An updating report on cancer among benzoylchloride manufacturing workers
Ind. Health, 15, 173–174 (1977)

Schiffmann, D., Eder, E., Neudecker, T., Henschler, D.
Induction of unscheduled DNA synthesis in HeLa cells by allylic compounds
Cancer Lett., 20, 263–269 (1983)

Simmon, V.F.
In vitro assays for recombinogenic activity of chemical carcinogens and related compounds with *Saccharomyces cerevisiae* D3
J. Natl. Cancer Inst., 62, 901–909 (1979a)

Simmon, V.F.
In vitro mutagenicity assays of chemical carcinogens and related compounds with *Salmonella typhimurium*
J. Natl. Cancer Inst., 62, 893–899 (1979b)

Simmon, V.F., Rosenkranz, H.S., Zeiger, E., Poirier, L.A.
Mutagenic activity of chemical carcinogens and related compounds in the intraperitoneal host-mediated assay
J. Natl. Cancer Inst., 62, 911–918(1979)

Skowronski, G., Abdel-Rahman, M.S.
Hepatotoxicity and teratogenicity of benzylchloride in rats
Am. Soc. Pharmacol. Exp. Ther. (ASPET), Annual Meeting, Indianapolis, Ind. paper 134, p. 50 (1984)

Skowronski, G., Abdel-Rahman, M.S.
Teratogenicity of benzyl chloride in the rat
J. Toxicol. Environ. Health, 17, 51–56 (1986)

Sorahan, T., Waterhouse, J.A.H., Cooke, H.A., Smith, E.B.M., Jackson, J.R., Temkin, L.
A mortality study of workers in a factory manufacturing chlorinated toluenes
Ann. Occup. Hyg., 27, 173–182 (1983)

Stekol, J.A.
Studies on the mercapturic acid synthesis in animals
IX. The conversion of benzyl chloride and S-benzylcysteine into benzylmercapturic acid in the organism of the dog, rabbit and rat
J. Biol. Chem., 124, 129 (1938)

Vernot, E.H., MacEwen, J.D., Haun, C.C., Kinkead, E.R.
Acute toxicity and skin corrosion data for some organic and inorganic compounds and aqueous solutions
Toxicol. Appl. Pharmacol., 42, 417–423 (1977)

Vinogradov, G.
Der Autosensibilisierungseffekt bei peroraler Aufnahme chemischer Stoffe in den Organismus (German translation from the Russian)
Vrach. Delo, 9, 100–102 (1979)

von Oettingen, W.F.
The halogenated aliphatic, olefinic, cyclic, aromatic and aliphatic-aromatic hydrocarbons including the halogenated insecticides, their toxicity and potential dangers
DHEW Publication No. 414, Washington D.C., US Government Printing Office, 300–302 (1955)
cited in IARC Monographs, Vol. 29

Walles, S.A.S.
Reaction of benzyl chloride with haemoglobin and DNA in various organs of mice
Toxicol. Lett., 9, 379–387 (1981)

Watrous, R.M.
Health hazards of the pharmaceutical industry
Br. J. Ind. Med., 4, 111–125 (1947)

Wong, O.
A cohort mortality study of employees exposed to chlorinated chemicals
Am. J. Ind. Med., 14, 417–431 (1988)

Yasuo, K., Fujimoto, S., Katoh, M., Kikuchi, Y., Kada, T.
Mutagenicity of benzotrichloride and related compounds
Mutat. Res., 58, 143–150 (1978)

Triethanolamine

1. Summary and assessment

Within 1 hour, 50–60% of a dose of triethanolamine (TEA) is absorbed from the gastro-intestinal tract and within 24 hours, 50% of the dose is excreted unchanged in the urine and 20% in the faeces. Information on the fate of the remaining amount is not available. On dermal application, maximum blood levels are reached after two hours in mice, and after 4 hours in rats.

Both pure and technical grade TEA administered orally to rats and guinea-pigs are of low acute toxicity (LD_{50} approximately 8 g/kg for both products in both species). Bleeding of the stomach epithelium occurs. In addition, absorption can lead to paralysis of the hind limbs of guinea-pigs. After neutralization with hydrochloric acid, technical grade TEA can be tolerated without damage at dose levels which, if given as the base, have a lethal effect. The constituents of TEA which are volatile at room temperature have no acute toxic effect in rats.

Symptoms of poisoning are evident in rats and mice after the administration of TEA in the drinking water for 2 weeks. Concentrations of 2% and less are tolerated. On repeated dermal application over 2 weeks, concentration-dependent effects are prominent.

After subacute inhalation of TEA aerosol, inflammation of the larynx occurs at and above concentrations of 125 mg/m^3 air.

Single applications of pure and technical grade TEA cause slight irritation of intact skin and clear inflammatory changes in hurt skin.

Instillation into rabbits' eyes causes slight, largely reversible inflammation of the conjunctiva, and the deeper layers of the eye may also be affected.

TEA is not sensitizing in the guinea maximization test.

On subchronic oral administration to rats and guinea-pigs over 3–4 months, paralysis and demyelinization of the peripheral nerves occurs, together with kidney damage and, to a lesser extent, liver damage. The kidney and liver effects may be reversible, depending on the dose. Anaemia has also been observed in rats. The lowest no effect level for rats is 80 mg/kg body weight. The main effect of dermal application is local damage. The no effect level by this route is 125–250 mg/kg body weight in rats, and >250 mg/kg body weight in mice.

TEA is inactive in various short-term tests (rec assay in *Bacillus subtilis*, Salmonella/microsome test with strains TA 98 and TA 100, *Escherichia coli* WP2, chromosome aberrations in CHL- and CHO-cells, cell transformation test, UDS test, SCE test). After incubation of TEA with sodium nitrite in an acidic medium (pH 3.5) a direct mutagenic action on *Bacillus subtilis* is found, an effect which is not seen after the addition of S9-mix. Also, after heating TEA with sodium nitrite, a direct mutagenic effect on various *Bacillus subtilis* strains is observed; the mutagenic activity of the heated mixture remains unchanged after 5 months.

After chronic life-time feeding of TEA-hydrochloride to ICL-ICR mice, there was a significant, dose-dependent, increase in the number of females with malignant tumours (predominantly of the lymphatic system). No tumours were observed in mice after dermal application of TEA. Chronic administration in the drinking water of rats for 2 years showed no evidence of carcinogenic activity.

In vitro, TEA and sodium nitrite may form the carcinogen N-nitrosodiethanolamine, under simulated gastric conditions, it is not known whether this chemical is a significant cause of tumour formation in the above oral administration study, or whether other nitroso-compounds are formed when the TEA-containing food is heated.

In a preliminary investigation of the reproductive toxicity of TEA in mice, there were no indications of foetotoxicity or teratogenic effects.

In man, slight skin irritation can be caused by TEA. Stronger irritation is likely to occur with broken skin.

A definite conclusion on the skin-sensitizing potential of TEA in man is not possible, but damaged or particularly sensitive skin may respond to TEA with a positive sensitization reaction. On the whole, TEA seems to be only a weak sensitizer. The report in the literature of allergic rhinitis from TEA exposure may prove to be an isolated case.

A 28-day inhalation study investigating possible neurotoxicity is currently being conducted on behalf of BG-Chemie.

Further long-term studies are scheduled (NTP, 1989).

2. Name of substance

2.1	Usual name	Triethanolamine
2.2	IUPAC-name	2,2′,2″-Nitrilotriethanol
2.3	CAS-No.	102-71-6

3. Synonyms, common and trade names

Nitrilo-2,2′,2″-triethanol
Nitrilotriethanol
2,2′,2″-Nitrilotrisethanol
Tris(2-hydroxyethyl)-amine
2,2′,2″-Trihydroxy-triethylamine
Trihydroxyethylamine
Daltogen
Sterolamide
Trolamine
Thiofaco-T-35
Tricolamin
TEA

4. Structural and molecular formulae

4.1	Structural formula	$(HO{-}CH_2{-}CH_2)_3N$
4.2	Molecular formula	$C_6H_{15}NO_3$

5. Physical and chemical properties

5.1	Molecular mass, g/mol	149.22
5.2	Melting point, °C	21–22 (CRC, 1981/82)
5.3	Boiling point, °C	360 (at 1013 hPa) (BASF, 1989)
5.4	Vapour pressure, hPa	5×10^{-5} (at 40 °C) (BASF, 1989) 13.3 (at 205 °C) (Sax, 1979)
5.5	Density, g/cm^3	1.1242 (at 20 °C) (CRC, 1981/82)
5.6	Solubility in water	Miscible (CRC, 1981/82)
5.7	Solubility in organic solvents	Miscible with methanol and acetone Solubility at 25 °C: 4.2% in benzene; 1.6% in ether; 0.4% in carbon tetrachloride; <0.1% in n-heptane (Windholz, 1983)

5.8 Solubility in fat	No information available
5.9 pH-value	10.5 (15 g/l water) (BASF, 1989)
5.10 Conversion factor	1 ppm $\hat{=}$ 6.19 mg/m^3 1 mg/m^3 $\hat{=}$ 0.16 ppm (at 25 °C and 1013 hPa)

6. Uses

Additive in lubricants, cutting oils and drilling oils and in cement; base for the manufacture of detergents, cosmetics, soaps, shoe polish, car cleaning products and household cleaners; intermediate for the manufacture of textile specialities and herbicides (Hammer et al., 1987; Windholz, 1983).

7. Experimental results

Pure triethanolamine has been found to be contaminated with small quantities (5 µg/kg) of N-nitrosodiethanolamine (NDEA) (Sommer et al., 1988). As technical grade triethanolamine may be contaminated with large amounts of diethanolamine, contamination from this source should also be taken into consideration. NDEA is a potent chemical carcinogen in laboratory animals (Preussmann et al., 1982).

According to information from manufacture, commercially available triethanolamine generally contains 0.1 to 0.5% diethanolamine, but products with a diethanolamine content of up to 12% are sold (BASF, 1990; Hüls, 1989).

7.1 Toxicokinetics and metabolism

After oral administration of TEA to male rats, 53% of the administered dose had been eliminated from the gastro-intestinal tract after 35 minutes and 63% after 65 minutes (determined with the aid of gas chromatography). Within 1 day of a single oral dose of 350 mg/rat, 53% of the dose was eliminated in the urine and 20% in the faeces as unchanged TEA. Information on the fate of the remaining amount was not provided. When 350 mg TEA was given repeatedly to male and female rats (5–6 times), excretion in the urine and faeces was constant during the treatment period. There was no difference between the sexes. Only small quantities of TEA-glucuronide were detectable in the urine (Naonori et al., 1982).

7.2 Acute and subacute toxicity

The acute oral toxicity of TEA was studied in rats and guinea-pigs (10 per dose in each case, strains not specified). Both highly purified and technical grade TEA were used (no precise details of purity for either product). The following LD_{50} values were determined (length of observation period not specified): highly purified TEA, rat 9 g/kg, guinea-pig 8 g/kg; technical grade TEA, rat 8 g/kg, guinea-pig 8 g/kg. At autopsy, both rats and guinea-pigs had bleeding in the stomach. In addition, the guinea-pigs showed paralysis of the hind limbs and pronounced choking which began an hour after administration. The toxicity and pathological effects were a consequence of the alkalinity of the product. After neutralization with hydrochloric acid, technical grade TEA could be tolerated without damage at dose levels which, if given as the base, would have been lethal (Kindsvatter, 1940).

In another study (number of animals not specified), an oral LD_{50} for rats of 9.11 (8.45–9.82) g/kg was reported (Smyth et al., 1951).

An oral LD_{50} value of ca. 7.2 g/kg was reported for Sprague-Dawley rats after a 14-day observation period. Apathy was seen as a sign of toxicity. Autopsy did not reveal any obvious effects (BASF, 1966).

Another author has reported an oral LD_{50} of 5200 (±720) mg/kg for rats (45 animals, strains not specified) and 5400 (±300) mg/kg for mice (70 animals) after a 3-week observation period. The absolute lethal dose for both species was 8000 mg/kg and the maximum tolerated dose was 2000 mg/kg. In most cases, death occurred within the first 3 days. Symptoms observed included hyperaesthesia to pain and tactile irritation, a transient increase in motor excitability in mice, sedation in rats and, as the experiment progressed, reduced reflex activity in both species. Most of the animals developed diarrhoea on day 2. The surviving animals appeared normal again by the end of the 2nd to 3rd week. Post-mortem examination revealed hyperaemia of the internal organs, congestion of the liver, kidneys and spleen and, occasionally, petechial bleeding in the endocardium. The relative weights of the lungs, liver, kidneys and spleen were increased, and that of the adrenal glands was decreased (Surupova, 1969).

After intraperitoneal injection in the mouse (numbers and strain not specified) the LD_{50} value was ca. 1.5 g/kg (14-day observation period). The signs of toxicity observed included convulsions; no further effects were found at autopsy (BASF, 1966).

In an inhalation hazard test, an 8-hour exposure of rats to airstreams enriched or saturated with TEA at 20 °C produced no signs of toxicity during the 14-day observation period. Autopsy revealed no obvious effects (BASF, 1966).

Groups of 5 male and 5 female Fisher-344 rats received TEA in their drinking water at levels of 8, 4, 2, 1 or 0.5% for 14 days. At 8%, deaths occurred and moribund animals had to be killed. By the end of the first week the animals were becoming emaciated, had brown crusty noses and reduced body weights. Water consumption was reduced, an effect which was also observed in rats in the 4% group. In the 8% group increases were seen in the erythrocyte count, the haemoglobin concentration and the haematocrit level, while in the 4% group there were significant reductions in the weights of the liver, thymus, heart and lungs. No obvious effects were seen on macroscopic and microscopic examination (Battelle, 1987).

In a similar study in B6C3F1 mice, groups of 5 males and 5 females received 8, 4, 2, 1 or 0.5% TEA in their drinking water for 14 days. All of the animals survived without showing symptoms of toxicity. Body weight gain was only temporarily reduced. However, reduced water consumption was seen in the 8 and 4% groups. A statistically significant reduction in thymus weight was seen in the 4% group. No obvious effects were seen on macroscopic and microscopic examination (Battelle, 1987).

Groups of 5 male and 5 female Fisher-344 rats inhaled TEA as an aerosol at concentrations of 2, 1, 0.5, 0.25 or 0.125 g/m^3 for 6 hours, 12 times within 16 days. All of the rats survived, but the body weight gain of those in the 2 g/m^3 group was reduced by 25% (males) and 30.9% (females). Blood composition was unaffected. The rats in the 2 g/m^3 group showed increased liver and kidney weights and a decrease in the thymus weight. On microscopic examination, inflammation of the laryngeal submucosa was seen at exposure levels down to 0.125 g/m^3 (Battelle, 1987).

The same study was carried out with groups of 5 male and 5 female B6C3F1 mice. The animals survived and showed no signs of toxicity. Body weight gain was reduced in all groups except for the males exposed to 2 g/m^3. The erythrocyte, haemoglobin and haematocrit levels were increased in both sexes in all groups, and leukopenia with relative neutrophilia was observed in all exposed males and in the high-dose females. The weights of the thymus, heart and lungs were increased. Microscopically, slight inflammation of the laryngeal submucosa was observed in the 0.25, 0.5, 1 and 2 g/m^3 groups (Battelle, 1987).

Neat TEA was applied 12 times within 16 days to the dorsal skin of Fisher-344 rats and B6C3F1 mice (number of animals and duration of application not specified) at doses of 0.1–2 g/kg and 0.2–3 g/kg, respectively. No deaths occurred. In the rats, necrotic inflammation of the epidermis and dermal fibrosis developed at the application site at doses of 0.6 g/kg and above. These local effects were not observed in the mice (Melnick et al., 1988).

In another study, groups of 5 male and 5 female Fisher-344 rats were treated dermally with neat TEA at doses of 0.141, 0.281, 0.563, 1.125 and 2.25 g/kg body weight/day for 14 days. No deaths occurred. Brown colouration of the application site was followed by inflammation, which was seen in all of the males at the 3 highest dose levels and in a few of the rats treated with 0.141 and 0.281 g/kg; in the females this local inflammation occurred in the 3 higher dose groups somewhat later. Body weight gain was reduced in males (–23.1%) and females (–9.1%) in the highest dose group (2.25 g/kg), as was the feed consumption. A reduction in the leucocyte count (ranging from 3.8 to 28.2%) was observed in all treated males; in contrast there was an increase (ranging from 1.4 to 27.5%) in the females. In the two higher dose groups the relative liver weight was increased in the females (12.7% and 6.4% above controls), and the relative kidney weight was increased in the males (18.6% and 9.5% above controls). Other effects seen in males in the high-dose group (2.25 g/kg) included reductions in the thymus weight (–27.1%) and lung weight (–31.2%) and increases in the heart weight (12.7%) and testis weight (16.8%). A threshold dose of 0.563 g/kg was recommended for a 90-day study (Battelle, 1985 a).

An analogous study was carried out in mice. Groups of 5 male and 5 female B6C3F1 mice received dermal applications of neat TEA at doses of 0.214, 0.427, 0.843, 1.686 and 3.37 g/kg body weight/day for 14 days. No deaths were observed. Local inflammation developed only in the males, mainly in the high-dose group but also occasionally in the groups treated with 1.686 and 0.427 g/kg. No skin irritation or inflammation was seen in the females. Body weight gain and feed consumption were not affected in either sex in any of the dose groups. No haematological changes of statistical significance were seen. Autopsy revealed no macroscopic changes in the internal organs and no changes in organ weight, except for reduced relative testis weights in the males treated with 1.686 or 0.472 g/kg (–10.9%

and –5.9%, respectively). Based on these results, a threshold dose of 3.37 g/kg was recommended for a 90-day study (Battelle, 1985b).

The repeated application of pure or technical grade TEA at a dose of 8 g/kg to the shaved skin of 10 guinea-pigs in each case (exposure time not specified, no indication of whether the applications were occlusive or semi-occlusive), caused the deaths of all of the guinea-pigs after 4–11 applications of technical grade TEA and 2–17 applications of pure TEA. Skin necrosis was evident; histological examination revealed cloudy swelling in the liver and kidneys and fatty degeneration in the liver (Kindsvatter, 1940).

7.3 Skin and mucous membrane effects

The irritant effect of various grades of TEA on the dorsal skin of white New Zealand rabbits was investigated (no information was provided on methods, exposure time, etc.). The materials tested were 98% pure TEA, TEA with less than 0.1% monoethanolamine, 2.7% diethanolamine and 87.4% triethanolamine, and TEA with 1.3% monoethanolamine, 6.3% diethanolamine, 74.2% triethanolamine and ca. 10% monoethoxy-triethanolamine. The different TEA samples showed variations in the strength of irritation from 1.4 to 1.6 (on a scale of 0 to a maximum of 8). Pure TEA was graded as 1.5. After 72 hours erythema was still present, but oedema was no longer visible. The irritancy of all 3 samples was classified as slight. Comparative tests of mono- (MEA), di- (DEA) and triethanolamine (TEA) on rabbit skin showed that the severity of the irritant effects decreased as follows: MEA > DEA > TEA (Dutertre-Catella et al., 1982).

Neat TEA on a patch was applied to the clipped dorsal skin of 2 rabbits for 1, 5 or 15 minutes. No irritant effects were observed. After a 20-hour semi-occlusive application, marked spotty redness and slight necrosis were seen after 24 hours. A week later the skin was still slightly red and marked flaking had occurred (BASF, 1966).

Repeated dermal application of TEA to the skin of guinea-pigs caused various degrees of irritation (no further details; Kharchenko and Ivanova, 1980).

In a 24-hour occlusive test on the clipped dorsal skin of white rabbits (collaborative study in 22 laboratories each using 8 animals) TEA was found to be not or only slightly irritating (Weil and Scala, 1971).

Neat TEA (0.02 ml) instilled into rabbits' eyes caused damage of grade 5 or more (whitish colouration of the cornea, iritis) on a scale of 1 to 10. Use of fluorescein revealed that over 63% of the cornea was necrotic. Less severe effects were evident with 0.005 ml TEA (details not reported; Carpenter and Smyth, 1946).

A comparative study in rabbit eyes was conducted with TEA (98% pure) and 2 technical grade products (No. 1: monoethanolamine <0.1%, diethanolamine 2.7%, triethanolamine 87.4%; No. 2: monoethanolamine 1.3%, diethanolamine 6.3%, triethanolamine 74.2%, monoethoxytriethanolamine ca. 10%). Three animals were used for each material. Pure TEA caused slight conjunctivitis, technical grade product No. 1 had no effect and product No. 2 caused corneal damage and inflammation of the conjunctiva in 1 rabbit (no details of dose, etc.). Comparative eye irritancy tests with MEA, DEA and TEA in rabbits showed that the severity of effects decreased as follows: MEA > DEA > TEA (Dutertre-Catella et al., 1982).

Groups of 6 New Zealand rabbits received applications of 98% TEA on the centre of the cornea at volumes of 0.01, 0.03 and 0.1 ml, and the eyes were observed for 21 days. The lowest volume (0.01 ml) had no effect on any of the eyes; at 0.03 ml slight irritation occurred, which cleared up after about 1 day; the largest volume (0.1 ml) caused conjunctival damage, and the average time taken for the lesions to disappear was 3 days (although in some eyes the effects could still be observed after 7 days, but not after 14 days). The authors considered that the lesions caused by TEA-treatment were negligible (Griffith et al., 1980).

TEA caused slight temporary effects in rabbits' eyes (no further details; Grant, 1974).

In another study in which 1 drop of TEA was instilled into the conjunctival sac of each of 2 rabbits, slight redness, slight oedema and slight clouding of the cornea occurred 1 hour later. After 24 hours the redness was worse, and after 8 days there was a scar on the upper eyelid in addition to slight clouding of the cornea. Conjunctival bleeding was observed at each reading (BASF, 1966).

7.4 Sensitization

According to a report which was not further substantiated, TEA induced skin sensitization in guinea-pigs (Kharchenko and Ivanova, 1980).

In contrast, in the maximization test (OECD method 406) 98.9% pure TEA showed no evidence of sensitization in guinea-pigs (Hoechst, 1988).

7.5 Subchronic and chronic toxicity

Groups of 24 albino rats (sex and strain unspecified) received pure or technical grade TEA daily (7 days a week) in their feed at doses of 1/5, 1/10, 1/20, and 1/40 of the oral LD_{50} ($\hat{=}$ 1.6, 0.8, 0.4 and 0.2 g/kg body weight). No control groups were used. 8 animals from each group were killed after 60 and 120 days of treatment, and the remaining 8 animals in each group (which had each received 120 doses) were killed after 3 months without treatment. Localized degeneration of the myelin sheath of the ischiatic nerve was found in all the rats after 60 or 120 doses (no comments were made on the dose/response relationship). Effects on the kidney (cloudy swelling) were observed at all dose levels after 120 days, and at all but the lowest dose level (0.2 g/kg/day) after 60 days. Effects on the liver (cloudy swelling and an increase in fibroblasts) were seen at ≥ 0.4 g/kg/day after 60 and 120 doses (Kindsvatter, 1940).

Similarly, groups of 24 guinea-pigs (sex and strain unspecified) received pure or technical grade TEA orally by stomach tube, 5 times a week, at the same dose levels as the rats of the study described above. Again no controls were used. Eight animals per group were killed after 60 and 120 doses, and the remaining 8 per group (which had received 120 doses) were killed after an observation period of 3 months. As in the rats, localized degeneration of the myelin sheath of the ischiadic nerve was observed in all dose groups after 60 and 120 doses (no details of the dose/response relationship were provided here either). After 60 and 120 doses, cloudy swelling was found in both the liver and the kidneys at the 2 highest dose levels (1/5 and 1/10 of the LD_{50}; 1.6 and 0.8 g/kg). Fatty degeneration was also seen in the liver. In the groups at the 2 lower dose levels (1/20 and 1/40 of the LD_{50}; 0.4 and 0.2 g/kg) no such effects were seen, even after the 3-month observation period. In both rats and guinea-pigs the slight effects observed in the liver and kidneys were reversible. There was no difference in the observed pathological effects of pure and technical grade TEA; rats and guinea-pigs reacted in the same manner. Repeated analysis of the urine (protein, total nitrogen, urea nitrogen) and blood (sugar, bile pigments, urea, haemoglobin) did not reveal any pathological effects in either species (Kindsvatter, 1940).

The subchronic oral toxicity of TEA (commercial product) was studied in Sherman rats (5 males and 5 females per dose level). Doses of 0.005 to 2.61 g/kg body weight were administered in the feed for 90 days. Weight loss was seen at dose levels of 1.27 g/kg or more, and deaths occurred from 0.73 g/kg. The latter dose level also produced histological changes in the liver and kidneys. The highest dose tested at which no toxic effects were seen was 0.08 g/kg (Smyth et al., 1951).

The tails of rats were immersed in a 13% solution of TEA for 1 hour daily, 6 times a week for 6 months. Functional changes were seen in the liver (an increase in alanine amino-transferase activity and a reduction in cholinesterase activity) and in the CNS (effects on muscle chronaxy, seen as "a sign of disruption of the dynamic equilibrium between the excitatory and inhibitory processes of the central nervous system"). A 6.5% TEA solution had no such effects. The toxicity of TEA was not increased when 1.4 mg TEA/l (maximum permitted concentration in reservoirs in the USSR) was administered in the drinking water in addition to the dermal application (Kostrodymova et al., 1976).

Groups of 8 rats were treated repeatedly by stomach tube with 1/10 (520 mg/kg = group 1), 1/20 (260 mg/kg = group 2) or 1/50 (104 mg/kg = group 3) of the acute oral LD_{50}. The study was carried out for 2 months with group 1 and for 4 months with the other groups. In group 1, 6/8 rats died after they had received a total of 6760 to 15,080 mg/kg (corresponding to 1- to 4-times the acute oral LD_{50}). Prior to death, the animals had ceased gaining weight, and had become irritable and aggressive. Reflex activity was generally depressed. The behaviour of the rats in groups 2 and 3 was not different from that of the controls, except for initial aggressiveness which lasted for 1 to 2 months. The rats in all dose groups showed a fall in erythrocytes and haemoglobin levels (erythrocytes: group 1 from 6.4 $\pm$ 0.7 to 5.1 $\pm$ 0.2, group 2 from 6.5 $\pm$ 0.1 to 4.7 $\pm$ 0.1 to 5.4 $\pm$ 0.3, group 3 from 9.0 $\pm$ 0.1 to 5.1 $\pm$ 0.2 million/µl; haemoglobin: Group 1 from 14.3 $\pm$ 1.4 to 7.4 $\pm$ 2.9, group 2 from 14.2 $\pm$ 0.6 to 8.5 $\pm$ 0.6, group 3 from 15.0 $\pm$ 0.9 to 10.2 $\pm$ 1.8 g%). At the end of the 2nd month, the reticulocyte count was increased in the rats in groups 1 and 2 (9 $\pm$ 3% and 11 $\pm$ 0.7%, respectively; controls 2 $\pm$ 0.3%). No changes were seen in the number of white blood cells. After 2 to 3 months the excretion of benzamidoacetic acid in the urine following administration of sodium benzoate was reduced in groups 2 and 3; after 3 months, residual nitrogen in the blood was increased (69.1 $\pm$ 4.4 and 68.7 $\pm$ 4.1 mg%, respectively; controls 49.0 $\pm$ 3.7 mg%). The authors therefore concluded that TEA caused changes in the red blood cells and impairment of the function of the liver and kidneys (Surupova, 1969).

To test the subchronic dermal toxicity of TEA, groups of 20 male and 20 female Fisher-344 rats were treated with 2, 1, 0.5, 0.25 or 0.125 g TEA/kg (99.6% pure) for 90 days. The highest dose was neat TEA; the lower doses were solutions of TEA in acetone at concentrations of 7–56%. The test substance was dropped onto the dorsal skin daily (weekdays only). The body weight of males and females in the highest dose group was significantly reduced ($p < 0.001$) by the end of the study. Clinically, the only treatment-related effect seen in the 3 highest dose groups was local inflammation at the application site, the extent of which was related to dose and concentration. The haematological and biochemical effects were not considered to be treatment-related. At autopsy, the relative liver and kidney weights were increased, particularly in the higher dose groups (liver 1.0 and 2.0 g/kg, kidneys 0.25, 0.5, 1.0 and 2.0 g/kg). The relative testis weight was also increased in males in the highest dose group. Histological examination of the skin revealed dose- and concentration dependent chronic active inflammation of the skin with acanthosis. No treatment-related effects were seen in the internal organs. The NOEL was 0.125 g/kg for males and 0.25 g/kg for females (Battelle, 1987).

An analogous study was carried out in mice. Groups of 20 male and 20 female B6C3F1 mice received dermal applications of 4, 2, 1, 0.5 or 0.25 g TEA/kg (99.6% pure) on their backs for 90 days. The treatment was carried out on weekdays. Concentrations of 7 to 56% in acetone were used, although the highest dose was neat TEA. No treatment-related deaths occurred and the body weight gain at the end of the study was equivalent to control values. Clinical findings were limited to local inflammatory changes at the application site in both sexes, and these were only seen at the highest dose level (4 g/kg). The leucocyte count and the corpuscular haemoglobin concentration were significantly increased in females in the high-dose group, and the haematocrit level was significantly decreased in the females given 2 g/kg. At the end of the study all dose groups showed a significant, dose-dependent reduction in serum sorbitol dehydrogenase activity. In addition, an increase in total serum protein and albumin occurred in the females given 2 g/kg and a significant reduction in alanine aminotransferase activity occurred in the females given 1 g/kg. At autopsy, the weights of numerous organs were found to be affected; there was a significant increase in the relative liver weights in both sexes at 4 g/kg and in the males at 2.0 and 0.25 g/kg; the relative kidney weights were significantly increased in both sexes at 4 g/kg and 2 g/kg and in females at 0.25 g/kg. Histologically, chronic inflammation and acanthosis of the skin were seen in males and females treated with 4 g/kg and in one female treated with 2 g/kg. No treatment-related effects were seen in the internal organs. With regard to local irritant effects, a NOEL of 1 g/kg was determined for skin inflammation in males and females, while minimal acanthosis still occurred at the lowest dose (0.25 g/kg). However, there was no clear dose- or concentration-dependency observed. A NOEL for systemic effects was not given, but was evidently below 0.25 g/kg (Battelle, 1987).

In the course of a carcinogenicity study, groups of 5 male and 5 female F-344 rats received 1 and 2% TEA or 0.5 and 1% TEA, respectively, in their drinking water for 2 years (for further details see Sect. 7.7). Chronic nephropathy was observed, particularly in the females, together with mineralization of the renal papilla, nodular hyperplasia of the pelvic mucosa and pyelonephritis with or without papillary necrosis. The shortened life expectancy of the females was attributed to these kidney effects (Maekawa et al., 1986).

7.6 Genotoxicity

7.6.1 In vitro

The mutagenic activity of purified TEA (no further details) was studied in various in vitro tests. No DNA damage was evident in a Rec assay in *Bacillus subtilis* (H17 Rec^+ and M45 Rec^-) at doses of 40 to 4000 µg TEA/plate. There was no information on the possible toxicity of the test substance in this study. The substance was also negative in the plate incorporation test in the *Salmonella typhimurium* indicator strains TA 98 and TA 100 (10 TEA doses from 1 to 20,000 µg/plate) and in *Escherichia coli* WP2 try^- (7 TEA doses from 10 to 10,000 µg/plate) with and without metabolic activation (S9-mix from PCB-induced rat livers; Inoue et al., 1982).

After exposure of Chinese hamster lung (CHL) cells to TEA (5 to 100 µg/ml) for 24 and 48 hours, no chromosomal aberrations were detected. According to the authors, slight cytotoxicity was observed at 100 µg/ml (Inoue et al., 1982; Hoshino and Tanooka, 1978).

TEA did not induce chromosomal aberrations in Chinese hamster ovary (CHO) cells at doses of up to 4030 µg/ml (without metabolic activation) or up to 10,070 µg/ml (with metabolic activation). Similarly, it caused no increase in sister chromatid exchange at doses of up to 1010 µg/ml (without metabolic activation) or up to 10,100 µg/ml (with metabolic activation; Galloway et al., 1987).

TEA (analytical grade) had no mutagenic activity in the *Bacillus subtilis* strain TKJ 5211, with or without metabolic activation (S9-mix from PCB-induced male Sprague-Dawley rats), at doses ranging from 6.75 to 27 mg/plate (Hoshino and Tanooka, 1978).

In a further study, TEA (88.2% pure) was tested in the *Salmonella typhimurium* strains TA 1535, TA 1537, TA 1538, TA 98 and TA 100, in *Escherichia coli* WP2 and WP2 uvrA, and in *Saccharomyces cerevisiae* JD1. It was also tested for chromosome-damaging effects in the rat liver cell lines RL_1 and RL_4. In the bacterial and yeast studies, the tests were carried out with and without metabolic activation. In the bacterial tests doses of 125, 250, 500, 1000, 2000 and 4000 µg/plate were used. It is not clear what dose levels were used in the studies in *Saccharomyces cerevisiae* and rat cells. TEA had no point-mutagenic or clastogenic effects in these tests (Dean et al., 1985).

TEA (purity unspecified) has also been tested in the primary rat hepatocyte unscheduled DNA synthesis assay (UDS test). A concentration of 1000 nl/ml caused extreme vacuolization in the cells and was cytotoxic (survival rate ca. 65%). Concentrations of 250 nl/ml and less were not cytotoxic. TEA was negative in this study at a dose range of 5 to 1000 nl/ml (Litton Bionetics, 1982 a).

TEA was also negative in another UDS test in rat hepatocytes (10^{-8} to 10^{-1} M; Anonymus, 1983).

7.6.2 In vivo

No information available

7.7 Carcinogenicity

In a chronic feeding study, groups of 40 male and 40 female ICR-ICL mice, which were 6 weeks old at the beginning of the study, received TEA hydrochloride (analytical grade) in their feed at concentrations of 0.3 and 0.03%. The authors did not calculate the doses in mg/kg body weight, but according to the so called Nelson table they were 450 and 45 mg/kg body weight. An appropriate control group was used. To incorporate the TEA into the powdered feed, both were heated to 100 °C for 40 minutes. The authors stated that the recovery of TEA in the feed at the conclusion of the study was nearly 100% (details not reported). TEA-treatment continued for the entire lifetime. The treated and control mice lived for equal lengths of time, the average survival time being 85 weeks for females and 65 weeks for males.

Table 1. Tumour incidence after chronic feeding of TEA to mice

% TEA in diet	Total number of malignant tumours/number of utilizable mice	Tumour incidence[a]	
Male			
0	1/35	2.9	
0.03	3/33	9.1	P>0.05
0.3	1/28	3.6	P>0.05
Female			
0	1/36	2.8	
0.003	10/37	27	P<0.001
0.3	13/36	36	P<0.01

[a] Tumour incidence= $\frac{\text{number of malignant tumours}}{\text{number of utilizable mice}} \times 100$

In the females fed TEA, the increase in malignant tumours compared with the controls was significant in both dose groups, and there was a dose/response relationship (see Table 1). In the females the tumours seen were mainly in the lymphoid tissues (lymphocytomas, lymphoblastomas, reticulum cell lymphomas, plasmocytomas of the thymus); tumours of these types were not seen in the males. Malignant tumours were also found in other organs, independent of sex. Exact details of macroscopic and histological findings were not provided (Hoshino and Tanooka, 1978).

A further study examined the carcinogenic effect on the mouse skin of pure TEA (1% impurities) and a technical grade TEA (up to 20% contaminants), and their possible co-carcinogenic (promoting) effect with methylcholanthrene. A 50% solution of the pure or technical grade product in acetone (volume not specified) was applied twice weekly to the dorsal skin of groups of 41 to 46 male CBAx$C_{57}BL_6$ mice (initial weight 16–20 g). The study duration was 18 months (group 1). In the promotion study the mice were treated once dermally with a 0.5% solution of 20-methylcholanthrene (MC) in acetone (volume not specified) and 3 weeks later were treated as for group 1 (group 2). A further group received only a single dermal application of MC (group 3). The parameters reported were: the time at which the first papilloma occurred and the latent period; the percentage of mice with papillomas out of the total number of surviving mice at the time when the first papilloma occurred; and the average number of papillomas per mouse. Neither pure nor technical grade TEA proved to be carcinogenic in this study. No visible effects or histologically detectable tumours were found on the skin. The incidence of tumours of the internal organs (lung adenomas, hepatomas) was no higher than the spontaneous tumour rate in this mouse strain. In the study on the promotional effect of TEA, papillomas occurred both in the study group and in the control group, but the incidences were not statistically significantly different from the incidence in mice treated only with MC (group 3; Kostrodymova et al., 1976).

Groups of 50 male and 50 female F-344/DuCrj rats received drinking water containing 1 or 2% TEA ad libitum for 2 years. The control group also consisted of 50 males and 50 females. As body weight gain was reduced in the males in week 2 and the number of deaths was higher than expected, the treatment was interrupted for 1 week in week 68, and from week 69 the drinking water concentrations were reduced by half (to 0.5 and 1% TEA). The total TEA intake of the rats after 2 years was calculated from the drinking water consumption at the end of the study: Control 0 g/rat, low-dose males 170 g/rat, high-dose males 358.1 g/rat, low-dose females 119.1 g/rat, high-dose females 231.8 g/rat (in the original paper these figures were given as mg/rat, but this is undoubtedly a mis-print). Based on an average weight for male rats of 420 g, the low dose in the males was calculated to be ca. 400 g/kg and the high dose ca. 850 g/kg. The corresponding values in the females (average weight 220 g) were ca. 540 g/kg for the low dose and ca. 1000 g/kg for the

Table 2. Tumor incidence in rats after chronic uptake of TEA with drinking water

Group	Male rats	Female rats
Control	48/48 (100%)	44/50 (88%)
Low dose	49/49 (100%)	36/48 (75%)
High dose	47/48 (98%)	37/47 (72%)

high dose. The tumour incidence is given in Table 2. In the males in all groups, testicular tumours occurred most frequently, followed by tumours of the haematopoietic organs, adrenal glands, pituitary gland, preputial gland and lungs. In the females, tumours of the uterus, haematopoietic organs, pituitary gland, mammary gland and adrenal glands were frequently observed. There was no significant increase in any specific tumour type compared with the control groups (calculated by means of the χ^2-test) in any of the dose groups, and all of the observed tumours corresponded histologically with the spontaneous tumour spectrum in the rat strain used. TEA had no carcinogenic effect under the chosen experimental conditions (Maekawa et al., 1986).

A test for cell-transforming activity of TEA in golden hamster embryo cells was negative at concentrations of 25 to 500 μg/ml (Inoue et al., 1980, 1982).

In another cell transformation test, TEA was tested in BALB/3T3-mouse fibroblasts without metabolic activation. At concentrations of 250 to 3125 nl/ml the survival rate of the cells ranged from over 90% to 10%. In this range, TEA had no cell-transforming effect (Litton Bionetics, 1982 b). A similar lack of activity was observed in the same test when a metabolic activation system (rat liver S9-mix) was added. TEA concentrations of 3.33 to 18.75 μl/ml were tested (Litton Bionetics, 1983).

In the USA, a dermal carcinogenicity study in rats and mice is in progress as part of the National Toxicology Program (NTP, 1989).

7.8 Reproductive toxicity

In a screening test for reproductive toxicity, 50 CD-1 mice received 1125 mg TEA/kg daily as an aqueous solution by stomach tube from day 6 to day 15 of pregnancy. The dams and pups were observed for 3 days after birth and were then killed. In this study, TEA was not toxic to the dams and had no effect on the number of live foetuses, the litter size, the birth weight of the pups or their survival time or weight gain. Neither was there any evidence of prenatal toxicity. As no maternal toxicity occurred, the authors recommended that the study be repeated with higher doses that would produce ca. 10% mortality in the dams (NTP, 1987).

In 3-day-old chicken embryos the ED_{50} for TEA for mortality and external malformations was found to be 2.6 μmol ($\hat{=}$ 388 μg) following a single injection into the air space of the egg. The incidence of malformations (mainly open coeloms) was relatively low (maximum 7%) with TEA compared with 80 other rubber chemicals (including 16 amines) tested (Korhonen et al., 1983 a, b).

7.9 Effects on the immune system

No information available.

7.10 Neurotoxicity

No information available.

7.11 Other effects

When TEA was incubated in the presence of nitrite under simulated gastric conditions, N-nitrosodiethanolamine was formed (Zingmark and Rappe, 1976).

The incubation of TEA with sodium nitrite [equal volumes of TEA (1 g/ml) and $NaNO_2$ (1 g/ml), 6.75 to 27 mg in total] at pH 3.5 resulted in a mixture that was clearly mutagenic (by a factor of 8) in the *Bacillus subtilis* strains TKJ 5211 and 6321 and HA 101. No mutagenic activity was seen in the presence of S9-liver homogenate. $NaNO_2$ alone was weakly mutagenic without S9-mix (by a factor of 2; the figures supporting this were not provided and there was no indication of the degree of variation of the reported results). After heating TEA with $NaNO_2$ (20 minutes in an autoclave at 120 °C; amounts used were 0.35–3.5 mg TEA with 0.43–4.3 mg $NaNO_2$), the mixture was both toxic and mutagenic to the *Bacillus subtilis* strains TKJ 5211 and 6321 and HA 101 without the addition of a metabolizing system. The mixture retained its activity after storage at room temperature for 5 days and for 5 months. Heating of TEA or $NaNO_2$ alone did not give rise to toxic or mutagenic products. A nitroso-compound (not further identified) was suggested as the mutagenic substance (Hoshino and Tanooka, 1978).

8. Experience in humans

TEA (purity not specified) was a slight irritant to intact human skin at concentrations greater than 50%. For damaged skin, the threshold concentration was 0.5% (TEA dissolved in ethanol; no data on test conditions; Frosch and Kligman, 1977).

TEA was a slight irritant when applied to the skin at concentrations of >5%. The strength of the irritant effect increased with concentration (CIR, 1983).

Skin irritation was also seen in a small proportion of exposed people at TEA concentrations of 1% (Iden and Schroeter, 1977).

Skin allergies were investigated in 578 workers at a rubber factory who were constantly exposed to a range of chemicals in the workplace air. Allergic effects were found in 283 of the subjects. Positive reactions to chemical allergens were found in 37 subjects, but only 2 of these were to TEA (Sidorenko et al., 1980).

Studied in 230 patients with industrial dermatoses, who had contact with cutting oils, revealed that TEA was implicated in many cases. Patch tests with a 10% aqueous solution of TEA produced a positive reaction in 42.7% of the patients (Alomar et al., 1985).

In dermatology clinics, about 1–4% of the patients treated, mainly eczema sufferers, had positive skin reactions when they were patch-tested with 1, 2 or 5% TEA in vaseline (Calas et al., 1978; Iden and Schroeter, 1977; Angelini et al., 1985; Fisher et al., 1971; Meneghini et al., 1971; Meneghini and Angelini, 1977).

In 1257 patients at a dermatology clinic (591 men and 766 women) with suspected contact eczema, skin tests with 10% aqueous TEA produced positive reactions (redness, infiltration and papulovesicles) in 41 cases (16 men and 25 women). It was assumed that these patients had been sensitized by using TEA-containing embrocations. A weak sensitizing effect of TEA in this particular group of people was thought to be probable (Scheuer, 1983).

A similar theory was put forward in a review article (Marghescu, 1983).

Two cases have been reported of female patients with recurrent eczema of the face and arms whose conditions were made worse by the use of E-45 cream (containing TEA). The patients were patch-tested with the "ICDRG" standard series, the normal "cosmetic battery" used in their skin clinic, their own cosmetics including E-45 cream, and finally with constituents of this cream. After 48 and 96 hours, a positive reaction to the cream and marked positive reactions to 5% and 2% TEA were seen. In the opinion of the authors, TEA should therefore be regarded as a possible contact sensitizer. The scarcity of reports however, implies that TEA is only a weak sensitizer (Jones and Kennedy, 1988).

Computer analysis of medical histories and skin test results from 5202 people tested for possible contact dermatitis due to cosmetics showed that TEA was not implicated as an allergen (Broeckx et al., 1987).

There is one case reported in the literature of an 8-year-old girl developing allergic rhinitis following TEA exposure. Positive tests included a prick test with TEA at 10^{-7}–10^{-4} mol, histamine liberation, and detection of specific IgE antibodies against TEA (Herman, 1982).

9. Threshold limit values

No information available.

References

Alomar, A., Conde-Salazar, L., Romaguera, C.
Occupational dermatoses from cutting oils
Contact Dermatitis, 12, 129–138 (1985)

Angelini, G., Vena, G.A., Meneghini, C.L.
Allergic contact dermatitis to some medicaments
Contact Dermatitis, 12, 263–269 (1985)

Anonymous
Final report on the safety assessment of triethanolamine, diethanolamine and monoethanolamine
J. Am. Coll. Toxicol., 2 (7), 183–233 (1983)

BASF AG, Gewerbehygienisch-Pharmakologisches Institut
Triethanolamin, gewerbetoxikologische Vorprüfung vom 17. 2. 1966

BASF AG
DIN-Sicherheitsdatenblatt (1989)

BASF AG
Communication to BG Chemie, 13. 3. 1990

Battelle, Columbus Laboratories, Columbus, Ohio 43201
Final report on the dermal repeated dose study of triethanolamine (CAS-No. 102-71-6) in Fisher-344 rats to National Toxicology Program (1985 a)

Battelle, Columbus Laboratories, Columbus, Ohio 43201
Final report on the dermal repeated dose study of triethanolamine (CAS-No. 102-71-6) in B6C3F1 mice to National Toxicology Program (1985 b)

Battelle, Columbus Laboratories, Columbus, Ohio 43201
Final report on the prechronic studies of triethanolamine (CAS-No. 102-71-6) in Fisher-344 rats and B6C3F1 mice
Vol. I of II to National Toxicology Program (1987)

Broeckx, W., Blondeel, A., Dooms-Gossens, A., Achten, G.
Cosmetic intolerance
Contact Dermatitis, 16, 189–194 (1987)

Calas, E., Castelain, P.Y., Piriou, A.
Epidemiology of contact dermatitis in Marseille
Ann. Dermatol. Venereol., 105, 345–347 (1978)

Carpenter, C.P., Smyth, H.F.
Chemical burns of the rabbit cornea
Am. J. Ophthalmol., 29, 1363–1372 (1946)

CIR (Cosmetic Ingredient Review)
Final report of the safety assessment for triethanolamine, diethanolamine, monoethanolamine
The expert panel of the Cosmetic Ingredient Review, Washington D.C. (1983)

CRC Handbook of Chemistry and Physics
62nd ed., C554
CRC-Press, Boca Raton, Florida 1981/82

Dean, B.J., Brooks, T.M., Hodson-Walker, G., Hutson, D.H.
Genetic toxicology testing of 41 industrial chemicals
Mutat. Res., 153, 57–77 (1985)

Dutertre-Catella, H., Nguyen, L.P., Huyen, V.N., Truhaut, R., Shechter, E.
Etude comparative de l'aggressivité cutanée et oculaire des éthanolamines (mono, di, tri et poly)
Arch. Mal. Prof., 43, 455–460 (1982)

NTP (National Toxicology Program)
Screening of priority chemicals for reproductive hazards, monoethanolamine, diethanolamine, triethanolamine;
Report-No. 87-377 (1987)

Fisher, A.A., Pascher, F., Kanof, N.B.
Allergic contact dermatitis due to ingredients of vehicles
Arch. Dermatol., 104, 286 (1971)

Frosch, P.J., Kligman, A.M.
Cutaneous Toxicity
eds. Drill, V.A., Lazar, P.
Academic Press Inc., New York, San Francisco, London, 133–146 (1977)

Galloway, S.M., Armstrong, M.J., Reuben, C., Colman, S., Brown, B., Cannon, C., Bloom, A.D., Nakamura, F., Ahmed, M., Duk, S., Rimpo, J., Margolin, B.H., Resnick, M.A., Anderson, B., Zeiger, E.
Chromosome aberrations and sister chromatid exchanges in Chinese hamster ovary cells: Evaluations of 108 chemicals
Environ. Mol. Mutagen., 10, 1–175 (1987)

Grant, W.M.
Toxicology of the eye
2nd ed., C.C. Thomas Publisher, Springfield, Illinois, USA, 1050 (1974)

Griffith, J.F., Nixon, G.A., Bruce, R.D., Reer, P.J., Bannan, I.A.
Dose-response studies with chemical irritants in the albino rabbit eye as a basis for selecting optimum testing conditions for predicting hazard to the human eye
Toxicol. Appl. Pharmacol., 55, 501–513 (1980)

Hammer, H., Körnig, W., Weber, T., Kieczka, H.
Ethanolamines and propanolamines
In: Ullmann's Encyclopedia of Industrial Chemistry
5th ed., Vol. A10, 1–22 (1987)
VCH Verlagsgesellschaft, Weinheim

Herman, J.J.
Intractable sneezing due to IgE mediated triethanolamine sensitivity
J. Allergy Clin. Immunol., 69, 158 (1982)

Hoechst AG, Pharma Forschung Toxikologie und Pathologie
Triethanolamin, Prüfung auf sensibilisierende Eigenschaften an Pirbright-White-Meerschweinchen im Maximierungstest
Unpublished study commissioned by BG Chemie (1988)

Hoshino, H., Tanooka, H.
Carcinogenicity of triethanolamine in mice and its mutagenicity after reaction with sodium nitrite in bacteria
Cancer Res., 38, 3918–3921 (1978)

Hüls AG
Communication to BG Chemie of 4. 10. 1989

Iden, D.L., Schroeter, A.L.
The vehicle tray revisited: The use of the vehicle tray in assessing allergic contact dermatitis by a 24-hour application method
Contact Dermatitis, 3, 122 (1977)

Inoue, K., Sunakawa, T., Takayama, S.
Studies of in vitro cell transformation and mutagenicity by surfactants and other compounds
Food Cosmet. Toxicol., 18, 289–296 (1980)

Inoue, K., Sunakawa, T., Okamoto, K., Tanaka, Y.
Mutagenicity tests and in vitro transformation assays on triethanol-amine
Mutat. Res., 101, 305–313 (1982)

Jones, S.K., Kennedy, C.T.C.
Contact dermatitis from triethanolamine in E-45® cream
Contact Dermatitis, 19, 230 (1988)

Kharchenko, T.F., Ivanova, T.P.
Hygienic evaluation of some bonding materials and chemical substances applied to skin (English translation)
Gig. Tr. Prof. Zabol., 7, 63–64 (1980)

Kindsvatter, V.H.
Acute and chronic toxicity of triethanolamine
J. Ind. Hyg. Toxicol., 22, 206–212 (1940)

Korhonen, A., Hemminki, K., Vainio, H.
Toxicity of rubber chemicals towards three-day chicken embryos
Scand. J. Work Environ. Health, 9, 115–119 (1983 a)

Korhonen, A., Hemminki, K., Vainio, H.
Embryotoxicity of 16 industrial amines to the chicken embryo
J. Appl. Toxicol., 3 (2), 112–117 (1983 b)

Kostrodymova, G.M., Voronin, V.M., Kostrodymov, N.N., Sysin, A.N.
The toxicity (in complex action) and the possibility of carcinogenic and cocarcinogenic properties of triethanolamines
(English translation)
Gig. Sanit., 3, 20–25 (1976)

Litton Bionetics, Inc., Kensington, Maryland 20895
Evaluation of triethanolamine No. 80/475 in the primary rat hepatocyte unscheduled DNA synthesis assay, final report
Submitted to BASF AG, Ludwigshafen/Rhein (1982 a)

Litton Bionetics, Inc., Kensington, Maryland 20895
Evaluation of triethanolamine No. 80/475 in the in vitro transformation of BALB/3T3 cells assay, final report
Submitted to BASF AG, Ludwigshafen/Rhein (1982 b)

Litton Bionetics, Inc., Kensington, Maryland 20895
Evaluation of triethanolamine No. 80/475 in the vitro transformation of BALB/3T3 cells with metabolic activation assay, final report
Submitted to BASF AG, Ludwigshafen/Rhein (1983)

Maekawa, A., Onodera, H., Tanigawa, H., Furuta, K., Kanno, J., Matsuoka, C., Ogiu, T., Hayashi, Y.
Lack of carcinogenicity of triethanolamine in F 344 rats
J. Toxicol. Environ. Health, 19, 345–357 (1986)

Marghescu, S.
Neuere Erkenntnisse über Arzneimittelwirkungen auf der Haut
Internist, 24, 329–333 (1983)

Melnick, R., Hejtmancik, M., Mezza, L., Ryan, M., Persing, R., Peters, A.
Comparative effects of triethanolamine (TEA) and diethanolamine (DEA) in short term dermal studies
The Toxicologist, 8 (1), 127 (1988)

Meneghini, C.L., Rantuccio, F., Lomuto, N.
Additives, vehicles and active drugs of topical medicaments as causes of delayed-type allergic dermatitis
Dermatologica, 143, 137–147 (1971)

Meneghini, C.L., Angelini, G.
Behavior of contact allergy and new sensitivities on subsequent patch tests
Contact Dermatitis, 3, 138–142 (1977)

Naonori, K., Toshiyuki, M., Kazutoshi, U., Katsumi, M., Takaichi, A.
Development of assay method in biological fluids and biological fate of triethanolamine
Yakuzaigaku, 42 (4), 342–348 (1982)

NTP (National Toxicology Program)
Fiscal Year 1988, Annual Plan, p. 124 (1988)

NTP (U.S. National Toxicology Program)
Chemical Status Report, 7. 7. 1989

Preussmann, R., Habs, M., Habs, H., Schmähl, D.
Carcinogenicity of N-nitrosodiethanolamine in rats at five different dose levels
Cancer Res., 42, 5167–5171 (1982)

Sax, N.I. (ed.)
Dangerous Properties of Industrial Materials
Van Nostrand Reinhold, New York (1979)

Scheuer, B.
Kontaktallergie durch Triethanolamin
Der Hautarzt, 34, 126–129 (1983)

Sidorenko, E.N., Buslenko, A.I., Bajda, N.A., Kozinceva, P.V., Iva-nova, S.I., Djacenko, E.I., Muchtarova, N.D., Titenkov, I.K.
Allergische Erkrankungen bei Arbeitern in der Gummiproduktion (German translation)
Vrach. Delo., 12, 14–16 (1980)

Smyth, H.F., Carpenter, C.P., Weil, C.S.
Range-finding toxicity data: List IV
Arch. Ind. Hyg. Occup. Med., 4, 119–122 (1951)

Sommer, H., Löffler, H.P., Eisenbrand, G.
A method to determine N-nitrosoethanolamines in alkanolamines
J. Soc. Cosmet. Chem., 39, 133–137 (1988)

Surupova, E.A.
Zur Toxikologie von Triethanolamin (German translation)
Gig. Priment. Polim. Mater. Izdelii Nikh., 1, 323–328 (1969)

Weil, C.S., Scala, R.A.
Study of intra- and interlaboratory variability in the results of rabbit eye and skin irritation tests
Toxicol. Appl. Pharmacol., 19, 276–360 (1971)

Windholz, M. (ed.)
The Merck Index, 10th ed., p. 1381
Merck & Co., Inc., Rahway, New Jersey (1983)

Zingmark, P.A., Rappe, C.
On the formation of N-nitrosodiethanolamine from a grinding fluid under simulated gastric conditions
Ambio, 5, 80–81 (1976)

Phenyl isocyanate

1. Summary and assessment

According to the available experimental data, phenyl isocyanate is of moderate acute toxicity on oral administration (with one exception) and on dermal application (LD_{50} rat oral 940–2750 mg/kg; LD_{50} rat dermal 5000 mg/kg or more; LD_{50} rabbit dermal >2000 mg/kg and ca. 7000 mg/kg). The chemical is however highly toxic by inhalation because of its relatively high vapour pressure (in an inhalation hazard test, all 10 rats died after an exposure of only 3 minutes). The 4-hour LC_{50} for phenyl isocyanate lies between 4 and 13 ppm. Under these conditions, delayed deaths occur. In the Alarie test, the concentration that reduces the respiratory frequency by 50% (RC_{50}) lies between 1.8 and 0.7 ppm, depending on the exposure time. Repeated inhalation exposure of rats for 3 weeks leads to histologically detectable damage to the respiratory tract, even at 0.05 ppm.

Liquid phenyl isocyanate is a severe skin irritant, and burns may occur in the eyes. The vapours also have a strong irritant effect.

In the Salmonella/microsome test, most studies provide no evidence of point-mutagenic activity, either with or without metabolic activation. Phenyl isocyanate does not cause chromosomal aberrations in mouse bone marrow.

Phenyl isocyanate has no embryotoxic effect in mice, but the study design which has produced this result is unsatisfactory.

In vitro, phenyl isocyanate inhibits acetylcholinesterase activity in erythrocytes and in whole blood, but this effect has been classified as relatively weak.

In summary, phenyl isocyanate is of moderate acute oral toxicity, but is of high inhalation toxicity. It is severely irritating to the skin and can cause burns in the eyes. Phenyl isocyanate vapours are also severely irritating. Cholinesterase activity is inhibited in vitro.

2. Name of substance

2.1	Usual name	Phenyl isocyanate
2.2	IUPAC-name	Phenyl isocyanate
2.3	CAS-No.	103-71-9

3. Synonyms, common and trade names

Isocyanatobenzene
Isocyanic acid, phenyl ester
Phenyl carbonimide
Phenylcarbimide
Carbanil
Mondur P
Phenylisocyanat

4. Structural and molecular formulae

4.1 Structural formula	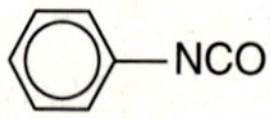
4.2 Molecular formula	C_7H_5NO

5. Physical and chemical properties

5.1 Molecular mass, g/mol	119.12
5.2 Melting point, °C	–31 (Solidification temperature) (Bayer, 1988)
5.3 Boiling point, °C	165 (at 1013 hPa) (Bayer, 1988)
5.4 Vapour pressure, hPa	2.5 (at 20 °C) (Bayer, 1988) 14 (at 50 °C) (Bayer, 1988) 133 (at 101 °C) (Bayer, 1988)
5.5 Density, g/cm^3	1.095 (at 20 °C) (Bayer, 1988)
5.6 Solubility in water	Hydrolyses (Bayer, 1988)
5.7 Solubility in organic solvents	No information available
5.8 Solubility in fat	No information available
5.9 pH-value	–
5.10 Conversion factor	1 ppm $\hat{=}$ 4.92 mg/m^3 1 mg/m^3 $\hat{=}$ 0.20 ppm (at 20 °C and 1013 hPa)

6. Uses

Intermediate for pesticides (Bayer, 1988). Used as a reagent for diamines and alcohols; used in the production of pharmaceuticals, optical brighteners, textile processing aids, plasticizers (Neumüller, 1985).

7. Experimental results

7.1 Toxicokinetics and metabolism
No information available.

7.2 Acute and subacute toxicity

To determine the oral LD_{50}, groups of 5 male and 5 female Sprague-Dawley rats (165 to 208 g) were given various single doses of phenyl isocyanate in polyethylene glycol 400 by stomach tube. The observation period was 14 days. An LD_{50} value of 1044 (805 to 1353) mg/kg was determined for the males, while for the females a value of 172 (139 to 210) mg/kg was determined. Therefore in this study phenyl isocyanate was 6 times more toxic to the females than the males. In all of the rats, symptoms such as lethargy and shortness of breath were seen within 20 minutes. The effects were reversed 24 hours later. The administration of lethal doses caused terminal convulsions. Post-mortems on the rats that died revealed gastro-intestinal inflammation. On dissection of the animals that survived, no macroscopic effects could be found (Mobay, 1975).

In another study, groups of 10 male and 10 female Wistar rats (160 to 200 g) were given single doses of phenyl isocyanate (ca. 98% pure) dissolved in groundnut oil in quantities ranging from 25 to 3250 mg/kg by stomach tube. The observation period was 14 days. An LD_{50} value of 2500 to 2750 mg/kg was determined for both male and female rats. The observed symptoms included dyspnoea, reeling, reduced motility, closed lids and, at high doses, weakened reflexes, lying on the stomach and cyanosis. The lowest dose without effect was 25 mg/kg. Following lethal doses, the rats died after 30 minutes to 24 hours. Autopsy of the animals that died revealed clay-coloured lungs, somewhat reddened kidney pelves, solid mucous membranes with a "tanned" appearance in the forestomach, reddened stomach, and pale discolouration of parts of the liver with slight marks on the lobes. The rats killed at the end of the observation period showed slight induration of the mucous membranes of the stomach (Bayer, 1981).

In a further study (no further details) an oral LD_{50} value for rats of 940 mg/kg was determined (Monsanto, 1983).

The oral LD_{50} has also been determined in male CFLP mice. Groups of 6 mice were given single oral doses of from 60 to 600 mg phenyl isocyanate/kg in sunflower oil, and were then observed for 14 days. The LD_{50} was 196 mg/kg (no further details; Nehéz et al., 1989).

The acute dermal toxicity of phenyl isocyanate (ca. 98% pure) was studied in groups of 5 male and 5 female Wistar rats (160 to 200 g) by the method of Noakes and Sanderson. Doses of 100 to 5000 μl/kg were used, the duration of exposure was 24 hours and there was a 14-day observation period. The neat chemical was thickened with 5 to 300 mg cellulose powder. The LD_{50} value was ca. 5000 mg/kg for males and >5000 mg/kg for females. Immediately after application the rats showed signs of pain, followed by a reduction in motility, closure of the eyelids and, in the males, increased aggression, dyspnoea, weakness of the hind-limbs and subsequent emaciation (which was marked in some cases). The symptoms began immediately or within 15 minutes of the start of application and lasted for 14 days. Locally, the skin was thickened, hardened and inflamed. Necroses formed 3 to 4 days after application, and healed with scars in the second week of observation. Autopsies of the rats that died revealed swollen and stained lungs, partly reddened kidney pelves and, in most cases, an empty gastro-intestinal tract. In the rats that were killed at the end of the study, those that had received doses in the lethal range had swollen lungs (Bayer, 1981).

To study the acute dermal toxicity of neat phenyl isocyanate, a single dose of 2000 mg/kg was applied to the abraded skin of 2 male and 2 female white New Zealand rabbits (2.6 to 3.0 kg). The occlusive application was for 24 hours, and the observation period was 14 days. There were no deaths and no signs of toxicity, and the dermal LD_{50} for rabbits is thus more than 2000 mg/kg. Autopsy of the rabbits revealed a dark ring-like discolouration at the base of the kidney cortex, granulation of the liver, darkening of the lungs and congestion of the spleen (Mobay, 1975).

In another study, groups of 3 female white New Zealand rabbits (3 to 4 kg) had neat phenyl isocyanate applied occlusively to their clipped skin for 24 hours. An LD_{50} value of 7130 (3740 to 13540) mg/kg was determined (no further details; Vernot et al., 1977).

The acute inhalation hazard from phenyl isocyanate was assessed in an inhalation hazard test at 21 to 22 °C, using groups of 5 male and 5 female Sprague-Dawley rats (175 to 220 g). An average nominal concentration of 2360 mg/m^3 was determined. All of the rats died within 1.25 hours of the beginning of exposure. Autopsy revealed haemorrhagic lungs with oedema (Mobay, 1975).

A further inhalation hazard test with phenyl isocyanate (ca. 98% pure) was carried out in groups of 5 male and 5 female Wistar rats (160 to 200 g) exposed for 3, 10 or 30 minutes at 20 °C, with a 14-day observation period. Even after exposure for 3 minutes all the rats died within 8 to 11 days. After longer exposure, death occurred within 24 hours (10 minutes exposure) or within an hour (30 minutes exposure). The symptoms observed included breathing difficulties and lying on the stomach and side. Locally, marked irritation of the eyes and nose occurred (redness, swelling, eye-watering). The body weight of rats that survived the first week of observation was clearly reduced. Autopsy revealed a dark-red liver-like appearance to the lungs after inhalation exposure for 10 or 30 minutes, and a clear liquid was found in the lungs and the pleural cavity. The spleen and the liver were pale, the gastro-intestinal tract was reddened and its contents reddish and slimy. Autopsy of rats exposed for 3 minutes revealed dark-red colouration and swelling of the lungs, which again appeared liver-like. The spleen and kidneys were pale-coloured (Bayer, 1981).

The LC_{50} for phenyl isocyanate was determined with groups of 4 male and 4 female albino rats (150 to 200 g) at each concentration. Depending on the method of analysis, values for the vapour after a 14-day observation period were 12.6 (8.4 to 19.0) ppm (HPLC) or 3.9 ppm ("Marcali" method). Results with the HPLC method were closer to the calculated values, particularly at higher concentrations. The deaths were delayed, occurring 8 to 12 days after exposure at concentrations of up to 80 ppm. Based on these results, phenyl isocyanate was classified as highly toxic (ICI, 1978).

In a study of the subacute inhalation toxicity of phenyl isocyanate, groups of 8 male and 8 female albino rats (150 to 200 g) inhaled 0.055 or 0.496 ppm phenyl isocyanate (as an aerosol in petroleum ether) for 6 hours/day, 5 days/week, for a total of 15 exposures. The concentration was determined analytically by the "Marcali" method. The body weight of the rats in the 0.5 ppm group was reduced on the 12th day, while that of the 0.055 ppm group remained unaffected. Feed and water consumption were not impaired. At the higher dose level, one male rat died after 9 days and one female after 12 days. The remaining animals in this group were killed on the 12th day, because 7 of them were moribund. Symptoms included crouching, pilo-erection, emaciation, hypothermia and shortness of breath. Chemical analysis of the blood (no further details) revealed no treatment-related effects, but there were signs of blood thickening at the higher dose level. At the lower dose level, lung function was normal with the exception of elevated respiratory resistance at the end of the third week of exposure. In the rats at the higher dose level, the respiratory volume and frequency and the pulmonary compliance were reduced, while respiratory resistance was increased on the 11th and 12th day. Macroscopic examination revealed pale and/or swollen lungs with red stains in some of the rats at the higher dose level. Red stains in the lungs were also found in a few of the rats in the lower dose group and in the petroleum ether control group. On histological examination, the rats in the higher dose group showed inflammatory changes of various degrees of severity in the nasal passages, the larynx, the trachea and the bronchial tree, as well as epithelial hyperplasia. The latter was accompanied by polyp formation, submucosal obstructive fibrosis and metaplasia of the squamous cells. In the lungs there was slight damage to the alveoli, with alveolar oedema, fibrin deposition, haemorrhages, acute inflammation, chronic inflammatory infiltration, fibrosis and epithelialization. In the animals of the 0.05 ppm group, the effects on the respiratory tract were similar, but minimal, and limited to the larynx, trachea and bronchial tree in 1 to 2 rats (ICI, 1979).

A no-effect level could not be established in this study, and from this it was inferred that a considerable safety factor is required in the setting of a threshold value (ICI, 1978).

In an Alarie test, groups of 4 Swiss-Webster mice (26–28 g) were exposed to phenyl isocyanate for periods of 10 and 30 minutes and 1, 2 and 3 hours. In this test, the sensory irritant effect before and during exposure is determined by plethysmography. It is expressed as the RC_{50}, the concentration that reduces the respiratory frequency by an average of 50%. For phenyl isocyanate this test gave a concentration- and time-dependent reduction in respiratory frequency, which was only slowly reversible. The RC_{50} values were 1.8 (1 to 4.6) ppm for 10 minutes, 1.2 (0.81 to 2) ppm for 30 minutes, 0.9 (0.43 to 1.6) ppm for 1 hour, 0.82 (0.51 to 1.2) ppm for 2 hours, and 0.73 (0.54 to 0.93) ppm for 3 hours (Sangha et al., 1981).

7.3 Skin and mucous membrane effects

The primary irritant effect of phenyl isocyanate was studied on the normal and abraded skin of 6 white New Zealand rabbits. A dose of 0.5 ml was applied occlusively for 4 hours, and the effects were assessed at 4, 24 and 48 hours and, if required, after 96 hours. The primary irritation index was 0.17 in accordance with the Federal Hazardous Substances Act, Section 191.11 (21CFR191.11). The substance was therefore classified as non-irritant (Mobay, 1975).

In a further test, the skin irritancy of phenyl isocyanate (ca. 98% pure) was determined on the hairless skin of the inner ear of white New Zealand rabbits (3 to 4 kg). In this case, 0.5 ml of the neat substance was applied to a cellulose patch and fixed with an adhesive dressing for 1, 2 or 4 hours. The observation period was 7 days. After exposure for 1 hour, slight reddening occurred which persisted for the entire observation period. The 2-hour exposure led to slight to moderate redness and the 4-hour exposure to marked or very marked redness and slight swelling. Based on these results, phenyl isocyanate was classified as a severe skin irritant (Bayer, 1981).

The eye irritancy of phenyl isocyanate was tested in a total of 8 rabbits, by the instillation of 0.1 ml of the neat substance into the conjunctival sac. In 5 rabbits the eye was rinsed with 300 ml water for 2 minutes after a 5-minute exposure period, while the eyes of 3 rabbits remained unrinsed. The effects were assessed after 1 hour and after 1, 2, 3 and 7 days, as well as after 7 to 14 days where necessary. The evaluation was carried out in accordance with the Federal Hazardous Substances Act, Section 191.12 (21CFR191.12). Based on the results obtained, phenyl isocyanate was classified as extremely irritating and corrosive. There was no fundamental difference between the findings in the rinsed and unrinsed eyes, but the reversibility of the effects appeared to be better in the rinsed eye after 14 and 21 days (Mobay, 1975).

In a further study on eye irritancy, 2 rabbits (3 to 4 kg) each had ca. 100 µl neat phenyl isocyanate (ca. 98% pure) instilled into the conjunctival sac. The observation period was 7 days. Both rabbits showed moderate reddening and swelling of the conjunctiva and slight diffuse clouding of the cornea. In one rabbit the slight diffuse corneal clouding progressed through a mother-of-pearl-like appearance to complete opacity. Based on these results, phenyl isocyanate was classified as severely irritating to the eyes (Bayer, 1981).

7.4 Sensitization

No information available.

7.5 Subchronic and chronic toxicity

No information available.

7.6 Genotoxicity

7.6.1 In vitro

The genotoxicity of phenyl isocyanate was studied in the Streptomycin-dependent Sd-4-73 strain of Escherichia coli at 0.01 to 0.025 ml/plate. Phenyl isocyanate showed no mutagenic activity under these conditions (Szybalski, 1958).

Phenyl isocyanate (100% pure) was tested for genotoxic activity in the Salmonella/microsome test. Doses of from 20 to 12,500 µg/plate were tested in strains TA 98, TA 100, TA 1535 and TA 1537. No bacteriotoxic effect was seen up to 2500 µg/plate. At this concentration and above, precipitation of the substance occurred. The study was carried out with and without the addition of a metabolizing system (S9-mix from rat-liver induced with Aroclor 1254). Phenyl isocyanate was not mutagenic in this study (Bayer, 1980).

A further mutagenicity test was carried out with phenyl isocyanate (analytical grade) in strains TA 98, TA 100 and TA 1537, with and without the addition of a metabolizing system (S9-mix from phenobarbital-induced rat liver). Phenyl isocyanate (no information on dose) did not induce any increase in revertants in this study and thus showed no point-mutagenic activity (Andersen et al., 1980).

Phenyl isocyanate (in DMSO) was studied in the Salmonella typhimurium strain TA 100 without metabolic activation at a concentration of 100 µg/plate. The revertant count was 295/plate (control 120/plate). The author concluded that phenyl isocyanate showed considerable mutagenic activity (Yamaguchi, 1980).

7.6.2 In vivo

The clastogenic activity of phenyl isocyanate in bone marrow cells was studied in groups of 10 male CFLP mice (ca. 30 g) after a single oral dose of 1/40 or 1/20 of the oral LD_{50} (ca. 5 or 10 mg/kg respectively). Sunflower oil was used as a solvent. The bone marrow preparation was carried out 24 and 48 hours later and 20 mitoses/mouse were evaluated. There was no increase in chromosomal aberrations after either 24 or 48 hours compared with 2 control groups (Nehéz et al., 1989). However, the results of the study are of limited value because the doses used were too low and the number of mitoses evaluated per mouse was insufficient.

In a micronucleus test, groups of 5 male and 5 female NMRI mice (8 to 12 weeks old at the beginning of the study) were given single intraperitoneal injections of phenyl isocyanate (99.9% pure) as a solution in paraffin oil at a dose of 30 mg/kg body weight. The dose was chosen on the basis of preliminary studies. One of the 40 treated mice died during the study, and others showed clear signs of toxicity such as apathy, ruffled fur, convulsions, dyspnoea and diarrhoea. Five males and 5 females were killed after 24, 48 and 72 hours, and the numbers of monochromatic erythrocytes/1000 polychromatic erythrocytes and of polychromatic erythrocytes with micronuclei were recorded. There was a change in the ratio of polychromatic to monochromatic erythrocytes (negative control 1000:1105, 24-hour group 1000:1572, 48-hour group 1000:2257, 72-hour group 1000:1699), but no change in the number of micronuclei-containing polychromatic erythrocytes in any of the groups. Therefore, in comparison with cyclophosphamide (20 mg/kg) which was included as a positive control, phenyl isocyanate showed no clastogenic activity (Bayer, 1990).

7.7 Carcinogenicity

No information available.

7.8 Reproductive toxicity

To investigate the embryotoxic effect of phenyl isocyanate pregnant mice of the Halle-AB-Jena and Halle-DBA strains were given single oral doses of 1/40 to 1/20 of the acute oral LD_{50} (ca. 5 and 10 mg/kg respectively) as a solution in olive oil on day 4, 7, 11 or 15 of pregnancy. Phenyl isocyanate had no noticeable effect on the total loss of implantations under these conditions (Nehéz et al., 1989). However, the study can be criticized as the doses were too low and the treatment was carried out on only one day of pregnancy.

7.9 Effects on the immune system

No information available.

7.10 Neurotoxicity

It has been reported that phenyl isocyanate inhibits human serum cholinesterase and bovine erythrocyte esterase activity in vitro. However, compared with other isocyanates, this effect was only weak. A 50% inhibition required a molar ratio of 50:1 or more (short report, no further details; Brown et al., 1981).

Phenyl isocyanate has been described as an inhibitor of human erythrocyte cholinesterase activity. In vitro, the concentrations that caused a 50% inhibition were 106 µM for erythrocyte cholinesterase and 130 μM for total blood cholinesterase. On the whole, inhibition by phenyl isocyanate was weak compared with other isocyanates. After incubation at 21 to 23 °C for a few days, a slow and limited reactivation of the inhibited enzyme occurred. The authors suggested that this inhibition of cholinesterase activity could be a factor in the development of the respiratory effects observed in about 5% of people exposed to isocyanates (Dewair et al., 1983).

7.11 Other effects

After incubation of phenyl isocyanate with chorionic gonadotropin at low temperatures (0 to –2 °C), the activity of the hormone was inhibited by more than 90%. The uterine weight of juvenile rats served as an indicator (Bischoff, 1943).

In vitro, the reaction of cytosine, adenine and guanine with phenyl isocyanate gives rise to the formation of the corresponding phenylcarbamyl compounds. After incubation of deoxyribonucleic acid (DNA) with phenyl isocyanate at 0 to 4 °C for 10 days, 4-N-phenylcarbamyl cytosine, 6-N-phenylcarbamyl adenine and 2-N-phenylcarbamyl guanine could be almost quantitatively isolated (Jones and Warren, 1970).

8. Experience in humans

See chapter 7.10.

9. Threshold limit values

As yet, no MAK or TLV values have been established for phenyl isocyanate.

However, it can be deduced from a report of the sensory irritant effect of the substance that 1/30 of the RC_{50} value for a 3-hour inhalation could serve as the empirical measurement for a TLV. The 3-hour RC_{50} value for phenyl isocyanate is 0.73 ppm, and so a TLV of 0.02 ppm has been suggested (Sangha et al., 1981).

References

Andersen, M., Binderup, M.L., Kiel, P., Larsen, H., Maxild, J.
Mutagenic action of isocyanates used in the production of polyurethanes
Scand. J. Work. Environ. Health, 6, 221–226 (1980)

Bayer AG, Institut für Toxikologie
Phenylisocyanat, Salmonella/Mikrosomen-Test zur Untersuchung auf punktmutagene Wirkung
Unpublished study, Report no. 9170 (1980)

Bayer AG, Institut für Toxikologie
Phenylisocyanat, Untersuchungen zur Gewerbetoxikologie
Unpublished study, Report no. 9694 (1981)

Bayer AG
DIN-Sicherheitsdatenblatt Phenylisocyanat (1988)

Bischoff, F.
Reaction of chorionic gonadotropin with phenylisocyanate
Endocrinology, 32, 260–262 (1943)

Brown, W.E., Green, A.H., Yen, C.
A study of isocyanates as active-site inhibitors of cholinesterase
Fed. Proc., 40, 1615 (1981)

Dewair, M., Baur, X., Fruhmann, G.
Inhibition of acetylcholinesterase from human erythrocytes by isocyanates
J. Occup. Med., 25, 279–282 (1983)

ICI (Imperial Chemical Industries Limited), Central Toxicology Laboratory
Status report on isocyanate toxicity programme for the International Isocyanate Institute (1978)

ICI (Imperial Chemical Industries Limited), Central Toxicology Laboratory
Status report on isocyanate toxicity programme for the International Isocyanate Institute (1979)

Jones, A.S., Warren, J.H.
The reaction of phenylisocyanate with purines, pyrimidines and desoxyribonucleic acid
Tetrahedron, 26, 792–794 (1970)

Mobay Chemical Corporation, Chemagro Agricultural Division
Acute toxicity studies of phenylisocyanate
Unpublished study, Report no. 44762 (1975)

Monsanto Co.
Toxicity information (1983)
cited in: Nehéz et al. (1989)

Nehéz, M., Fischer, G.W., Nehéz, I., Scheufler, H., Dési, I.
Investigations on the acute toxic, cytogenetic and embryotoxic activity of phenylisocyanate and diethoxyphosphoryl isocyanate
Ecotoxicol. Environ. Safety, 17, 258–263 (1989)

Neumüller, O.A. (ed.)
Römpps Chemie Lexikon
8th ed., vol. 4, p. 3140
Franckh'sche Verlagshandlung, Stuttgart (1985)

Sangha, G.K., Matijak, M., Alarie, Y.
Comparison of some mono- and diisocyanates as sensory irritants
Toxicol. Appl. Pharmacol., 57, 241–246 (1981)

Szybalski, W.
Special microbiological systems. II. Observations on chemical mutagenesis in microorganisms
Ann. N.Y. Acad. Sci., 76, 475–489 (1958)

Vernot, E.H., MacEwen, J.D., Haun, C.C., Kinkead, E.R.
Acute toxicity and skin corrosion data for some organic and inorganic compounds and aqueous solutions
Toxicol. Appl. Pharmacol., 42, 417–423 (1977)

Yamaguchi, T.
Mutagenicity of isothiocyanates, isocyanates and thioureas on *Salmonella typhimurium*
Agric. Biol. Chem., 44 (12), 3017–3018 (1980)

4-Chlorophenyl isocyanate

1. Summary and assessment

4-Chlorophenyl isocyanate is of low acute toxicity [LD_{50} rat oral male 335, female 138 mg/kg; LC_{50} (4 hours) rat 113 mg/m^3]. In addition to irritant effects on the eyes, inhalation (one time) of 4-chlorophenyl isocyanate vapours (45 mg/m^3 and more) causes bronchitis, pneumonia and pleuritis in rats, the extent of the respiratory damage being dependent on the vapour concentration. Damage to the kidneys, spleen and cardiac muscle is also suspected after exposure to lethal concentrations. A no-effect level is not reported. The same effects are observed after exposure to an enriched atmosphere over 10 minutes at 20° C. The exposure over 3 minutes under the same conditions causes no death.

There is no evidence of toxicity after repeated subacute oral daily administration of 100 mg/kg over 14 days in rats.

A single application of 4-chlorophenyl isocyanate causes minimal skin irritation. Repeated administration may result in reddening and xerosis of the skin, but these effects recede on cessation of exposure.

Instillation of the chemical into the eyes causes severe inflammation with ulceration of the cornea and connective tissues, effects which recede without causing permanent damage.

There are no indications that 4-chlorophenyl isocyanate causes skin sensitization.

Subchronic inhalation exposure of low concentrations (0.03 mg/m^3) over 80 days, which do not damage the mucous membranes, results in an increase in a number of parameters in rats, including the serum globulin fraction, blood eosinophilic granulocytes and 17-ketosteroid secretion in the urine. These parameters return to normal in the post-observation period. Exposure to 0.0015 mg/m^3 has not revealed these changes. In a further subchronic inhalation study 1.2–1.4 mg/m^3 (exposure 4 hours daily, 6 time/week over 4 months) has been regarded as the toxic border line concentration for rats and mice.

In man, eczema can be observed after repeated contact with 4-chlorophenyl isocyanate, which recedes after exposure had ceased. Concentrations as low as 0.8 mg/m^3 cause eye irritation in volunteers.

The odour threshold for this chemical is 0.015 mg/m^3. Concentrations of 0.0029 mg/m^3 cause variations in the EEG (there are no data on the test method for determining the latter values).

The principal toxic effect of 4-chlorophenyl isocyanate and its vapours is severe irritation of the eyes and respiratory tract.

2. Name of substance

2.1	Usual name	4-Chlorophenyl isocyanate
2.2	IUPAC-name	4-Chlorophenyl isocyanate
2.3	CAS-No.	104-12-1

3. Synonyms, common and trade names

p-Chlorophenylisocyanate
4-Chlorphenylisocyanat
Isocyanic acid
p-chlorophenylester
PCPJ
4-Chlorophenyl isocyanursäure

4. Structural and molecular formulae

4.1 Structural formula

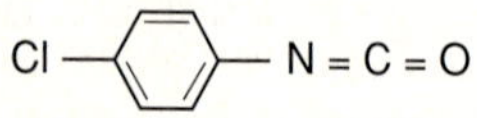

4.2 Molecular formula C_7H_4NOCl

5. Physical and chemical properties

5.1	Molecular mass, g/mol	153.57
5.2	Melting point, °C	28 (Sax, 1979)
5.3	Boiling point, °C	106.5 (Sax, 1979)
5.4	Vapour pressure, hPa	1 (at 20 °C) (Hoechst, 1986) 1.33 (at 35 °C) (Hoechst, 1986) 13.3 (at 78 °C) (Hoechst, 1986)

5.5 Density, g/cm^3	1.26 (at 30 °C) (Hoechst, 1986)
5.6 Solubility in water	Insoluble
5.7 Solubility in organic solvents	Toluene, mono- and dichlorobenzene, carbon tetrachloride, ethyl acetate (Frolova, 1967)
5.8 Solubility in fat	No information available
5.9 pH-value	–
5.10 Conversion factor	1 ppm $\hat{=}$ 6.37 mg/m^3 1 mg/m^3 $\hat{=}$ 0.16 ppm (at 25 °C and 1013 hPa)

6. Uses

Intermediate in the production of pharmaceuticals and pesticides (Sax and Lewis, 1987; Bayer, 1981).

7. Experimental results

7.1 Toxicokinetics and metabolism
No information available.

7.2 Acute and subacute toxicity

The results of acute toxicity studies by various routes of administration are summarized in Tables 1, 2 and 3.

Rats given a single oral dose of 4-chlorophenyl isocyanate became lethargic (Mobay, 1975) and lost weight (Frolova, 1966). Deaths occurred within 24 hours (most within 2 hours) of administration (Mobay, 1975). Autopsy of the animals that died during the study revealed inflammation of the gastro-intestinal tract. No pathological changes in the internal organs were seen on post-mortem examination of the rats killed at the end of the 14-day observation period (Mobay, 1975).

In a study in rats, an LD_{50} value of 63 mg/kg was established following intraperitoneal administration, but there was no indication of the toxic effect or of the findings at autopsy (Bayer, 1960).

No local damage was seen in rats or rabbits in dermal toxicity studies. At autopsy, a red coloration of the kidney cortex was found in rabbits (Mobay, 1975).

After acute inhalation exposure of rats and mice to 4-chlorophenyl isocyanate, there were marked irritant effects on the eyes and mucous membranes of the upper respiratory tract, as well as watery eyes, salivation, breathing difficulties and gasping for breath. A concentration-dependent reduction in weight gain was seen during the observation period. Autopsy of the animals that died a few days after exposure revealed that the lungs had a liver-like consistency (hepatization), and pulmonary oedema and pleuritis were observed. Dystrophy of the kidneys, spleen and heart muscle was also seen (Frolova, 1966, 1967; Mobay, 1975; Bayer, 1981).

In rabbits exposed for 40 minutes to 4-chlorophenyl isocyanate, a change in the breathing rate was seen at a threshold level of 0.0018 to 0.0020 mg/l (1.8 to 2 mg/m^3; Frolova, 1966, 1967).

Another inhalation study reported on the pathological and histological findings following acute or repeated exposure to 4-chlorophenyl isocyanate. 20 to 25 minutes after the beginning of a 2-hour exposure period at 0.1 mg/l (100 mg/m^3, observation period 3 months) white rats (strain not specified) produced colourless secretions from their mouths and noses and had difficulty breathing. Within 48 hours of the end of exposure 14/49 rats had died and after 7–14 days 45/49 rats were dead. Histopathological examination of the animals that died in the first 2 days revealed fibrous necrotic tracheitis, bronchitis, pulmonary oedema and hyaline membranes on the walls of the respiratory tract. In the rats that died later (after 1 to 2 weeks), panbronchitis, bronchitis obliterans, bronchiolitis and focal pneumonia were observed (Voznesenskaja, 1968).

In a further study, rats were exposed to 4-chlorophenyl isocyanate at concentrations of 0.025–0.03 mg/l (25–30 mg/m^3) for 4 hours/day for 17 days. Almost all of the rats (numbers not specified) died after 1 to 2 weeks. Pathological and histological examination revealed bronchitis, bronchiolitis, pneumonia and pulmonary oedema, as well as the first signs of carnification of the lungs and lymph congestion (Voznesenskaja, 1968).

In a subacute study, a daily dose of 100 mg/kg was administered orally (as a 1% oily solution) to 10 rats (no details of strain or sex) for 14 days. No effects were observed (Bayer, 1960).

7.3 Skin and mucous membrane effects

No irritation was evident after a 4-hour semi-occlusive application of 0.5 ml 4-chlorophenyl isocyanate to the intact or abraded skin of 6 white rabbits [evaluated according to the Federal Hazardous Substance Act, Section 191.11 (21 CFR 191.11); Mobay, 1975].

When 4-chlorophenyl isocyanate was applied semi-occlusively to the skin of the rabbit ear, slight redness and swelling were seen after 8 hours and marked irritant effects after 24 hours of exposure (Bayer, 1960).

A very general report, which provides no detailed information, states that a single application of 4-chlorophenyl isocyanate to animal skin caused no toxic effects. Repeated application produced slight dermatitis (hyperaemia and xerosis), but the skin returned to normal very quickly after the end of the experiment (Frolova, 1966).

7.4 Sensitization

The shaved dorsal skin of 10 male Hartley guinea-pigs was treated with 0.1 ml 4-chlorophenyl isocyanate, 4 times within 10 days. On the third application, 0.2 ml Freund's adjuvant was injected intradermally close to the application site. After a further 2 weeks the test substance was applied to the clipped skin of one flank, and the skin reaction (redness, oedema) was evaluated after 24 and 48 hours. There was no evidence of skin sensitization in any of the guinea-pigs (Rao et al., 1981).

In an 80-day inhalation study in rats (continuous exposure), there were increased levels of eosinophilic granulocytes in the blood (26 to 42% above the initial value) and of γ-globulin in the serum from the second week of exposure, at a concentration of 0.03 mg/m^3 (see also section 7.5). These effects declined in the second half of the study period, but were nevertheless viewed by the authors as a possible indication of allergy (Zibireva, 1967).

7.5 Subchronic and chronic toxicity

11 mice inhaled concentrations of 0.02 mg/l (20 mg/m^3) for 2 hours a day for 45 days. They showed weight loss, loss of appetite and some dyspnoea. 6 out of 11 mice died during the study (Frolova, 1966).

In another study by the same authors, mice and rats (strain, sex and group size not specified) were exposed to concentrations of 0.0014 mg/l (1.4 mg/m^3, mouse) and 0.0012 mg/l (1.2 mg/m^3, rats) for 4 hours daily, 6 times a week for 4 months. Neither species developed any symptoms of toxicity. Although the mice showed signs of irritation and were over-excited during the first 5 to 10 minutes, these effects occurred only at the beginning of the study. During the 2nd and 3rd month, the weight of the exposed mice was below that of the controls ($p=0.05$), while in the 4th month it matched that of the controls. Histological examination of the organs of both species (no details) revealed no damage that could be attributed to the inhalation of 4-chlorophenyl isocyanate (Frolova, 1966, 1967).

Male albino rats (strain and group size not specified) inhaled concentrations of 0.0015 mg/m^3 or 0.03 mg/m^3 continuously for 80 days. No effects were seen in the low-dose rats. In the 0.03 mg/m^3 group there was an increase in total globulins in the blood due to the increase in γ-globulin; the eosinophils in the blood were increased in the first half of the study (26 to 42% above the initial value), but the eosinophil count and γ-globulin levels returned to normal later in the study. Increased excretion of 17-ketosteroids in the urine subsequently occurred. These effects were interpreted as a possible sensitizing effect caused by 4-chlorophenyl isocyanate. In addition, a fall in the vitamin C levels in various organs was observed during the study, together with a decrease in SH-groups and an increase in pyrovate in the liver, an increase in serum sialic acid (acetylated

Table 1. Acute toxicity of 4-chlorophenyl isocyanate

Species	Sex	Exposure route	Observation period (days)	LD_{50} (mg/kg)	References
Rat	♂	Oral	14	335 (232–484)	Mobay, 1975
(Sprague-Dawley)	♀	Oral	14	138 (85–225)	
Rat	♂	Oral	–	>500 <1000	Bayer, 1960
Rat	–	Oral	–	4710	Sax, 1979
Mouse	–	Oral	14	530	Frolova, 1966
Mouse	–	Oral	14	450	Izmerov, 1982
Rat	♂	i.p.	–	63	Bayer, 1960
Rat	–	Dermal	–	>1000 (2 and 4 hours)	Bayer, 1960
Rabbit (New Zealand)	♂, ♀	Dermal	14	>2000 (24-hour exposure)	Mobay, 1975
Rabbit	–	Dermal	–	<300	Izmerov, 1982

Table 2. Acute inhalation toxicity of 4-chlorophenyl isocyanate (LC_{50}-determination, 4 hours)

Species	Sex	Exposure	Observation period (days)	LC_{50} (mg/m^3)	References
Rat (Wistar)	♂	Inhalation	21	113–272	Bayer, 1981
	♀	(4 hours)	21	ca. 113	
Mouse	–	Inhalation (2 hours)	25	53	Frolova, 1966, 1967

Table 3. Acute inhalation toxicity of 4-chlorophenyl isocyanate (inhalation hazard test)

Species (Strain)	Sex	Exposure duration	Results: dead/ total animals	Time of occurrence of death	Observation period (days)	References
Rat (Wistar)	♂,♀	3 minutes	0/5	–	15	Bayer, 1981
Rat (Wistar)	♂	10 minutes	3/5	8–10 days	15	Bayer, 1981
	♀	10 minutes	3/5	8–15 days	15	
Rat (Wistar)	♂	30 minutes	5/5	1–9 days	15	Bayer, 1981
	♀	30 minutes	5/5	1–14 days	15	
Rat	♂	6 hours[a]	5/5	4–6 hours	–	Mobay, 1975
	♀	6 hours[a]	5/5	5–96 hours	–	

[a] Average concentration of 4-chlorophenyl isocyanate in the inhalation system 1.67 g/m^3

neuraminic acid) and a reduction in urinary coproporphyrin. All of these effects disappeared during the 3-week observation period, which indicates their functional nature (Zibireva, 1967; Pushkina et al., 1967).

7.6 Genotoxicity

No information available.

7.7 Carcinogenicity

No information available.

7.8 Reproductive toxicity

No information available.

7.9 Effects on the immune system

No information available.

7.10 Neurotoxicity

No information available.

7.11 Other effects

4-Chlorophenyl isocyanate inhibited the growth of Ehrlich ascites tumours when it was injected intraperitoneally into mice on 3 consecutive days at doses of 20 to 30 mg/kg/day (Moos et al., 1971).

8. Experience in humans

Out of 4 people who had had repeated contact with 4-chlorophenyl isocyanate, 1 developed itchy erythema and xeroses on the backs of the hands. These effects cleared up after exposure ended (Frolova, 1966).

A threshold concentration of 0.008 mg/l (0.8 mg/m^3) was determined in human volunteers. The subjects mainly complained of discomfort in the eyes (Frolova, 1967).

An odour threshold of 0.015 mg/m^3 was determined in humans. At a concentration of 0.0029 mg/m^3 changes in the EEG occurred, and sensitivity of the eyes to light was observed at 0.0068 mg/m^3 (details of study methods and concentration determination not given; Zibireva, 1967).

9. Threshold limit values

Validated threshold limit values are not available. A maximum permitted concentration in the workplace of 0.0015 mg/m^3 is recommended in the USSR (Zibireva, 1967).

References

Bayer AG, Toxikologisch-gewerbehygienisches Labor
m-Chlorphenylisocyanat, p-Chlorphenylisocyanat, 3,4-Dichlorphenylisocyanat
Unpublished report (1960)

Bayer AG, Institut für Toxikologie
p-Chlorphenylisocyanat, Akute Inhalationstoxizität
Unpublished report no. 9695 (1981)

Frolova, I.N.
Maximum permissible concentration of p-chlorphenyl isocyanate in factory air
Gig. Sanit., 31, 481–483 (1966)

Frolova, I.N.
Toxikologische Charakteristik der bei der Herbizidherstellung vorkommenden Isocyanate (German translation)
Gig. Tr. Prof. Zabol., 11, 23–26 (1967)

Hoechst AG
Communication of 7. 8. 1986

Izmerov, N.F., Santosky, I.V., Sidorov, K.K.
Toxicometric parameters of industrial toxic chemicals under single exposure
Centre of International Projects GKNT, Moscow (1982)

Mobay Chemical Corporation, Research and Development
Acute toxicity studies of para-chlorophenyl isocyanate
Unpublished report 44761 (1975)

Moos, G.E., Maguire, I.A., Kitchlew, T.Z., Swyers, W.A., Volk, P.Z., Croft, I.R., Quigley, M.I., Fries, I.R., Oser, N.A., Anderson, L.I.
Inhibition of growth of Ehrlich ascites tumors in ICR/HA Swiss mice by isocyanates
Cancer Res., 31, 937–941 (1971)

Pushkina, N.N., Zibireva, I.A., Khikmatullaeva, S.H.S.
The effect of low concentrations of thiophene and chloroisocyanates on the ascorbic acid content in the organs of rats
Gig. Sanit., 32, 121–124 (1967)

Rao, K.S., Betso, J.E., Olson, K.J.
A collection of guinea pig sensitization test results, grouped by chemical class
Drug Chem. Toxicol., 4, 331–351 (1981)

Sax, N.I. (ed.)
Dangerous Properties of Industrial Materials
5th ed., p. 498
van Nostrand Reinhold Company, New York (1979)

Sax, N.I., Lewis, R.J. (eds.)
Hawley's Condensed Chemical Dictionary
11th ed., p. 270
van Nostrand Reinhold Company, New York (1987)

Voznesenskaja, G.A.
Morphologische Veränderungen in den Atmungsorganen von Versuchstieren bei Parachlorphenylisocyanat-Intoxikation
(German translation)
Gig. Tr. Prof. Zabol., 12, 59–61 (1968)

Zibireva, I.A.
Relative toxicity of microconcentrations of two chloroisocyanates (the para- and meta-isomers)
Gig. Sanit., 32, 3–10 (1967)

Diisopropanolamine

1. Summary and assessment

Experiments in laboratory animals show that up to about 25% of a dermal application of diisopropanolamine is absorbed, with about 12% of the dose excreted in the urine and a further 12% remaining in the tissues (but not in the fat). After intravenous administration, about 90% of the dose is excreted in the urine within 12 hours.

Diisopropanolamine is of low acute toxicity (LD_{50} rat oral 6720 mg/kg). On subacute oral administration to rats in the drinking water for 2 weeks, 600 mg/kg body weight/day is tolerated without adverse effects. Diisopropanolamine is a severe eye irritant and a weak skin irritant.

In the Salmonella/microsome test, diisopropanolamine shows no point-mutagenic activity.

In humans, combined diisopropanolamine patch-test application and UVA/UVB-irradiation does not induce allergic or photo-allergic reactions. In tests of several sun-protection creams containing 1% diisopropanolamine, isolated cases of irritation have been seen in volunteers, and one case of sensitization has been observed.

Like other secondary amines, diisopropanolamine may be contaminated with N-Nitrosodiisopropanolamine (Spiegelhalder et al., 1978). N-Nitrosodiisopropanolamine is a carcinogen in mice, rats, hamster, guinea pigs and rabbits (Preussmann and Stewart, 1984).

2. Name of substance

2.1	Usual name	Diisopropanolamine
2.2	IUPAC-name	Bis(2-hydroxypropyl)amine
2.3	CAS-No.	110-97-4

3. Synonyms, common and trade names

1,1'-Iminobis-2-propanol
1,1'-Iminodi-2-propanol
Bis(2-propanol)amine
Dipropyl-2,2'-dihydroxyamine
Diisopropanolamine S

4. Structural and molecular formulae

4.1 Structural formula

```
   OH           OH
   |            |
CH3CHCH2NHCH2CHCH3
```

$CH_3CH(OH)CH_2NHCH_2CH(OH)CH_3$

4.2 Molecular formula $C_6H_{15}NO_2$

5. Physical and chemical properties

5.1 Molecular mass, g/mol: 133.20

5.2 Melting point, °C: ca. 35–38 (BASF, 1987)

5.3 Boiling point, °C: 245–250 (BASF, 1987)

5.4 Vapour pressure, hPa: <1 (at 20 °C) (BASF, 1987); 3 (at 100 °C) (BASF, 1987)

5.5 Density, g/cm^3: 1.0 (at 40 °C) (BASF, 1987)

5.6 Solubility in water: Miscible (BASF, 1987)

5.7 Solubility in organic solvents: No information available

5.8 Solubility in fat: No information available

5.9 pH-value: 11.4 (100 g/l water) (BASF, 1987)

5.10 Conversion factor: 1 ppm $\hat{=}$ 5.53 mg/m^3; 1 mg/m^3 $\hat{=}$ 0.18 ppm (at 20 °C and 1013 hPa)

6. Uses

Intermediate in the manufacture of drugs, pesticides, dyes, preservatives and disinfectants; catalyst for the production of polyurethane foam; purification of industrial gases (Klink and Gelbke, 1980).

7. Experimental results

7.1 Toxicokinetics and metabolism

Four female Fischer-344 rats had 19.5 mg/kg ^{14}C-labelled diisopropanolamine in acetone applied to the skin in the shoulder area. After the solvent had evaporated, the area was covered occlusively for 48 hours. After 48 hours, about 50% of the applied radioactivity was found at the application site and a further 25% on the skin of the surrounding area. Of the radioactivity absorbed (about 25%), 12% was excreted in the urine and less than 1% in the faeces or expired air. The other 12 to 12.5% diisopropanolamine remained in the tissues. No storage in the fat was detected. When 4 female Fischer-344 rats were injected intravenously with 19 mg ^{14}C-labelled diisopropanolamine in aqueous solution, more than 70% of the radioactivity was eliminated from the blood during the first 6 hours. About 90% of the dose was recovered from the urine within 12 hours (CIR, 1987).

7.2 Acute and subacute toxicity

The National Institute for Occupational Safety and Health (NIOSH) reported an oral LD_{50} for diisopropanolamine in rats of 6720 mg/kg (no further details; NIOSH, 1978).

A single oral dose of 2000 mg diisopropanolamine/kg did not give rise to any signs of toxicity in rats. After the administration of 3960 mg/kg to 2 rats, both died within 24 hours (no further details; CIR, 1987).

Groups of 5 male and 5 female Sprague-Dawley rats were given 5000 mg/kg of a sun-screening agent that contained 1% diisopropanolamine, as a single dose by stomach tube. One rat had diarrhoea 2 hours after administration. The animals were observed for 14 days and showed no other signs of toxicity during this time. On histological examination no lesions were observed (CIR, 1987).

In an inhalation hazard test, rats inhaled air enriched with diisopropanolamine vapour at room temperature. 12 animals tolerated exposure for 8 hours without symptoms (BASF, 1965).

In order to study the subacute toxicity of diisopropanolamine, groups of 5 male and 5 female CDF-Fischer-344 rats were given doses of 0, 100, 300, 600, 1200 and 3000 mg/kg body weight for 2 weeks in their drinking water. At the highest dose level, 2 males died within 2 weeks. A marked loss of body weight related to a considerable reduction in feed and water consumption was observed. Autopsy revealed acute inflammation and degeneration of the kidneys and bladder, together with generalized atrophy of the liver. In the 1200 mg/kg dose group, a slight reduction in feed and water intake occurred. Weight loss was only observed in the males. The relative kidney weight was increased, but only 1 male showed changes to the kidneys similar to those at the highest dose level. No toxic effects were observed in the lower dose groups (CIR, 1987).

7.3 Skin and mucous membrane effects

An 80% aqueous preparation of diisopropanolamine caused moderate skin irritation in rabbits after a 20-hour exposure period, while no irritation occurred after a 15-minute exposure period (BASF, 1965).

Diisopropanolamine caused slight skin irritation and severe eye irritation (no further details; NIOSH, 1978).

After application of neat diisopropanolamine to the intact abdominal skin of rabbits, hyperaemia and marked necrosis were observed. Application to abraded skin caused weak hyperaemia, oedema and slight denaturation (no details of duration of exposure). A 10% aqueous solution of diisopropanolamine was applied to the intact ear skin of 10 rabbits, the intact abdominal skin of 10 further rabbits and the abraded abdominal skin of 2 rabbits (no details of duration of exposure). The 10% solution had no effect on the skin of the ear, but application to the intact abdominal skin led to slight hyperaemia and vesicle formation. The abraded skin showed slight hyperaemia, weak oedema and slight denaturation. In a 4-hour test carried out in accordance with the Federal Hazardous Substances Act, diisopropanolamine was not corrosive (CIR, 1987).

A facial sun-protection product containing 1% diisopropanolamine gave a mean primary irritation index of 1.33, and was classified as a weak irritant, after occlusive application of 200 mg to 6 New Zealand rabbits for 50 hours. UV-irradiation after exposure for 2 hours followed by further application of the product for 48 hours gave a phototoxic irritation index of 1.5, which was classified as weakly phototoxic. A further study with 0.2 ml of a 1% diisopropanolamine-containing sun-protection agent gave the same results (CIR, 1987).

To study the eye irritancy of neat diisopropanolamine, 4 rabbits each had 50 mg instilled into the conjunctival sac. This induced moderate corrosion of the eyelids, the eyeball and the cornea, which was improved after 22 days, but cataracts and clouding of the cornea were still present. Based on these findings, diisopropanolamine was classified as a severe eye irritant (CIR, 1987).

In another study, 50 mg neat diisopropanolamine in the eye likewise caused severe irritation that was still not completely reversed after 8 days (BASF, 1965).

A sun-protection product containing 1% diisopropanolamine was tested for its eye irritancy. Nine albino rabbits had 0.1 ml instilled into the conjunctival sac. In 6 of the rabbits, the eyes were not rinsed, while in the remaining 3 they were rinsed with 20 ml water after 4 seconds. The findings were recorded after 1 hour, and 1, 2, 3, 5 and 7 days. No local effects were observed in the unrinsed eyes, while slight irritation occurred in the rinsed eyes after 1 hour (average irritation score on the Draize scale 1.3 out of a maximum of 110). The product was classified as non-irritant. A further study in 6 rabbits with no rinsing of the eyes gave the same results (CIR, 1987).

7.4 Sensitization
No information available.

7.5 Subchronic and chronic toxicity
No information available.

7.6 Genotoxicity

7.6.1 In vitro
The genotoxic potential of diisopropanolamine was tested in the Salmonella/microsome test in strains TA 97, TA 98, TA 100, TA 1535 and TA 1537. The assays were carried out with and without metabolic activation (S9-mix from the livers of male Sprague-Dawley rats and Syrian hamsters that had been induced with Arochlor 1254). In a preliminary test in *Salmonella typhimurium* TA 100, the bacteriotoxic concentration was determined, and this served as the highest dose for the subsequent mutagenicity test. In this study, diisopropanolamine showed no point-mutagenic activity either with or without metabolic activation (Mortelmans et al., 1986).

7.6.2 In vivo
No information available.

7.7 Carcinogenicity
No information available.

7.8 Reproductive toxicity
No information available.

7.9 Effects on the immune system
No information available.

7.10 Neurotoxicity
No information available.

7.11 Other effects
No information available.

8. Experience in humans

In a repeated patch-test, 25 male and female volunteers had 0.2 ml of a 2% aqueous solution of diisopropanolamine applied to the skin on their backs for 24 hours/day on 3 consecutive days/week for 3 weeks. After treatment, the application sites were irradiated 3 times with a combination of UVA- and UVB-rays, at a dose which caused minimal erythema. Thereafter, they were treated only with UVA-rays for 6 weeks (at a dose that did not cause erythema), and diisopropanolamine was then applied as patches to 2 sites on the back. One patch remained in place for 24 hours and the site was irradiated at patch removal; the other patch was kept on for 48 hours, and the site was examined for signs of contact dermatitis after removal. Diisopropanolamine did not cause allergic or photoallergic dermatitis (CIR, 1987).

In a further study, 0.05 ml of a facial sun-protection cream that contained, among other substances, 1% diisopropanolamine, was applied to the skin on the backs of 10 volunteers under occlusive cover for 48 hours. No irritation was observed either 2 or 24 hours after the patch was removed (CIR, 1987).

In a test involving 24 volunteers, 0.5 ml of a facial sun-protection cream that contained 1% diisopropanolamine was applied under semi-occlusive cover for 24 hours/day for a period of 22 days. The irritant effects observed were classed as minimal (no further details; CIR, 1987).

121 volunteers took part in a further patch-test series with repeated exposure to a facial sun-protection cream that contained 1% diisopropanolamine. For a period of 3.5 weeks, 0.5 ml was applied under semi-occlusive cover for 24 hours/day and for 72 hours at the weekends. Two weeks after the final application, a challenge patch was applied for 48 hours to a previously untreated site. Sensitization to the sun-protection cream was induced in one of the volunteers (CIR, 1987).

In a further study in 203 volunteers, 0.2 ml of a facial sun-protection cream containing 1% diisopropanolamine was applied to the skin on their backs under occlusive cover for 24 hours. The application site was then examined for irritation. 24 hours later, a further patch was applied for 24 hours and this procedure was repeated for 10 working days. After a 13-day treatment-free interval, a patch was applied for 48 hours to test for sensitization. A second challenge patch was applied 8 days later for 48 hours. During the induction period, 12 volunteers showed irritation of varying degrees of severity. The sun-protection cream induced sensitization in one volunteer. The authors concluded from these results that diisopropanolamine is a safe component in cosmetics under present conditions of use and concentration (CIR, 1987).

9. Threshold limit values

No information available.

References

BASF AG, Gewerbehygienisch-Pharmakologisches Institut
Gewerbetoxikologische Vorprüfung, Study No. XIV 411
Unpublished report (1965)

BASF AG
DIN-Sicherheitsdatenblatt Diisopropanolamin (1987)

CIR (Cosmetic Ingredient Review)
Final report on safety assessment of diisopropanolamine, triisopropanolamine, isopropanolamine, and mixed isopropanolamine
J. Am. Coll. Toxicol., 6, 53–77 (1987)

Klink, W., Gelbke, H.P.
Propanolamine
in: Ullmanns Encyklopädie der technischen Chemie
Verlag Chemie, Weinheim, vol. 19, p. 433–442 (1980)

Mortelmans, K., Harworth, S., Lawlor, T., Speck, W., Tainer, B., Zeiger, E.
Salmonella mutagenicity tests: II. Results from the testing of 270 chemicals
Environ. Mutagen., 8, 1–119 (1986)

NIOSH (National Institute for Occupational Safety and Health)
cited in: Klink, W., Gelbke, H.P. (1980)

Preussmann, R., Stewart, B.
N-Nitroso Carcinogens
in: Chemical Carcinogens, C.E. Searle (ed.), p. 643–828
Am. Chem. Soc. Monograph, no. 182, Am. Chem. Soc., Washington, D.C. (1984)

Spiegelhalder, B., Eisenbrand, D., Preussmann, R.
Verunreinigung von Aminen mit N-Nitrosaminen
Angew. Chemie, 90, 379–380 (1978)

Triethylene tetramine

1. Summary and assessment

Triethylene tetramine is of low acute toxicity on oral administration and moderate toxicity on dermal application (LD_{50} rat oral 2778–4940 mg/kg, LD_{50} rabbit dermal 550 and 820 mg/kg). The acute inhalation hazard of the volatile fraction at room temperature is slight to moderate in rats. In animal studies, acute inhalation of the chemical in aerosol form leads to irritation of the mucous membranes.

Subacute oral administration of triethylene tetramine to rats for 7 days in the feed causes weight loss and changes in the liver and kidney weights. The highest dose with no such effect is 490 mg/kg body weight.

After subacute dermal application of triethylene tetramine to rats and guinea-pigs (1 drop/animal daily, 17 to 55 times), some of the animals show severe irritation at the application site, as well as weight loss. Deaths have occurred in the treated guinea-pigs. Morphologically, the prominent findings in these species are fatty degeneration of the liver and inflammatory changes at the application site. Alterations in enzyme activity and other biochemical parameters also occur. There is no fundamental difference between the effects on pregnant and non-pregnant animals. It is unclear whether the general toxic effects and deaths are primarily due to the chemical's local or systemic action.

Triethylene tetramine is strongly alkaline and in laboratory animals causes severe irritation of the skin and eyes, which can lead to necrosis.

It induces skin sensitization in guinea-pigs and mice.

In a 10-month subchronic oral study in rats, the "threshold dose for chronic toxicity" is said to be 0.8 mg/kg body weight.

Triethylene tetramine shows clear point-mutagenic activity in the Salmonella/microsome test. Point mutations have also been induced in CHO cells treated with the chemical, but a second study provides inconclusive findings. Positive results have been produced in the SCE test and the UDS test. Triethylene tetramine therefore has clear point-mutagenic activity in vitro, while it is not point-mutagenic in vivo in the SLRL test in Drosophila. The chemical is not clastogenic in the mouse micronucleus test in vivo following oral or intraperitoneal administration.

A carcinogenicity study involving life-long dermal application of triethylene tetramine provides no indication of an increased incidence of local or other tumours, but the doses used were too low for this to be convincing.

Triethylene tetramine shows clear embryotoxic and teratogenic activity in rat and chicken embryos. This appears to be due mainly to the chelating properties of the chemical and the resulting copper deficiency. Copper supplementation markedly reduces this effect in the rat. In another study, triethylene tetramine was not embryotoxic or teratogenic. In rabbits, triethylene tetramine does not cause embryotoxic or teratogenic effects even at maternally toxic dose levels. In contrast to the rat, there is no reduction in the copper content of the serum and urine.

Human experience is based mainly on its therapeutic use in Wilson's disease and from observations in occupational medicine.

In the treatment of Wilson's disease, a symptom of which is increased copper levels in the liver, brain and kidneys, triethylene tetramine is an alternative to penicillamine (in cases of intolerance) for the promotion of copper excretion. Most publications state that oral doses of up to 2.3 g/day are well tolerated over prolonged periods. A few pregnancies in treated patients have gone to term without complications and with no signs of embryotoxic or teratogenic effects.

Occupational experiences with triethylene tetramine relate primarily to its skin irritant and sensitizing properties in the manufacture of epoxy resins, where it is used as a hardener. Triethylene tetramine is a relatively potent skin sensitizer, and a case of recidivating allergic asthma has been described. Liver damage is a possible systemic effect. Serum monoamine oxidase activity is increased in exposed workers, indicative of increased amine metabolism in the connective tissue.

In summary, triethylene tetramine is of low to moderate acute toxicity, and is slightly toxic after oral administration for longer periods. It is a severe skin irritant and also induces skin sensitization. It shows clear point-mutagenic activity in vitro. There is no evidence of carcinogenic activity following dermal application. The reproductive toxicity in rats very probably arises indirectly from copper deficiency. In occupational medicine, the main concerns are skin irritation and skin sensitization.

2. Name of substance

2.1	Usual name	Triethylene tetramine
2.2	IUPAC-name	3,6-Diazaoctane-1,8-diamine
2.3	CAS-No.	112-24-3

3. Synonyms, common and trade names

Araldite HY951
Bis(2-aminoethyl)-ethylenediamine
N,N'-Bis(2-aminoethyl)-1,2-ethanediamine
Hardener 951
Hardener T
HY951
TETA

4. Structural and molecular formulae

4.1	Structural formula	$H_2N-(CH_2)_2-NH-(CH_2)_2-NH-(CH_2)_2-NH_2$
4.2	Molecular formula	$C_6H_{18}N_4$

5. Physical and chemical properties

5.1	Molecular mass, g/mol	146.24
5.2	Melting point, °C	ca. –35 (Bayer, 1988)
5.3	Boiling point, °C	ca. 280 (Bayer, 1988)
5.4	Vapour pressure, hPa	<0.01 (at 20 °C) 13.33 (at 144 °C) 400 (at 240 °C) (Axel et al., 1974)
5.5	Density, g/cm^3	0.9818 (at 20 °C) (Axel et al., 1974)
5.6	Solubility in water	Miscible (Bayer, 1988)

5.7 Solubility in organic solvents	No information available
5.8 Solubility in fat	No information available
5.9 pH-value	ca. 10.7 (10 g/l water) (Bayer, 1988)
5.10 Conversion factor	1 ppm $\hat{=}$ 6.07 mg/m^3 1 mg/m^3 $\hat{=}$ 0.17 ppm (at 20 °C and 1013 hPa)

6. Uses

Hardener for epoxy resins; intermediate in the production of wetting agents, emulsifiers, textile processing aid and additive for lubricants and motor fuels (Axel et al., 1974). Used in medicine as a chelating agent (Haslam et al., 1980; Walshe, 1982; Epstein and Sherlock, 1980).

7. Experimental results

7.1 Toxicokinetics and metabolism
No information available.

7.2 Acute and subacute toxicity

To determine the acute oral toxicity, groups of 5 male Wistar rats (90–120 g) were given single doses ranging from 1 to 8 g triethylene tetramine/kg body weight as an aqueous preparation by stomach tube. The observation period was 14 days. An approximate LD_{50} of 4340 (3810–4940) mg/kg was calculated by the method of Thompson (Smyth et al., 1949).

In another study, groups of 3 rats were given single doses of 1000, 2500, 3750 or 5000 mg triethylene tetramine/kg body weight as an aqueous solution by stomach tube. Within 24 hours, all 3 rats given 5000 mg/kg and 2/3 rats given 3750 mg/kg had died. Typical symptoms of toxicity were not observed. The LD_{50} was therefore about 3750 mg/kg (Bayer, 1957).

An oral LD_{50} of 2.83 (2.05 to 3.89) ml/kg was reported for male Wistar rats in a further study with neat triethylene tetramine (CHF, 1976).

An oral LD_{50} of 1600 mg triethylene tetramine/kg was determined in mice, while the value determined in rabbits was 5500 mg/kg (no further details; Stavreva, 1979).

Intraperitoneal injection of rats with 375 mg/kg body weight as an aqueous solution led to the deaths of all 5 animals. At 200 mg/kg 2/5 rats died and at 100 mg/kg 1/3 rats died, while 3 rats survived 50 mg/kg. The 200 mg/kg dose caused breathing difficulties. An LD_{50} value of 200 mg/kg was determined (Bayer, 1957).

Female albino mice (25–30 g) were given single intraperitoneal injections of triethylene tetramine as an aqueous solution adjusted to pH 7.0 $\pm$ 0.2 with hydrochloric acid. 10 mice were used at each dose and the observation period was 14 days. An LD_{50} of 604.26 (537.0–679.30) mg/kg was reported. Symptoms observed included convulsions which lasted for up to 20 minutes. Death occurred within 2 days, and post-mortems on the dead mice revealed congestion of the internal organs (Srivastava and Katiyar, 1988).

A dermal LD_{50} of 820 (720–940) mg/kg body weight was determined for triethylene tetramine in an occlusive test with the neat material applied to the clipped skin of rabbits (no further details). The observation period was 14 days (Smyth et al., 1949).

A further study of the acute dermal toxicity in groups of 4 male albino rabbits gave an LD_{50} value of 0.561 (0.264–1.19) ml/kg for the neat material (CHF, 1976).

The acute inhalation hazard for triethylene tetramine was determined in groups of 6 male albino rats in an inhalation hazard test. Air was passed through the test material in a fritted bottle at room temperature for periods of time falling in a geometric series with a constant ratio of 2, up to a maximum of 8 hours. The exposure time that was survived by all rats after a 14-day observation period was reported to be 4 hours (Smyth et al., 1949).

In another inhalation hazard test at 21 °C all 6 rats survived a single 8-hour exposure without symptoms (CHF, 1976).

In a further study of acute inhalation toxicity, 10 ml of a 40% (v/v) solution of triethylene tetramine (Hardener T) in ethanol was sprayed into a 400 l chamber containing 1 rabbit, 1 guinea-pig, 2 rats and 4 mice. The duration of exposure was 1 hour. The animals showed slight irritation of the mucous membranes and breathing difficulties, but recovered very quickly at the end of the experiment (no further details; Bayer, 1957).

The same protocol and the same number of animals were used in a subacute inhalation study, but 0.4 ml triethylene tetramine (Hardener T) in 5 ml ethanol (8%, v/v) was sprayed into the chamber. The animals were exposed for 1 hour on each of 10 consecutive

Table 1. Changes in some clinical-chemical parameters in the serum and the amniotic fluid of non-pregnant and pregnant rats after subacute dermal application of triethylene tetramine (Dobryszycka et al., 1974).

	Non-pregnant rats (serum)	Pregnant rats (serum)	Pregnant rats (amniotic fluid)
Total protein (g/100 ml)	Reduced (6.37/5.49)[a]	Unchanged	Unchanged
Seromucoid (mg/100 ml)	Increased (98.33/142.90)[a]	Unchanged	Unchanged
Sialic acid (mg/100 ml)	Unchanged	Increased (64.83/76.69)[a]	Unchanged
Haptoglobin (mg/100 ml)	Increased (15.55/45.61)[a]	Reduced (61.33/33.29)[a]	Unchanged
Lactate dehydrogenase (U)	Increased (234.60/490.00)[a]	Increased (255.00/338.00)[a]	Unchanged
Leucylnaphthylamidase (IU)	Increased (31.88/42.74)[a]	Unchanged	Increased (3.36/10.00)[a]
γ-Glutamyltranspeptidase (IU)	Unchanged	Unchanged	Unchanged
Aspartate aminotransferase (U)	Reduced (126.73/74.00)[a]	Increased (76.16/128.60)[a]	Unchanged
Alanine aminotransferase (U)	Reduced (49.33/22.75)[a]	Unchanged	Unchanged
Alkaline phosphatase (U)	Increased (38.89/52.50)[a]	Reduced (30.28/11.84)[a]	Unchanged
Acid phosphatase (U)	Unchanged	Increased (6.10/22.09)[a]	Unchanged
Acetylcholinesterase (U)	Unchanged	Not measured	Unchanged

[a] Controls/treated animals

days. No signs of irritation or toxicity were observed (no further details; Bayer, 1957).

In a study of the subacute oral toxicity of triethylene tetramine, groups of 5 male Harlan-Wistar rats (30 days old at the beginning of the study) were given 2.81, 1.16 or 0.47% triethylene tetramine in their feed for 7 days, while groups of 5 females of the same strain and age received 3.02, 1.31 or 0.51%. This was equivalent to daily intakes of 2.98, 1.23 and 0.5 g/kg body weight, respectively, in the males and 2.63, 1.38 and 0.47 g/kg body weight, respectively, in the females. The highest dose caused a marked reduction in body weight and a reduction in the absolute and relative liver weights, while the relative kidney weights were increased in both sexes. An increase in the relative kidney weights also occurred at the middle dose. The lowest dose caused no changes in body weight or in the relative organ weights. No deaths occurred in any of the groups. The highest average dose without effect was 0.49 g/kg body weight (CHF, 1976).

To test the subacute dermal toxicity of triethylene tetramine, 1 drop (ca. 50 mg) was rubbed into the clilpped dorsal skin of each of 10 pregnant and 10 non-pregnant Wistar rats (initial weight ca. 190 g) daily for 17 days. A further 10 pregnant and 10 non-pregnant rats served as controls. At the end of the study, the body weights were clearly reduced in both treated groups. Histological examination revealed hyperaemia of the liver and kidneys and inflammatory changes at the application site. In the non-pregnant rats, the respective activities of glutamate-oxalate transaminase and glutamate-pyruvate transaminase in the liver were increased from 26.14 to 38.67 and from 14.88 to 20.18 U/g tissue. In the kidneys, γ-glutamyltranspeptidase activity was increased from 8.75 to 12.05 U/g tissue, while brain acetyl cholinesterase activity was reduced from 150 to 109 U/g tissue. In the pregnant rats, there was a reduction in glutamate-oxalate transaminase activity in the liver from 27.7 to 18.03 U/g tissue, while the remaining parameters were unaffected (Woyton et al., 1975).

The same authors measured a variety of parameters in the serum and amniotic fluid using the same protocol (groups of 10 rats, dermal treatment for 17 days) and the same doses. The results are presented in Table 1. Various effects were seen in the serum, although these did not follow any pattern, while in the amniotic fluid only the activity of leucyl-naphthylamidase was significantly increased. The body weights of the treated pregnant and non-pregnant rats were also clearly reduced in this study. Symptoms observed included emaciation, apathy and loss of appetite. From the 5th application onwards, skin inflammation occurred, with erythema, oedema and erosions (Dobryszycka et al., 1974).

A similar study was conducted in guinea-pigs (ca. 450 g) by the same investigators. Initially, 1 drop of triethylene tetramine (ca. 50 mg) was rubbed on to the clipped dorsal skin of each of 11 pregnant and 11 non-pregnant animals daily for 10 days, starting on the 10th day of pregnancy for the pregnant guinea-pigs. 11 untreated animals were used as controls. During the course of the experiment, 7 guinea-pigs in each treatment group died. From the 11th day of the study, therefore, the remaining animals were only treated every 2nd day for a further period of 45 days. At the end of the study, the body weights in the treatment groups were markedly reduced from the initial 450 g to 180 g (non-pregnant animals) and 200 g (pregnant animals). All of the guinea-pigs had severe skin reactions at the application site. Post-mortems carried out the day after the last application revealed fatty liver degeneration, brain oedema and hyperaemia of the kidneys in all of the treated animals and in those that had died prematurely. Histologically, fatty degeneration of the liver, hyperaemia of the kidneys, hyperaemia and oedema of the brain and inflammation and necrosis of the treated skin were observed. No differences were discernible between the pregnant and non-pregnant animals. In the former, diffuse necrotic foci with focal calcification were observed in the placenta. In the uterus, a lack of fetal ovum was detected in 7 cases and presence of mortified foetuses in 4 cases (Szacki et al., 1974). Altogether, the value of the study is limited because of the small number of animals that could be evaluated.

In an analogous study, 9 pregnant and 10 non-pregnant guinea-pigs (initial weight ca. 450 g) each had 1 drop (ca. 50 mg) of triethylene tetramine rubbed on to the clipped dorsal skin daily for 55 days. Treatment of the pregnant animals commenced on day 10 of pregnancy. Groups of 6 pregnant and 5 non-pregnant guinea-pigs served as controls, but as they could not be distinguished from each other in the study results they were combined into one group. During the study, 6 controls and 2 pregnant treated animals died. On the day after the last treatment, enzyme assays were carried out on tissues from the liver, kidneys and brain. Glutamate-oxalate transaminase activity was significantly increased from 19000 to 28400 U/g tissue in the livers of the non-pregnant treated animals. In the pregnant treated animals, there was a significant increase in γ-

glutamyltranspeptidase activity in the kidneys from 0.84 to 1.24 U/g tissue. Otherwise, there were no significant effects (Dobryszycka et al., 1975). However, the value of these findings is limited because of the small number of animals and the high mortality in the control group.

7.3 Skin and mucous membrane effects

Application of neat triethylene tetramine to the skin of 5 rabbits caused necrosis (no further details; Smyth et al., 1949).

In another study, 0.01 ml neat triethylene tetramine applied dermally to 2 rabbits (non-occlusive, exposure time not specified) caused necrosis in both animals. A 10% aqueous solution did not cause skin irritation in 5 rabbits (CHF, 1976).

Neat triethylene tetramine (1 g/kg) and a 25% aqueous solution (0.05 g/kg) caused severe irritant effects on the shaved abdominal skin of rats (no further details; Bayer, 1957).

Intracutaneous injection of 0.1 ml of a 0.5–1% un-neutralised solution or a 2–3% neutralised solution led to signs of skin necrosis in guinea-pigs (no further details; Pletscher et al., 1954).

In rabbits' eyes (5 animals), 5 µl concentrated triethylene tetramine caused necrosis (visualised by means of fluorescein) covering 63–87% of the surface of the cornea (no further details; Smyth et al., 1949).

Necrosis of the cornea caused by triethylene tetramine has also been reported by other authors (no further details; Pletscher et al., 1954).

In another study, severe corneal damage and iritis were seen after instillation of 0.005 ml neat triethylene tetramine into the eyes of 5 rabbits, and slight corneal damage (affecting 15% of the surface) was seen after instillation of 0.5 ml of a 40% aqueous solution (CHF, 1976).

7.4 Sensitization

To test the sensitizing potential of triethylene tetramine in a maximization test, 15 guinea-pigs were first treated intradermally with a 0.5% aqueous solution (w/v) of a commercial product (amount not specified), and subsequently (interval not specified) the same concentration was applied dermally. 2 weeks after the 2nd treatment, a challenge was carried out with a 2% (w/v) aqueous solution. After a 24-hour occlusive exposure (patch test) the reaction was evaluated; 80% of the animals had a positive reaction with redness and swelling at the application site. Of the animals treated with triethylene tetramine, 67% were also sensitized to diethylene triamine (Thorgeirsson, 1978).

In another study, 99.5% pure triethylene tetramine and the by-products contained in the technical grade product, tris(2-aminoethyl)amine, N,N'-bis(2-aminoethyl)piperazine and N-(2-piperazin-1-yl-ethyl)ethylenediamine, were tested for their ability to induce sensitization in the mouse ear test and in the guinea-pig maximization test. Groups of 10 female 4-week-old BALB/c mice received 10 µl of the substance in an ethanol/water/Tween 80® mixture (4:3:1, final concentration 10%) on days 0, 2, 4, 7, 9 and 11, applied to the clipped skin of the thorax and abdomen. On day 15 a challenge was carried out with 25 µl of the test substance (2.5 and 5%) applied to the ear. Ear thickness was measured after 0, 24 and 48 hours in a blind study. A 0.3% oxazolone solution served as a positive control. All test substances caused a statistically significant ($p < 0.05$ or < 0.001) increase in ear thickness. The most effective was N-(2-piperazin-1-yl-ethyl)ethylene-diamine, which induced a reaction in 6/10 mice. 4 out of 10 mice reacted to triethylene tetramine, while all 10 reacted to the positive control (Maisey et al., 1988).

In the guinea-pig maximization test conducted by the same authors, groups of 10 female guinea-pigs (Dunkin-Hartley, 4 weeks old, 300–350 g) were given 6 intradermal injections of 0.1 ml of a 0.5% aqueous solution together with 0.1 ml Freund's adjuvant followed, 1 week later, by a 48-hour occlusive application of triethylene tetramine (0.35 ml of a 0.5% solution in mineral oil). A challenge with an epidermal application of 0.1 ml of a 2% triethylene tetramine solution in mineral oil was carried out 21 days later. The exposure period was 24 hours. The reaction was evaluated 1 to 3 hours after removal of the patch and again 24 and 48 hours later. Chlorodinitrobenzene served as a positive control. Positive reactions to triethylene tetramine were seen in 9/10 guinea-pigs. Once again, the by-product N-(2-piperazin-1-yl-ethyl)ethylenediamine had the most marked effect (10/10 positive reactions). The reaction to chlorodinitrobenzene was also positive in all 10 guinea-pigs (Maisey et al., 1988).

7.5 Subchronic and chronic toxicity

Rats were given daily oral doses of 1/10 or 1/20 LD_{50} (corresponding to 430 and 215 mg/kg body weight, respectively) for 4 months. These doses were reported to cause excitation of the central nervous system. In the blood, there were reductions in the levels of haemoglobin, protein and hippuric acid, and in the activities of catalase and peroxidase (no further details; Stavreva, 1979).

7.6 Genotoxicity

7.6.1 In vitro

Triethylene tetramine was tested in the Salmonella microsome strains TA 1535 and TA 100 with and without metabolic activation (S9-mix from Clophen A50-induced rat liver). The substance was shown to be a direct mutagen (no further details of dose and revertant numbers; Hedenstedt, 1978).

In a further test in the Salmonella strain TA 100, and in *Escherichia coli*, triethylene tetramine likewise induced point-mutations (0.07 revertants/nmol). This short report contained no further details (Hulla et al., 1981).

In the course of mutagenicity testing of a series of rhodium-complex compounds and their ligands, triethylene tetramine was tested in a limited experiment. The study was carried out in the Salmonella strains TA 92, TA 100 and TA 98 (apparently without metabolic activation), but only the results in TA 92 were reported. The revertant count in this strain was 0.07/nmol (Warren et al., 1981).

A more comprehensive study was carried out in the Salmonella strains TA 1535, TA 1537, TA 1538, TA 98 and TA 100, with and without metabolic activation. Purified triethylene tetramine hydrochloride was tested. The doses used were between 1 and 10,000 µg/plate. Without metabolic activation, triethylene tetramine caused a dose-dependent increase in the mutation rate in all strains except TA 1537. The threshold dose was between 100 and 1000 µg/plate (TA 1535, TA 1538), about 100 µg/plate (TA 98) and between 10 and 100 µg/plate (TA 100; Heinz and Schröder, 1981).

In another study, triethylene tetramine (technical grade, no further details) was tested in the Salmonella strains TA 100, TA 1535, TA 1537 and TA 98 in a pre-incubation test with and without metabolic activation (S9-mix from Arochlor 1254-induced rat and hamster livers). The concentrations used were 33 to 10,000 µg/plate. A dose-dependent direct mutagenic effect was found in all strains from about 33 µg/plate, the effect being weakest in TA 1537. Bacteriotoxicity was noted in a few strains from 3333 µg/plate (Mortelmans et al., 1986).

Two technical-grade products (sample A 56.4% and sample B 68.5%) were tested in the Salmonella strains TA 98, TA 100, TA 1535, TA 1537 and TA 1538 with and without metabolic activation

(S9-mix from Arochlor 1254-induced rat liver). The concentrations tested were 0.03 to 2.0 mg/plate (sample A) and 3.0 mg/plate (sample B) whithout activation and 0.1 to 5.0 mg/plate with activation. Sample A induced dose-dependent mutations in all strains except TA 1535 without metabolic activation. With metabolic activation, a marked dose-dependent positive effect was noted in strains TA 98, TA 100 and TA 1535. Sample B was a dose-dependent mutagen in all 5 strains without S9-mix and in all strains except TA 1538 with S9-mix (UCC, 1987 a, b).

Various purity grades of triethylene tetramine were tested for point-mutagenic activity in the CHO test in Chinese hamster ovary cells. Triethylene tetramine with a purity of 79.15% caused a significant increase in mutations at volume concentrations of 80×10^{-2}% to 2.5×10^{-2}% with and without metabolic activation (S9-mix from Arochlor 1254-induced rat liver), but without activation there was no clear dose-effect relationship (UCC, 1981 a).

In contrast, a 99.42% pure linear triethylene tetramine caused no statistically significant increase in the mutation frequency in the CHO test at volume concentrations between 80×10^{-2}% and 2.5×10^{-2}% with or without metabolic activation. However, because of the steep dose-effect curve for cytotoxicity, the authors considered the results to be inconclusive (UCC, 1981 b).

Both aforementioned products were also studied in the SCE test with CHO cells and in the UDS test with rat hepatocytes. The 79.15% pure product caused a statistically highly significant increase in the sister chromatid exchange rate in CHO cells at volume concentrations from 40×10^{-2}% to 1.25×10^{-2}% without metabolic activation. With metabolic activation the effect was comparatively lower, but the top dose similarly induced a highly significant increase (UCC, 1981 a).

Results with the 99.42% linear triethylene tetramine were similar to those with the 79.15% product, but the authors considered that further studies were necessary (UCC, 1981 b).

Another SCE test was carried out with technical grade triethylene tetramine (56.4% pure) in CHO cells from Chinese hamsters. Without metabolic activation, a concentration of 0.2 mg/ml was without effect; 0.3 and 0.4 mg/ml led to a significant increase in SCEs/chromosome. With metabolic activation a significant increase in SCEs occurred only at the lowest test concentration of 0.5 mg/ml, higher levels of 0.6 and 0.8 mg/ml being without effect. The respective increases, with and without metabolic activation, were only 1.3-fold and 1.4-fold above the solvent controls (UCC, 1987 c).

In the UDS test on rat hepatocytes, 79.15% pure triethylene tetramine caused a significant increase in the rate of ^{3}H-thymidine incorporation at volume concentrations from 100×10^{-2}% to 0.1×10^{-2}% (UCC, 1981 a).

The 99.42% pure linear triethylene tetramine produced the same result in the UDS test at volume concentrations from 100×10^{-2}% to 0.1×10^{-2}% (UCC, 1981 b).

7.6.2 In vivo

The mutagenic activity of triethylene tetramine (as the purified dihydrochloride) was studied in vivo in the micronucleus test. Groups of 10 NMRI or 10 Charles River CD1 mice received single oral doses of 1500, 3000 or 6000 mg/kg body weight or single intraperitoneal injections of 130, 190 or 250 mg/kg body weight. Triethylene tetramine was not clastogenic in either experiment (Heinz and Schröder, 1981).

Another micronucleus test was carried out with a technical grade triethylene tetramine (purity 68.5%) in male and female Swiss Webster mice by single intraperitoneal injection. The doses used were 185, 370 and 600 mg/kg body weight (LD_{50} mouse i.p. 740 mg/kg body weight). Even the highest dose caused no increase in micronuclei in the peripheral polychromatic erythrocytes (UCC, 1987 d).

The SLRL test in *Drosophila melanogaster* gave negative results (no further details; NTP, 1986).

7.7 Carcinogenicity

In order to test the carcinogenic effect of triethylene tetramine, 25 µl of a 5.39% aqueous solution was applied to the dorsal skin of 50 male C3H/HeJ mice (corresponding to ca. 1.25 mg/mouse) 3 times weekly for their entire lives. The sample contained 79.15% triethylene tetramine, 4.03% Tris-(aminoethylamine), 8.08% diaminoethyl piperazine, 8.34% piperazinoethylethylenediamine and traces of 7 other higher amines. After 18 months, 10 mice were killed prematurely and histologically examined. The average survival time of the treated mice was 627 days, while that of the controls was 626 days. At the end of the study, one papilloma of the lower lip was seen in the treated group and another animal developed dermatitis at the application site. In the control group, one mouse had a skin adenoma and another developed skin hyperplasia. Thus, in this study, triethylene tetramine showed no carcinogenic activity (De Pass et al., 1987). However, the dose tested (calculated ca. 30 mg/kg) and the concentration appear very low compared with the acute toxicity data for mice (LD_{50} oral 1600 mg/kg, LD_{50} i.p. 604 mg/kg), so that the likelihood of tumours arising in this study was low.

7.8 Reproductive toxicity

In a prenatal study, female Sprague-Dawley rats (190–200 g) were given triethylene tetramine (purity >99%, as the hydrochloride) in their daily feed at levels of 0.17% (5 rats), 0.83% (9 rats) or 1.66% (5 rats), from day 0 to day 21 after mating. These concentrations were equivalent to about 170, 830 and 1670 mg/kg body weight/day. The control group comprised 7 rats. At the highest dose level the feed intake of the dams was reduced, and at the two higher dose levels maternal weight gain was reduced (control +130 g, 0.83% +107 g, 1.66% +90 g). The average litter size/rat was the same in all groups (10 foetuses/rat), but the foetal weight at the highest dose level was significantly reduced (control 5.16 g, 1.66% 4.62 g, $p<0.01$). Likewise the length of the foetuses was reduced (control 3.9 cm, 1.66% 3.4 cm, $p<0.001$). There was a dose-dependent increase in dead, abnormal and resorbed foetuses (see Table 2).

The abnormal foetuses showed massive haemorrhages and oedema and, at the highest dose level, reduced ossification of the spine and phalanges. Trace element analysis revealed a dose-dependent reduction in the copper levels in the plasma of the dams at the two highest dose levels ($p<0.001$), in the livers of the dams at all dose levels ($p<0.01$ and <0.001), in the placentas of the dams at the 2 higher dose levels ($p<0.01$) and in the foetal liver tissue at the

Table 2. Prenatal toxicity of triethylene tetramine

Dose	Rats	Implantations (n)	Dead foetuses (n)	Alive foetuses (n)	Abnormal foetuses (n)	Resorbed foetuses (%)
0	7	73	0	73	0	0
0.17%	5	52	3	49	0	5.8
0.83%	9	93	7	86	22	8.7
1.66%	5	48	9	39	39	18.8

2 higher dose levels ($p<0.01$). There was also a dose-dependent increase in the zinc concentration in the kidneys of the dams at all concentrations ($p<0.01$ and <0.001), in the muscles of the dams at the 2 higher dose levels ($p<0.01$), in the whole foetuses at all dose levels ($p<0.001$) and in the foetal livers at all dose levels ($p<0.001$; Keen et al., 1983).

In a further study, groups of 8 female Sprague-Dawley rats (190–200 g) received feed containing 0.83 or 1.67% triethylene tetramine (purity >99%) for the entire duration of pregnancy (days 0 to 21). At the same time, half of the animals received copper in the diet at a concentration of 5 µg/g, the other half at 50 µg/g. Maternal weight gain at the top dose of triethylene tetramine was significantly reduced, independent of the dietary copper concentration. Both foetal weight and length were reduced at this dose, again independent of the copper concentration. In contrast, increased dietary copper levels led to a marked reduction in foetal anomalies. The results are presented in Table 3. Observed abnormalities included marked haemorrhages, oedema and, in a few foetuses, hydronephrosis and domed skulls. The reduction in the prenatal toxicity of triethylene tetramine by means of high-dose copper was accompanied by an increase in the copper level in the maternal and foetal tissues. At the same time, the zinc level in these rats was less markedly increased than when a lower copper level was given. The authors concluded from these findings that the primary mechanism for the prenatal toxicity of triethylene tetramine involves copper deficiency (Cohen et al., 1983).

In another study, female Sprague-Dawley rats (initial weight 180–200 g) were given 75, 325 or 750 mg triethylene tetramine/kg body weight (purity >98%) by stomach tube as a solution in distilled water, from days 6 to 15 of pregnancy. In the second half of the experiment the dams showed a slight reduction in feed consumption, but this was not dose-dependent. Apart from increased body weight at the highest dose level, the foetuses showed no treatment-related effects. In the lowest dose group and in the control group occasional anomalies and/or malformations were found. One foetus in the low-dose group had a unilateral internal hydrocephalus, while one foetus in the control group had an encephalocele. Neither these effects nor the occasional sternebrae anomalies seen in all dose groups were considered to be treatment-related (Ciba-Geigy, 1984).

Triethylene tetramine was applied dermally (occlusive) to 4 groups of 22 New Zealand rabbits for 6 hours daily on days 6 to 18

Table 3. The effect of copper on the prenatal toxicity of triethylene tetramine (Cohen et al., 1983)

Triethylene tetramine (%)	Copper (µg/g)	Litter size (n)	Implantations (n)	Alive foetuses (n)	Dead foetuses (n)	Abnormal foetuses (n)	Resorbed foetuses (%)[a]	Abnormal foetuses (%)[b]	Total (%)[c]
0	5	3	29	27	2	0	6.9	0	6.9
0.83	5	3	31	30	1	0	3.2	0	3.2
1.67	5	4	44	39	5	27	11.4	69.2	72.7
0	50	4	40	36	4	0	10.0	0	10.0
0.83	50	4	46	45	1	0	2.2	0	2.2
1.67	50	5	51	46	5	3	9.8	6.5	15.7

[a] $\frac{\text{Dead foetuses}}{\text{Implantations}} \times 100$

[b] $\frac{\text{Abnormal foetuses}}{\text{Alive foetuses}} \times 100$

[c] $\frac{\text{Abnormal + dead foetuses}}{\text{Implantations}} \times 100$

of pregnancy at doses of 5, 50 or 125 mg/kg body weight (in 2 ml distilled water in each case). The material was about 95% pure. Decreased maternal weight gain was seen at the highest dose level and 2 rabbits died (9.1%). At 125 and 50 mg/kg marked skin irritation was seen, although this was somewhat reversed during the treatment-free phase (up to day 29 of pregnancy). In the low-dose group, slight skin irritation occurred which was completely reversible. The copper content of the serum and urine of the treated dams was not different from the controls. There was no difference in the number of corpora lutea, the total number of foetuses/litter, the number of alive or dead foetuses/litter or the percentage of pre-implantation losses. The percentage of alive foetuses, the sex ratio and the foetal body weight were likewise unchanged. No treatment-related external, visceral or skeletal malformations or variations were discernible. Triethylene tetramine was thus toxic to the dams at a dose of 125 mg/kg in this study but was not embryotoxic or teratogenic at any dose tested (UCC, 1988).

Technical grade triethylene tetramine (in acetone) was injected in the inner shell membrane of hens' eggs (White Leghorn) that had been incubated for 3 days. The doses used were 0.35, 0.7, 1.4 and 2.7 μmol/egg, each in a volume of 5 μl. The eggs were then incubated further, and any dead embryos were examined for malformations. On day 11 the embryos were removed, and the resultant findings are presented in Table 4. Malformations observed included eye defects, open coeloms, short backs and necks, wing defects and oedema. The ED_{50} for embryotoxicity of triethylene tetramine was

Table 4. Prenatal toxicity of triethylene tetramine in hens' eggs

Dose (μmol/ egg)	Treated eggs	Premature deaths (before day 5)	Malformed embryos (days 6–14)	Malformed survivors (day 14)
0.35	30	1	0	2
0.70	30	2	0	3
1.40	30	10	8	4
2.70	20	20	0	0
Acetone	100	1	1	0

arithmetically 1.1 µmol/egg and for total mortality 1.3 µmol/egg. The dose/effect curve was thus very steep (Korhonen et al., 1983).

7.9 Effects on the immune system

No information available.

7.10 Neurotoxicity

After daily oral administration of 4 mg or 0.8 mg triethylene tetramine/kg body weight to rats for 10 months, increased nervous excitation and stimulation of tactile reflexes was reported to occur. Furthermore, disturbances in liver function were observed, primarily inhibition of the activity of nicotinamide coenzyme and increased cytochrome oxidase activity. The author reported that the "threshold dose for chronic toxicity" was 0.8 mg/kg (no further details; Stavreva, 1979).

7.11 Other effects

Triethylene tetramine acts as a chelating agent and binds metal ions, and this property has been the subject of several studies.

Groups of 17 female Fischer-344 rats (140–190 g) were injected intramuscularly with 0.75 mmol triethylene tetramine/kg body weight (as the tetrahydrochloride, purified by recrystallization) and, within 1 minute, 0.068 or 0.10 mmol $^{63}NiCl_2$/kg were injected intraperitoneally or 0.068 mmol/kg intramuscularly. After 10, 20 and 40 minutes and 1, 1.5, 2, 6 and 24 hours, the nickel content of the blood was determined. The nickel content of the urine and faeces was determined at intervals of 6 hours for 5 days after nickel administration. Triethylene tetramine reduced the nickel concentration in the plasma and increased nickel excretion in the urine. Urinary nickel excretion within 6 hours was 70±7% of the administered dose in the rats given triethylene tetramine and 36±23% in the controls ($p<0.01$). In the liver of the treated rats there was 3.5 times as much nickel as in the controls; equivalent figures in the other organs were 0.72 times in the kidneys, 0.27 times in the spleen, 0.22 times in the lungs and 0.12 times in the heart (Sunderman et al., 1976).

In another study, the influence of triethylene tetramine on copper excretion was investigated. Norwegian hooded rats (ca. 300 g) were each given 100 mg triethylene tetramine (as the hydrochloride) in 5 g of feed (pulverised and mixed to a paste with water) for 3 days; the urine was then collected and its copper content determined. Triethylene tetramine caused an increase in copper excretion (22 measurements) from 65.1±2.9 nmol to 309.5±22.2 nmol/24 hours (Gibbs and Walshe, 1977).

3 female mongrels (17–23 kg) were each given 150 mg triethylene tetramine (as the tetrahydrochloride) in gelatine capsules twice daily for 23 days. Prior to treatment and again 9, 15 and 23 days after treatment had started, the copper content of the urine and serum was determined, while that of the serum was also determined at 7 days. Urinary copper excretion increased significantly from 119.5±56.7 µg/24 hours to 663.0±291.3 µg/24 hours ($p<0.05$), while the serum copper level remained unchanged. The zinc and iron levels in the serum and the urine were not affected (Allen et al., 1987).

8. Experience in humans

Triethylene tetramine is used therapeutically in medicine in the treatment of Wilson's disease, if the usual treatment with penicillamine leads to intolerance reactions. Use is made of the copper-binding and -excreting effect of triethylene tetramine, as this disease is characterized by increased levels of copper in the liver, kidneys and brain. Several case-studies on the use of triethylene tetramine in Wilson's disease have been published, only a few of which will be mentioned here.

A patient initially received the usual treatment with D-penicillamine. Due to increasing signs of intolerance, her therapy was changed to triethylene tetramine (purified, as the dihydrochloride). She then received 2.3 g twice daily and, after 3 days, 1.15 g twice daily over an observation period of 2.5 years. Copper excretion in the urine was about 10 times higher than without triethylene tetramine-therapy. The treatment was tolerated without side-effects (Haslam et al., 1980).

20 patients with Wilson's disease received 400 to 800 mg triethylene tetramine dihydrochloride orally, 3 times daily, over periods ranging from 14 to 120 months, without signs of intolerance. In addition to increased copper excretion in the urine and a reduction in serum copper levels, there was also a reduction in the serum iron content from 16.9 to 10.7 µmol/l in a few patients. Among the 20 patients there were 6 complication-free pregnancies in 4 of the women. All 6 children developed normally up to the age of 5, when the observation period ceased (Walshe, 1982).

On the other hand, side-effects have also been described following therapy with triethylene tetramine (highly purified, no by-products detectable). 4 patients with primary biliary liver cirrhosis were given up to 1200 mg daily in gelatine capsules. Acute rhabdomyolysis occurred in 1 patient only 48 hours after the first dose, and after 3 weeks of treatment, side-effects appeared in 3/4 patients, including gastro-intestinal complaints and skin rashes. After cessation of the triethylene tetramine-therapy, rapid improvement occurred in all cases; renewed therapy produced the same symptoms. The authors considered triethylene tetramine to be unsuitable for the treatment of primary biliary liver cirrhosis but, in the treatment of Wilson's disease where penicillamine-intolerance exists, it is the alternative therapy of choice (Epstein and Sherlock, 1980).

Numerous occupational medicine reports concern the skin irritant and sensitizing potential of triethylene tetramine from its use as a hardener for epoxy resins.

In the plastics department of a condenser factory in which casting resin and triethylene tetramine were processed without protective measures being taken, skin rashes developed within a few weeks to months of the beginning of operation. Of the 20 employees, 8 had slight skin effects (itchy irritation, erythema, papules) and 6 had marked skin problems (papulovesicular weeping eczema on the arms and the genital and groin areas, oedematous swelling of the face). The remaining 6 workers showed no skin effects. After exposure ceased, recovery was rapid. Epicutaneous patch tests with triethylene tetramine, casting resin (ethoxylin resin) and various control allergens were carried out in the 20 workers. Of the 6 employees with severe skin problems, 5 reacted to triethylene tetramine and 6 to casting resin. On the 8 employees with slight skin changes, none reacted to triethylene tetramine, but 3 reacted to casting resin. The 6 subjects without skin problems did not react to either triethylene tetramine or casting resin. 6 of the 20 workers showed signs of liver function disturbance, for which a contributing effect of triethylene tetramine could not be excluded (Pletscher et al., 1954).

A year later, 14 further cases were reported of skin complaints in women after handling casting resin (Araldite) and Hardener 951 (triethylene tetramine). 12 of these individuals were seborrhoics, and it was concluded by the author that seborrhoic patients are particularly at risk (Welcker, 1955).

Another study investigated 11 electronics factories, in which a total of 228 workers were in contact with hardener (triethylene tetramine) and casting resin. Of these, 164 (43%) had dermatoses, of which 21% were slight and 22% were marked (0–3 and >3 days off work, respectively). Workers returning to their jobs after a break showed a recurrence of eczema. The eczema occurred on the face (55 cases), the upper extremities (34 cases), both the face and the upper extremities (53 cases) or additionally on other parts of the body (15 cases). In 7 cases the location could no longer be ascertained. In sensitization tests (no further details) there were 32 positive skin reactions, 16 to araldite resin, 5 to triethylene tetramine and 11 to both. The concentration of triethylene tetramine in the air at the workplace under normal conditions was below the registration level of 0.15 µg/l air (Grandjean, 1957).

In another synthetic resin processing business, 20 people were exposed to Araldite resin and Hardener 951 (which mainly contains triethylene tetramine) for at least 6 months, but generally for 13 to 18 months. 12 of these were examined 2 to 4 times at intervals of 6 months. After 1 year of exposure a significant decrease in lymphocytes occurred in the blood, while at the same time there was an increase in neutrophilic granulocytes. 7 subjects developed eczema (no further details). Subjective symptoms included loss of appetite, head and stomach pains, fatigue, weakness and eye irritation (Zielhuis, 1961).

Dermatitis was observed in 126 out of 422 workers at another factory. Skin tests were carried out on 99 patients. A positive reaction to triethylene tetramine (1% in water) was observed in 55.1% of these cases. The average latent period before the appearance of skin complaints (localized on the hands and face) was 18.5 months (Krajewska and Rudzki, 1976).

In a group of 135 epoxy resin workers, 23 had work-related dermatoses on the hands and/or forearms. Patch tests with the resin, isophorone diamine, triethylene tetramine and xylenediamine were carried out in all of these workers. Similar patch tests were carried out in the 112 workers without dermatitis, of whom only 2 reacted to triethylene tetramine. Overall, only 1.5% of the 135 workers reacted to triethylene tetramine, the majority of the positive reactions (18.5%) being due to the epoxy resin (Van Putten et al., 1984).

A case of asthma has been reported after contact with triethylene tetramine and synthetic resin. Initially the individual developed cold-like symptoms (runny nose, headache, watering eyes) about 5 hours after commencing work. 6 months after the initial contact, an asthma attack occurred after work. On return to work after a break for hospital treatment, severe asthma attacks recurred. The subject experienced no problems at weekends or when work with triethylene tetramine was discontinued. Skin tests with a 5%

alcoholic solution of triethylene tetramine and a 70% casting resin solution in acetone were negative. In contrast, cold-like symptoms were observed after 30 minutes in an inhalation challenge test with a mixture of resin and hardener. These symptoms were similar to those which occurred at work, and lasted for up to 1 hour. Lung function (respiratory volume) was reduced after inhalation for 5 minutes and had not returned to normal 7 hours later (Fawcett et al., 1977).

In Poland, 447 patients who suffered from eczema after industrial contact with epoxy resin and triethylene tetramine were tested with the resin (Epidian 5) and 5 different concentrations of triethylene tetramine. The authors reached the conclusion that in Poland there were more cases of sensitization to triethylene tetramine than to the epoxy resin. The latent period was longer with triethylene tetramine than with the resin (Rudzki et al., 1981).

Cross-reactions between triethylene tetramine, ethylenediamine and diethylenetriamine have also been reported. Of 1544 patients with no record of industrial contact with epoxy resin systems, 28 showed a positive reaction to ethylenediamine (1% in paraffin). When 400 patients from the main group were tested with triethylene tetramine (1% in water), the results were all negative. A further 137 patients who had been occupationally exposed to epoxy resins and hardeners were tested with ethylenediamine and triethylene tetramine, and a large number of them were also tested with diethylenetriamine (1% in water). Of these 137 patients, 23 reacted to ethylenediamine and triethylene tetramine, while 40 reacted to diethylenetriamine and triethylene tetramine. Similar cross-reactions were also observed in guinea-pigs. Of 8 animals that were sensitized to triethylene tetramine, one reacted to diethylenetriamine and another to both diethylenetriamine and ethylenediamine (Rudzki and Krajewska, 1976).

In another study involving 32 patients who were allergic to ethylenediamine, 12 also experienced skin reactions to a 1% solution of triethylene tetramine (no further details; Balato et al., 1986).

In an investigation of 542 cases of industrial allergic contact dermatitis reported to a Finnish skin clinic between 1974 and 1983, 71 were attributed to contact with epoxy resin systems (resin plus hardener), of which 19 were due to various hardeners, including 3 that were attributed specifically to triethylene tetramine (Jolanki et al., 1987).

Serum monoamine oxidase activity was determined in 15 people who had contact with triethylene tetramine, and was found to be increased in comparison with that of a control group of the same size (33.5±6.4 compared with 28.9±7.9 units). This increase was thought to be indicative of increased amine metabolism in the connective tissue. No observations were made on exposure levels (Yano, 1987).

9. Threshold limit values

No information available.

References

Allen, K.G.D., Twedt, D.C., Hunsaker, H.A.
Tetramine cupruretic agents: A comparison in dogs
Am. J. Vet. Res., 48, 28–30 (1987)

Axel, H., Stechl, H.H., Adelsberger, K., Gräfje, H.
Aliphatische Amine
in: Ullmanns Encyklopädie der technischen Chemie
4th Edition, Volume 7, p. 380–382
Verlag Chemie, Weinheim (1974)

Balato, N., Cusano, F., Lembo, G., Ayala, F.
Ethylenediamine dermatitis
Contact Dermatitis, 15, 263–265 (1986)

Bayer AG, Geschäftsbereich Organica
DIN-Sicherheitsdatenblatt Triethylentetramin (1988)

Bayer AG, Toxikologisches und gewerbehygienisches Laboratorium
Untersuchung von E 570 und Härter T
Unpublished report (1957)

CHF (Chemical Hygiene Fellowship)
Carnegie-Mellon Institute of Research, Carnegie-Mellon University
Triethylene tetramine, range finding toxicity and 7-day dietary inclusion studies
Special Report 39–54 (1976)

Ciba-Geigy Ltd.
Report on TK 10458 (Triethylene tetramine) teratology study in rats
Unpublished report No. 830035 (1984)

Cohen, N.L., Keen, C.L., Lönnerdahl, B., Hurley, L.S.
The effect of copper supplementation on the teratogenic effects of triethylenetetramine in rats
Drug Nutr. Interact., 2, 203–210 (1983)

DePass, L.R., Fowler, E.H., Weil, C.S.
Dermal oncogenicity studies on various ethyleneamines in male C3H mice
Fundam. Appl. Toxicol., 9, 807–811 (1987)

Dobryszycka, W., Warwas, M., Woyton, A., Woyton, J., Szacki, J.
Serum proteins and enzymes in pregnant rats treated with epoxy resin or triethyleneamine stabilizer
Arch. Toxicol., 33, 73–80 (1974)

Dobryszycka, W., Kulpa, J., Woyton, A., Woyton, J., Szacki, S., Dzioba, A.
Influence of industrial toxic compounds on pregnancy
Arch. Immun. Ther. Exp., 23, 867–870 (1975)

Epstein, O., Sherlock, S.
Triethylenetetramine dihydrochloride toxicity in primary biliary cirrhosis
Gastroenterology, 78, 1442–1445 (1980)

Fawcett, I.W., Newman Taylor, A.J., Pepys, J.
Asthma due to inhaled chemical agents – epoxy resin systems containing phthalic acid anhydride, trimellitic acid anhydride and triethylenetetramine
Clin. Allergy, 7, 1–14 (1977)

Gibbs, K., Walshe, J.M.
The effect of certain chelating compounds on the urinary excretion of copper by the rat: observations on their clinical significance
Clin. Sci. Mol. Med., 53, 317–320 (1977)

Grandjean, E.
Das Risiko von Dermatosen durch kalthärtende Äthoxylinharze
Z. Präventivmed., 2, 77–98 (1957)

Haslam, R.H.A., Sass-Kortsak, A., Stout, W., Berg, M.
Treatment of Wilson's disease with triethylenetetramine dihydrochloride
Dev. Pharmacol. Ther., 1, 318–324 (1980)

Hedenstedt, A.
Mutagenicity screening of industrial chemicals; seven aliphatic amines and one amide tested in the Salmonella/microsomal assay
Mutat. Res., 53, 198–199 (1978)

Heinz, N., Schröder, H.F.
Untersuchungen zur Abschätzung des Mutagenitätsrisikos von Triethylentetramin
Arzneimittelforschung, 31, 950–953 (1981)

Hulla, J.E., Rogers, S.J., Waren, G.R.
Mutagenicity of a series of polyamines
Environ. Mutagen., 3, 332–333 (1981)

Jolanki, R., Estlander, T., Kanerva, L.
Occupational contact dermatitis and contact urticaria caused by epoxy resins
Acta Derm. Venereol. (Stockh.), 134, 90–94 (1987)

Keen, C.L., Cohen, N.L., Lönnerdal, B., Hurley, L.S.
Teratogenesis and low copper status resulting from triethylenetetramine in rats
Proc. Soc. Exp. Biol. Med., 173, 598–605 (1983)

Korhonen, A., Hemminki, K., Vainio, A.
Embryotoxicity of sixteen industrial amines to the chicken embryo
J. Appl. Toxicol., 3, 112–117 (1983)

Krajewska, D., Rudzki, E.
Sensitivity to epoxy resins and triethylenetetramine
Contact Dermatitis, 2, 135–138 (1976)

Maisey, J., Purchase, F., Robbins, M.C., Miller, K.
Evaluation of the sensitivity potential of 4 polyamines present in technical triethylenetetramine using 2 animal species
Contact Dermatitis, 18, 133–137(1988)

Mortelmans, K., Haworth, S., Lawlor, T., Speck, W., Tainer, B., Zeiger, E.
Salmonella mutagenicity tests: II. results from the testing of 270 chemicals
Environ. Mutagen., 8(7), 1–119 (1986)

NTP (National Toxicology Program)
Annual Plan for Fiscal Year 1986, NTP-86-086, 72 (1986)

Pletscher, A., Schuppli, R., Reipert, R.
Über Gesundheitsschäden durch Gießharze
Z. Unfallmed. Berufskr., 47, 163–176 (1954)

Rudzki, E., Krajewska, D.
Cross-reactions between ethylenediamine, diethylenetriamine and triethylenetetramine
Contact Dermatitis, 2, 311–313 (1976)

Rudzki, E., Krajewska, D., Grzywa, Z., Napiorkowska, T.
Contact allergy to epoxide resin hardeners
Med. Pr., 32(1), 59–62 (1981)

Smyth, H.F., jr., Carpenter, C.P., Weil, C.S.
Range-finding toxicity data list III
J. Ind. Hyg. Toxicol., 31, 60–62 (1949)

Srivastava, A., Katiyar, S.S.
Evaluation of LD_{50} of some macrocyclic drugs and their linear analogues used as chelating drugs in metal intoxication
Chemosphere, 17, 839–844 (1988)

Stavreva, M.
Toxicity and mechanism of action of triethylenetetramine (TETA) used as siccative for anticorrosive epoxide and protective coatings
Khig. Zdraveopaz., 22(2), 179–182 (1979)

Sunderman, F.W., jr., Kasprzak, K., Horak, E., Gitlitz, P., Onkelinx, C.
Effects of triethylenetetramine upon the metabolism and toxicity of $NiCl_2$ in rats
Toxicol. Appl. Pharmacol., 38, 177–188 (1976)

Szacki, J., Woyton, J., Dzioba, A., Rabczynski, J., Woyton, A.
Influence of industrial toxic compounds on pregnancy, II
Arch. Immunol. Ther. Exp., 22, 123–128 (1974)

Thorgeirsson, A.
Sensitization capacity of epoxy resin hardeners in the guinea pig
Acta Derm. Venereol. (Stockh.), 58, 332–336 (1978)

UCC (Union Carbide Corporation)
Bushy Run Research Center, Pennsylvania
Triethylenetetramine (TETA), in vitro mutagenesis studies:
3-test battery
Project Report 43–127 (1981 a)

UCC (Union Carbide Corporation)
Bushy Run Research Center, Pennsylvania
Triethylenetetramine – linear (TETA linear), in vitro mutagenesis studies: 3-test battery
Project Report 44-11 (1981 b)

UCC (Union Carbide Corporation)
Bushy Run Research Center, Pennsylvania
Triethylenetetramine – Sample A, Salmonella/microsome (Ames) bacterial mutagenicity assay
Project Report 50-9 (1987 a)

UCC (Union Carbide Corporation)
Bushy Run Research Center, Pennsylvania
Triethylenetetramine – Sample B, Salmonella/microsome (Ames) bacterial mutagenicity assay
Project Report 50-43 (1987 b)

UCC (Union Carbide Corporation)
Bushy Run Research Center, Pennsylvania
Triethylenetetramine – Sample A, in vitro genotoxicity studies: sister chromatid exchanges assay
Project Report 50-99 (1987 c)

UCC (Union Carbide Corporation)
Bushy Run Research Center, Pennsylvania
Triethylenetetramine (TETA), in vivo mouse micronucleus study
Project Report 50-122 (1987 d)

UCC (Union Carbide Corporation)
Bushy Run Research Center, Pennsylvania
Triethylenetetramine: developmental toxicity evaluation after cutaneous application in New Zealand white rabbits
Project Report 50-127 (1988)

Van Putten, P.B., Coenraads, P.J., Nater, J.P.
Hand dermatoses and contact allergic reactions in construction workers exposed to epoxy resins
Contact Dermatitis, 10, 146–150 (1984)

Walshe, J.M.
Treatment of Wilson's disease with trientine (triethylene tetramine dihydrochloride)
The Lancet, 1982, 643–647 (1982)

Warren, G., Abbott, E., Schultz, P., Bennett, K., Rogers, S.
Mutagenicity of a series of hexacoordinate rhodium (III) compounds
Mutat. Res., 88, 165–173 (1981)

Welcker, A.
Gewebeekzem durch Arbeit mit Gießharz
Dermatol. Wochenschr., 132, 871–876 (1955)

Woyton, J., Szacki, J., Woyton, A., Warwas, M., Dobryszycka, W.
Tissue enzyme changes in pregnant rats treated topically with epoxy resin or triethylenetetramine stabilizer
Toxicol. Appl. Pharmacol., 32, 5–10 (1975)

Yano, E.
Increased activity of monoamine oxidase by epoxy resin hardeners
Toxicol. Lett., 37, 27–32 (1987)

Zielhuis, R.L.
Systemic toxicity from exposure to epoxy resins, hardeners, and styrene
J. Occup. Med., 3, 25–29 (1961)

Hydrazobenzene

1. Summary and assessment

After oral administration to rats, hydrazobenzene is eliminated unchanged in the urine, together with benzidine, aniline, two hydroxy-derivatives of benzidine and two other unidentified metabolites. After intraperitoneal injection, o- and p-aminophenol appear in the urine.

Hydrazobenzene is of low acute oral toxicity (LD_{50} rat oral 301 mg/kg). Preliminary studies show that dietary administration to rats and mice for 4 weeks is fatal at and above concentrations of 1000 mg/kg of food.

Hydrazobenzene induces point-mutations in strain TA 100 in the Salmonella/microsome assay after metabolic activation, but the results are predominantly negative in strains TA 98, TA 1535, TA 1537 and TA 1538, and in *Escherichia coli*. After metabolic activation the chemical induces chromosomal aberrations and increases sister chromatid exchange in Chinese hamster ovary (CHO) cells. Hydrazobenzene also inhibits testicular DNA synthesis in mice.

Technical grade hydrazobenzene is carcinogenic to rats and mice after long-term oral administration. In male rats there is a significant dose-related increase in hepatocellular carcinomas and Zymbal gland carcinomas, whilst in female rats, neoplastic nodules are observed in the liver and adenocarcinomas in the mammary glands. Hydrazobenzene also causes a significant increase in the incidence of hepatocellular carcinomas in female mice. Increased tumour formation is seen in carcinogenicity tests on rats and mice treated dermally or subcutaneously, and in mice (strain A) treated by intraperitoneal injection. In addition, the rats show an increased incidence of Zymbal gland carcinoma, a tumour which rarely occurs spontaneously. However, the tests involving dermal or subcutaneous treatment are generally inadequately documented.

Technical grade hydrazobenzene may contain a number of impurities, including benzidine. One out of 16 samples from one manufacturer has been shown to contain 25 μg benzidine/g of hydrazobenzene (Ciba-Geigy, 1982). Similarly, a sample of the hydrazobenzene used in the NCI study (1978) contained benzidine at a concentration of 40–50 μg/g (BIA, 1984). A further analysis of

10 production samples showed an average concentration of 74±11 μg of benzidine/g of hydrazobenzene. However, this value is regarded as artificially high, due to the presence of aniline (Hüls, 1989 c). Benzidine is carcinogenic in man (included in the list of MAK values for the first time in 1966 and in Category III A 1 of the same list since 1976). Benzidine may also be formed in the metabolic breakdown of hydrazobenzene.

In the Soviet Union, the maximum permissible concentration in the workplace is 0.1 mg/m^3 of air.

In a study of 189 Czechoslovakian workers engaged in benzidine production, where hydrazobenzene is used as a raw material, 20 cases of bladder cancer have been observed (10.6%). However, these are more likely to be due to benzidine exposure than to the hydrazobenzene.

Isolated cases of irritating cystitis with urinary urge and haematuria have previously been described following overexposure to hydrazobenzene, but no bladder cancers have been observed based on documentation extending over 75 years.

2. Name of substance

2.1	Usual name	Hydrazobenzene
2.2	IUPAC-name	1,2-Diphenylhydrazine
2.3	CAS-No.	122-66-7

3. Synonyms, common and trade names

N,N'-Diphenylhydrazine
Hydrazodibenzene
N,N'-Bianiline

4. Structural and molecular formulae

4.1 Structural formula

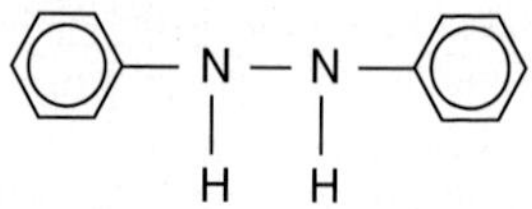

4.2 Molecular formula $C_{12}H_{12}N_2$

5. Physical and chemical properties

5.1 Molecular mass, g/mol	184.24
5.2 Melting point, °C	ca. 125 (Hüls, 1989 a)
5.3 Boiling point, °C	No information available
5.4 Vapour pressure, hPa	No information available
5.5 Density, g/cm^3	1.16 (at 20 °C) (Hüls, 1989 a)
5.6 Solubility in water	<0.01 g/l (at 20 °C) (Hüls, 1989 a)
5.7 Solubility in organic solvents	Dissolves readily in alcohol and ether (Neumüller, 1977)
5.8 Solubility in fat	No information available
5.9 pH-value	No information available
5.10 Conversion factor	1 ppm $\hat{=}$ 7.65 mg/m^3 1 mg/m^3 $\hat{=}$ 0.13 ppm (at 25 °C and 1013 hPa)

6. Uses

Manufacture of pharmaceuticals (Hüls, 1989 b)

7. Experimental results

7.1 Toxicokinetics and metabolism

After oral administration of 200 or 400 mg hydrazobenzene/kg body weight to rats, hydrazobenzene, benzidine, aniline, two hydroxy-derivatives of benzidine and two further unidentified metabolites were found in the urine by thin layer chromatography. Following intraperitoneal administration of 100 or 200 mg hydrazobenzene/kg body weight, hydrazobenzene, aniline, benzidine, p-aminophenol and o-aminophenol were detected in the urine. After intravenous or intratracheal application, only one metabolite was detected in the urine, and this appeared to be of a phenolic nature (no further details; Dutkiewicz and Szymanska, 1973).

7.2 Acute and subacute toxicity

The oral LD_{50} for hydrazobenzene in rats was 301 mg/kg body weight (no further details; cited in NIOSH, 1985).

A 4-week feeding study (with a 2-week observation period) was carried out in groups of 5 male and 5 female Fischer-344 rats and the same number of B6C3F1 mice, in order to establish the maximum tolerated dose for a carcinogenicity study. The concentrations of technical-grade hydrazobenzene were 70, 140, 280, 550, 1080, 2140, 3010 and 4230 mg/kg feed for male rats and mice, and 0.8 (rats only), 3, 11, 20, 40, 150, 1040, 7310 and 51,380 mg/kg feed for female rats and mice. Appropriate control groups were employed. Two of the 5 male rats in the 1080 mg/kg feed group died, and at higher concentrations, all of the male and female rats died. No substance-related pathological changes were found. One out of 5 male mice died in the 3010 mg/kg feed group and 2/5 in the 4230 mg/kg feed group. 4 out of 5 female mice died in the 7310 mg/kg feed group, and all 5 females given 51,380 mg/kg feed. Bleeding of the gastro-intestinal tract was the only pathological change in the mice (NCI, 1978).

7.3 Skin and mucous membrane effects

No information available.

7.4 Sensitization

No information available.

7.5 Subchronic and chronic toxicity

The following non-neoplastic effects were seen in carcinogenicity studies in rats and mice (study protocol described in Sec. 7.7; NCI, 1978):

In the course of the study, a slight decrease in body weight occurred in male rats in the high-dose group. Female rats showed a slight decrease in body weight after 46 weeks in the low-dose group, and after 22 weeks in the high-dose group. There was no difference in survival time between treated and untreated male rats, while in the female rats there was a significant reduction in the survival time of the high-dose group compared with the controls (Cox test, $p<0.001$). In week 100 of the study, 25/50 rats in the high-dose group were still alive, compared with 43/50 in the control group. There was no reduction in survival time in the low-dose group.

In mice there were no changes in body weight in the low-dose group compared with controls. In the high-dose group, male and female mice showed a reduction in body weight to 20–25 g (controls 35–45 g) from week 28. No other clinically conspicuous effects occurred. Survival of the male and female mice in the high-dose group was significantly less than that of the controls from week 70 (treated males 33/50, treated females 26/50, compared with control males 39/50, control females 38/50). No shortening of survival time was seen in the low-dose group.

7.6 Genotoxicity

7.6.1 In vitro

Technical-grade hydrazobenzene was studied in a pre-incubation test in the *Salmonella typhimurium* strains TA 1535, TA 1537, TA 98 and TA 100, with and without metabolic activation (S9-mix from Aroclor 1254-induced livers of male Sprague-Dawley rats and male Syrian hamsters). The doses ranged from 3.3 to 333.3 µg/plate. Hydrazobenzene induced point mutations only in strain TA 100, from 33.3 µg/plate, in the presence of a metabolic activation system. No mutagenic activity was observed in the other strains either with or without metabolic activation (Haworth et al., 1983).

Hydrazobenzene (at least 65% pure) was investigated along with 62 other substances in a spot test in *Salmonella* strains TA 98, TA 100, TA 1535, TA 1537 and TA 1538, and in a plate-incorporation test in *Escherichia coli* WP2uvrA. The tests were conducted with and without metabolic activation (S9-mix from Aroclor 1254-induced livers of rats, mice and hamsters). The concentrations were between 0.1 and 6666.6 µg/plate. Again, hydrazobenzene induced point mutations in strain TA 100 after metabolic activation at concentrations of 10 to 333.3 µg/plate. The results were predominantly negative in the other *Salmonella* strains, and were clearly negative in *Escherichia coli* (Dunkel et al., 1985).

The effect of hydrazobenzene on chromosomes and sister chromatid exchange was studied in vitro in Chinese hamster CHO cells (CHO-W-B1), with and without metabolic activation (S9-mix from Aroclor 1254-induced rat liver). Doses used in the chromosome aberration test were 1.4 to 42 µg/ml. Without metabolic activation the highest dose (42 µg/ml) had a questionable effect, whilst in the presence of a metabolic activation system doses of 14 and 42 µg/ml showed a significant positive effect ($p \leq 0.05$). In the SCE test, doses of between 1.4 and 15 µg/ml were used. Hydrazobenzene was negative up to the highest dose (14 µg/ml) in the absence of metabolic activation, but was positive with metabolic activation at all dose levels (5, 10 and 15 µg/ml; $p \leq 0.05$). Hydrazobenzene thus induced chromosomal aberrations and increased the rate of sister chromatid exchange in this study (Galloway et al., 1987).

7.6.2 In vivo

The effect of hydrazobenzene was studied in a short-term test of the inhibition of testicular DNA synthesis in mice by potential mutagens and carcinogens. Male mice received an intraperitoneal injection of 100 mg hydrazobenzene/kg and an injection of ^{3}H-thymidine, 3.5 hours and 30 minutes, respectively, before they were killed. The incorporation of ^{3}H-thymidine into testicular DNA was then measured. Hydrazobenzene reduced thymidine incorporation by 72% ($p<0.01$; Seiler, 1977).

7.7 Carcinogenicity

In an early study, 52 female Sherman rats (about 150 g) each received weekly injections of 60 mg technical-grade hydrazobenzene (in olive oil) throughout their lives (cumulative dose 6.4 g). 31 rats survived for more than 300 days (controls 28/50). In contrast to benzidine which was tested at the same time, no liver tumours and only one Zymbal gland tumour occurred after 366 days (Spitz et al., 1950).

A long-term feeding study in rats (Fischer-344) and mice (B6C3F1) was carried out with technical-grade hydrazobenzene. The study groups and control groups (one for each dose level) consisted of 50 females and 50 males (except for one control group with 47 female mice and one control group with 49 male rats). The concentrations in the feed were 80 and 300 mg/kg in male rats, 40 and 100 mg/kg in female rats, 80 and 400 mg/kg in male mice and 40 and 400 mg/kg in female mice. The animals received this diet for 78 weeks. Observation periods were 28–30 weeks for rats and 17–18 weeks for mice. In rats, the administration of hydrazobenzene in the diet increased the development of liver tumours in both sexes. The incidence of neoplasms of the Zymbal glands in the ear canal (a tumour which rarely occurs spontaneously; Baker et al., 1979) was increased in the males, and there was an increase in mammary adenocarcinomas in the females. Hepatocellular carcinomas were found in 5/49 males in the low-dose group ($p=0.031$), in 31/49 males in the high-dose group ($p<0.001$) and in 1/95 control males. No liver carcinomas were observed in the female rats, but in 6/50 animals in the high-dose group, neoplastic nodules occurred (control 0/47; $p=0.013$). Tumours of the Zymbal glands and the skin of the ears occurred in 1/95 control males, 2/50 males in the low-dose group and 7/49 males in the high-dose group ($p=0.007$), and in 0/98 control females, 1/50 females in the low-dose group and 2/50 females in the high-dose group. Eight of these tumours were squamous epithelial carcinomas, 1 was a squamous epithelial papilloma and 2 were adenocarcinomas (histology of 2 tumours not specified). Adenocarcinomas of the mammary glands occurred in 0/50 control females, 3/50 females in the low-dose group and 6/50 females in the high-dose group ($p=0.013$). Statistical evaluation adjusted for age was by the Fisher exact test. In mice, an increased incidence of hepatocellular carcinomas was seen in the females (20/43 in the high-dose group, 4/39 in the low-dose group and 3/97 in the controls). The increased tumour rate in the high-dose group was statistically significant ($p<0.001$; Fisher exact test, adjusted for age). There was no indication of a carcinogenic effect of hydrazobenzene in male mice (NCI, 1978).

Other authors subsequently calculated the average tumour-causing dose (TD_{50}) for the individual types of tumour in the NCI study. These were 38.5 mg/kg body weight/day for Zymbal gland tumours (male rats), 26.0 mg/kg body weight/day for liver tumours (female mice), 3.70 mg/kg body weight/day for liver tumours (male rats) and 11.40 mg/kg body weight/day for mammary gland tumours (female rats). The TD_{50} for all target organs together was 3.55 mg/kg body weight/day for male rats (Gold et al., 1986).

In a long-term study involving 91 male and female rats (strain not specified), hydrazobenzene was injected subcutaneously once a week, initially at a dose of 60 mg/rat in 0.3 ml sunflower oil and then at 40 mg/rat in 0.5 ml sunflower oil (corresponding to about 300 and 200 mg/kg body weight, respectively). The treatment period was 588 days and the total dose per rat during this time was 3.8 g hydrazobenzene. The first neoplasm (a Zymbal gland carcinoma) occurred on day 187 of the study, after the rats had received 1.3 g hydrazobenzene. At this time, 53 rats were still alive (29 males and 24 females). By the end of the study, which lasted 692 days, 10 further tumours had developed (1 uterine adenocarcinoma, 2 mammary carcinomas, 1 mammary adenoma, 2 Zymbal gland tumours, 2 liver adenomas, 1 spleen angio-endothelioma, 1 reticuloma). No data were supplied on the control group (Pliss, 1974).

In a further study by the same author, male and female rats (strain not specified) received hydrazobenzene in 0.5 ml sunflower oil in their feed, five times weekly at a dose of 30 mg/rat (about 150 mg/kg body weight). The chemical was administered for 590 days, and each rat received a total of 12.57 g hydrazobenzene in its feed. With an average latent period of 566 days, tumours were detected in 21 rats (5 Zymbal gland tumours, 6 liver tumours of which 4 were adenomas and 2 were haemangiomas, 4 mammary tumours, 3 uterine carcinomas, 2 kidney tumours and 1 leukosis). Again, there was no information on the control group (Pliss, 1974).

The same investigator also tested hydrazobenzene in mice, administering a dose of 5 mg (about 200 mg/kg) in 0.5 ml sunflower oil subcutaneously to 60 mice once a week for 512 days (about 72 weeks). The total dose per mouse was 370 mg. The first tumour (a sarcoma at the injection site) was detected on day 265. At this time 30 mice were still alive (29 males and 1 female). After 365 days 22 mice remained, 3 of which were still alive after 548 days. In total, 11 mice developed tumours (2 sarcomas at the injection site, 5 lung adenomas, 3 liver tumours, 1 leukosis). Spontaneous tumours were said to have occurred in 17% of the control mice, but no further details were given (Pliss, 1974).

In a further study by the same author, hydrazobenzene dissolved in benzene was applied topically to mice (2 mg/mouse in 0.05 ml benzene, 3 times per week for 442 days), providing a total dose of 360 mg hydrazobenzene. No changes were detectable at the application site between the shoulder blades. The first tumour was observed on day 179 of the study (skin cancer on the hind leg). At this time 12 females and 29 males were still alive. After 1 year 3 females and 13 males were still alive, and 4 males survived for more than 1.5 years. The following tumours occurred in the mice: 1 skin cancer, 2 liver haemangiomas, 3 leukoses and 3 lung adenomas. The same control group was apparently used as for the study previously described, in which 17% of the mice had tumours (no further details). In these studies, the high loss of animals during the time before the appearance of the first tumours is striking. According to Pliss, this can be attributed to infectious disease in addition to the chemically-related effects, although no further details were given (Pliss, 1974). On the whole, the studies of Pliss are inadequately reported.

Another long-term study was carried out with 50 rats (25 males and 25 females, strain not specified) given technical grade hydrazobenzene. The test substance was collected from the manufacturer and consisted of 55% hydrazobenzene. The rats received weekly subcutaneous injections of 20 mg (in 0.5 ml sunflower oil). Fifty injections were made in one year. Thereafter, the rats were observed until they died naturally or through tumour formation. When the first tumour was detected 19 rats were still alive,

4 of which developed tumours (1 sarcoma at the injection site, 1 Zymbal gland carcinoma, 1 renal carcinoma and 1 uterine hyperplasia of the endometrium). The average latent period was 603±45 days. In the 50 control animals, 36 of which survived for 630 days, 1 mammary fibroadenoma was observed. Using the same study protocol and control group, the authors tested a benzidine-containing mixture (27.2% benzidine sulphate), benzidine being an impurity that may be found in hydrazobenzene. The rats were injected subcutaneously with 15 mg of this mixture of substances once a week. After an average latent period of 599±39 days, 5 tumours were diagnosed in the 14 surviving animals (1 sarcoma at the site of injection, 3 Zymbal gland carcinomas, 1 metastasized carcinoma of not specified origin; Kurlyandsky et al., 1976).

A mixture of chemicals containing benzidine and hydrazobenzene was administered (15 and 20 mg/rat) using the same protocol and control group as before. 10 tumours were found in the 14 surviving animals after an average latent period of 506±15 days (4 sarcomas at the injection site, 2 Zymbal gland carcinomas, 1 hepatoma, 1 mammary carcinoma and 2 mammary fibroadenomas). The control animals were injected with 0.5 ml sunflower oil. In this group, 1 mammary fibroadenoma occurred in the 26 surviving animals. The authors noted that the administration of benzidine and hydrazobenzene together led to a higher tumour rate (71.4%) than either substance alone (35.7% and 21% respectively). It should be borne in mind that the substance tested was not available in a chemically pure form, but was always a mixture of substances (Genin et al., 1975; Kurlyandsky et al., 1976).

Hydrazobenzene (purity not specified) was tested for its ability to induce lung tumours in strain A mice, a strain which is particularly susceptible to these tumours (spontaneous occurrence beginning at the age of 3–4 months, and nearing 100% after 24 months). Groups of 10 male and 10 female mice were given intraperitoneal injections three times a week for 8 weeks at doses of 200, 100 or 50 mg/kg (in tricaprylin). The mice then remained untreated for a further 16 weeks. After a total of 24 weeks, the tumours were evaluated. At the highest dose (200 mg/kg body weight) there was a significant increase in the lung tumour incidence (alveolar and bronchial adenomas) in the male mice with respect to the percentage of tumour-bearing surviving animals (67%; solvent control 13%) and the number of tumours per mouse (0.89%, $p \leq 0.05$; solvent control 0.167%). In the females given the same dose, only the percentage of tumours per surviving mouse

(0.56%; solvent control 0.11%) was significantly increased ($p \leq 0.05$; Maronpot et al., 1986).

7.8 Reproductive toxicity
No information available.

7.9 Effects on the immune system
No information available.

7.10 Neurotoxicity
No information available.

7.11 Other effects
No information available.

8. Experience in humans

From 1940 to 1960, benzidine was manufactured by the East Bohemian chemical works under relatively poor conditions of industrial hygiene. During the process, hydrazobenzene was produced as an intermediate. In 1960, the operation was transferred to a new, modern building. The workplace concentrations measured there from 1961 to 1965 were between 0.006 and 3 μg/l air for hydrazobenzene, and were thus below the highest permissible level in the USSR of 10 μg/l air. From a total of 329 people who had been exposed since 1940, 189 were followed up. In these, 20 cases of bladder cancer were found (10.6%). The average exposure time was 8 years (Kuzelová et al., 1969). It is, however, more likely that benzidine caused these bladder carcinomas than hydrazobenzene.

In 1951, bladder papillomatosis was reported in a 47-year-old patient who had been occupationally exposed to trinitro-toluene for 6 years and subsequently to benzidine and hydrazobenzene for $3^3/_4$ years. He had also been in contact with other intermediates to a lesser extent. At the time of diagnosis the man had had no exposure for a year. It is very unlikely that hydrazobenzene was the causative agent (Marhold, 1951).

Some years ago, there were reports of isolated irritative cystitis with incontinence, haematuria, and a feeling of pressue in the area of the bladder and kidneys amongst workers exposed to high concentrations of hydrazobenzene. Bladder cancers were not associated with hydrazobenzene exposure (Ciba-Geigy, 1985).

Documentation which goes back to 1914 provides no evidence that hydrazobenzene is carcinogenic to man (Korallus, 1985, 1989).

9. Threshold limit values

In 1990, the limit for hydrazine derivatives was 0.1 mg/m^3 air in the USSR (Anonymous, 1990).

References

Anonymous
Valeurs limités d'exposition professionnelle aux substances dangereuses de l'ACGIH, de la RFA et de l'URSS
Cah. Notes Doc., 138, 162 (1990)

Baker, H.J., Lindsey, J.R., Weisbroth, S.H. (eds.)
The laboratory rat, Vol. I, p. 337
Academic Press, New York (1979)

BIA (Berufsgenossenschaftliches Institut für Arbeitssicherheit, St. Augustin)
Letters to BG Chemie, dated 23. 2. 1984 and 13. 3. 1984

Ciba-Geigy AG, Company Medical Department, Grenzach
Letter to BG Chemie dated 29. 12. 1982

Dunkel, V.C., Zeiger, E., Brusick, P., McCoy, E., McGregor, D., Mortelmans, K., Rosenkranz, H.S., Simmon, V.F.
Reproducibility of microbial mutagenicity assays: II. Testing of carcinogens and non-carcinogens in Salmonella typhimurium and Escherichia coli
Environ. Mutagen., 7 (5), 1–248 (1985)

Dutkiewicz, T., Szymanska, J.
Chromatographic determination of hydrazobenzene metabolites in rats
Bromatol. Chem. Toksykol., 6, 323–327 (1973)
(Polish work, only available as an abstract)

Galloway, S.M., Armstrong, M.J., Reuben, C., Colman, S., Brown, B., Cannon, C., Bloom, A.D., Nakamura, F., Ahmed, M., Duk, S., Rimpo, J., Margolin, B.H., Resnick, M.A., Anderson, B., Zeiger, E.
Chromosome aberrations and sister chromatid exchanges in chinese hamster ovary cells: Evaluations of 108 chemicals
Environ. Mol. Mutagen., 10 (10), 1–175 (1987)

Genin, V.A., Medvedovsky, A.G., Voronin, V.M.
Stronger carcinogenic activity with joint effect of hydrazine-benzene and benzidine-sulphate (translation from Russian)
Gig. Tr. Prof. Zabol., 4, 28–31 (1975)

Gold, L.S., Ward, J.M., Bernstein, L., Stern, B.
Association between carcinogenic potency and tumour pathology in rodent carcinogenesis bioassays
Fundam. Appl. Toxicol., 6, 677–690 (1986)

Haworth, S., Lawlor, T., Mortelmans, K., Speck, W., Zeiger, E.
Salmonella mutagenicity test results for 250 chemicals
Environ. Mutagen., 5 (1), 3–142 (1983)

Hüls AG, Marl
Safety data sheet of 17. 8. 1989 a

Hüls AG, Marl
Letter to BG Chemie dated 26. 4. 1989 b

Hüls AG, Marl
Letter to BG Chemie dated 6. 12. 1989 c

Korallus, U., BAYER AG (Medical Department)
Letter to BG Chemie dated 16. 9. 1985

Korallus, U., BAYER AG (Medical Department)
Letter to BG Chemie dated 11. 8. 1989

Kurlyandsky, B.A., Medvedovsky, A.G., Genin, V.A., Voronin, V.M., Mashbits, F.D.
Experimental study on a combined action of some diphenylamino derivatives with a view of preventing occupational newgrowths of the urinary bladder (English translation)
Gig. Tr. Prof. Zabol., 5, 34–38 (1976)

Kuzelová, M., Kunor, V., Hurt, K.
Überwachung von bei der Benzidin-Herstellung beschäftigten Arbeitskräften (German translation from Czech)
Prac. Lék., 21 (7), 310–313 (1969)

Marhold, J.
A case of tumour of the bladder following exposure to benzidine (In Czech with English summary)
Prac. Lék., 3, 272–274 (1951)

Maronpot, R.R., Shimkin, M.B., Witschi, H.P., Smith, L.H., Cline, J.M.
Strain A mouse pulmonary tumor test results for chemicals previously tested in the National Cancer Institute, carcinogenicity tests
J. Natl. Cancer Inst., 76 (6), 1101–1112 (1986)

NCI (National Cancer Institute)
Bioassay of hydrazobenzene for possible carcinogenicity
Technical Report Series No. 92, NCI-CG-TR-92 (1978)

Neumüller, O.A. (ed.)
Römpps Chemie Lexikon
8th Edition, p. 1784
Frankh'sche Verlagshandlung, Stuttgart (1983)

NIOSH (National Institute for Occupational Safety and Health)
Registry of Toxic Effects of Chemical Substances, 1983–84
Suppl., p. 1024, Cincinnati, Ohio (1985)

Pliss, G.B.
Carcinogenic properties of hydrazobenzene
(translation from Russian)
Vopr. Onkol., 20, 53–57 (1974)

Seiler, J.P.
Inhibition of testicular DNA synthesis by chemical mutagens and carcinogens. Preliminary results in the validation of a novel short term test
Mutat. Res., 46, 305–310 (1977)

Spitz, S., Maguigan, W.H., Dobriner, K.
The carcinogenic action of benzidine
Cancer, 3, 789–804 (1950)

1,4-Diaminoanthraquinone

1. Summary and assessment

According to the available data, 1,4-diaminoanthraquinone is moderately toxic on acute administration (LD_{50} rat oral ca. 1800 mg/kg, LD_{50} mouse i.p. ca. 640 mg/kg) and is not irritating to the skin or eyes.

In the Salmonella/microsome test, 1,4-diaminoanthraquinone induces point mutations mainly in the frameshift strains TA 1537 and TA 98 and in bacteriophage T4D.

In mouse T-lymphocytes in vitro, 1,4-diaminoanthraquinone causes marked immunodepression of mastocytoma cells.

In a retrospective mortality study in humans exposed to substituted anthraquinones, there is no increase in the total number of deaths or in the number of cancer deaths.

2. Name of substance

2.1	Usual name	1,4-Diaminoanthraquinone
2.2	IUPAC-name	1,4-Diaminoanthraquinone
2.3	CAS-No.	128-95-0

3. Synonyms, common and trade names

1,4-Diaminoanthrachinon
1,4-diamino-9,10-anthracene-dione

4. Structural and molecular formulae

4.1 Structural formula

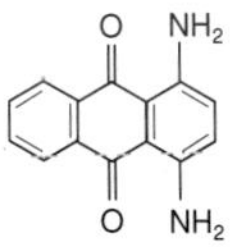

4.2 Molecular formula $C_{14}H_{10}N_2O_2$

5. Physical and chemical properties

5.1	Molecular mass, g/mol	238.2
5.2	Melting point, °C	245–251 (BASF, 1990) 268 (Bien et al., 1985)
5.3	Boiling point, °C	No information available
5.4	Vapour pressure, hPa	No information available
5.5	Density, g/cm^3	No information available
5.6	Solubility in water	Insoluble (BASF, 1978)
5.7	Solubility in organic solvents	Slightly soluble in ethanol, soluble in dimethylformamide (BASF, 1978)
5.8	Solubility in fat	No information available
5.9	pH-value	No information available
5.10	Conversion factor	1 ppm $\hat{=}$ 9.88 mg/m^3 1 mg/m^3 $\hat{=}$ 0.10 ppm (at 25 °C and 1013 hPa)

6. Uses

Intermediate for use in the manufacture of anthraquinone dyes (Bien et al., 1985).

7. Experimental results

7.1 Toxicokinetics and metabolism

No information available.

7.2 Acute and subacute toxicity

To determine the acute oral toxicity of 1,4-diaminoanthraquinone, male and female Sprague-Dawley rats received a single dose of the chemical by stomach tube as a 12% or 20% aqueous suspension in 0.5% carboxymethylcellulose. The observation period was 7 days. Signs of toxicity included dyspnoea and violet-coloured urine. At autopsy, diarrhoea was observed as well as general colouration of the internal organs. The approximate LD_{50} was 1800 mg/kg (BASF, 1972).

The acute intraperitoneal LD_{50} of 1,4-diaminoanthraquinone was determined in male and female NMRI mice after a 7-day observation period. The chemical was administered as a 12% or 20% aqueous suspension in 0.5% carboxymethylcellulose by a single injection into the abdominal cavity. Symptoms observed included dyspnoea, apathy and lying on the stomach, as well as violet colouration of the extremities, ears and tails. The LD_{50} was about 640 mg/kg. Autopsy revealed general colouration of the internal organs and intra-abdominal deposits of the chemical (BASF, 1972).

In an inhalation risk test, 12 Sprague-Dawley rats tolerated inhalation of the volatile fraction of 1,4-diaminoanthraquinone at 20 °C for 8 hours without any deaths or signs of toxicity. No abnormalities were seen at autopsy (BASF, 1972).

7.3 Skin and mucous membrane effects

The primary skin irritancy of 1,4-diaminoanthraquinone as an 80% aqueous preparation was investigated in 2 rabbits (white Viennese) by 20-hour semi-occlusive application. After 24 hours and eight days, violet residues were seen but there were no signs of inflammation (BASF, 1972).

To test the eye irritancy of 1,4-diaminoanthraquinone, 50 mg of the chemical was instilled into the conjunctival sac of each of 2 white Viennese rabbits. After 1 hour slight reddening was seen and there were residues of the substance in the eye. The slight reddening was still evident after 24 hours, but was no worse than that caused by talc. After 8 days, the eyes had returned to normal (BASF, 1972).

7.4 Sensitization

No information available.

7.5 Subchronic and chronic toxicity

No information available.

7.6 Genotoxicity

7.6.1 In vitro

The ability of 1,4-diaminoanthraquinone to induce point mutations was studied in the Salmonella test in strains TA 1535, TA 1538, TA 1978, TA 100 and TA 98, in the absence of a metabolic activation system. The concentrations used were 10–1000 µg/plate. The chemical did not induce point mutations at any of the concentrations tested (Tamaro et al., 1975).

Another study was carried out in the *Salmonella typhimurium* strain TA 98 at doses of 15, 50 and 150 µg/plate, with and without metabolic activation. A significant increase in the number of revertants was found from 15 µg/plate, both in the presence and absence of a metabolic activation system (Yoshikawa et al., 1976).

1,4-Diaminoanthraquinone was studied in the Salmonella/microsome test in strains TA 1535, TA 100, TA 1537, TA 1538 and TA 98, with and without metabolic activation. Concentrations of 100, 500, 1000 and 2000 µg/plate were tested. The results were negative in strains TA 1535 and TA 100. Positive results were seen in strains TA 1537, TA 1538 and TA 98, particularly with metabolic activation (Brown and Brown, 1976).

A further study tested the ability of 1,4-diaminoanthraquinone to induce point mutations in the Salmonella test in strains TA 1535, TA 100, TA 1537, TA 1538 and TA 98 at doses of 10, 20 and 40 µg/plate. The number of revertants did not increase at any of the doses tested (Shahin and von Borstel, 1978).

Another study also failed to establish point-mutagenicity in the Salmonella/microsome test in strains TA 1535, TA 100, TA 1538 and TA 98, with and without metabolic activation, at doses of 100, 500 and 1000 µg/plate. Inhibition of growth occurred in TA 100 at 1000 µg/plate (Venturini and Tamaro, 1979).

The point-mutagenic activity of 1,4-diaminoanthraquinone was also tested in strains TA 1537 and TA 98 at doses of 100–2500 µg/plate, with and without metabolic activation. No positive reaction was observed in the absence of metabolic activation. With metabolic activation, however, doses of 100 µg/plate or more resulted in an increase in the number of revertants in both strains by factors of 3.5 (TA 98) and 5.5 (TA 1537). No bacteriotoxic effect was observed at any dose level (BASF, 1982).

Another investigator tested the point-mutagenic activity of 1,4-diaminoanthraquinone in the Salmonella/microsome test in strains TA 1535, TA 1537, TA 1538, TA 98 and TA 100, with and without metabolic activation. The doses used were 1.25 to 5000 µg/plate. No mutagenic effect was seen in strains TA 1535 or TA 100 at any dose level. In contrast, clear dose-dependent mutagenicity was seen in the frameshift strains TA 1537, TA 1538 and TA 98 after metabolic activation. Strain TA 1538 was the most sensitive, a concentration of 2.5 µg/plate causing a 3.3-fold increase in the number of revertants. At 500 µg/plate, the number of revertants was 12.5 times higher than the control level. In the absence of a metabolic activation system, no mutagenic activity was seen in the frameshift strains (Henry, 1983).

In *Saccharomyces cerevisiae* (strain XV185-14C), 1,4-diaminoanthraquinone was negative at doses of 20, 40 and 100 µg/plate (Shahin and von Borstel, 1978).

A positive mutagenic effect was seen in bacteriophage T4D at doses of 12.8, 30.5 and 61 μg/ml (with 32.8, 23.7 and 22.4 mutants/10^4 surviving phages, respectively), while lower doses (0.3 to 9.6 μg/ml) and higher doses (107 to 291 μg/ml) had no mutagenic effect. It was notable that at the active dose levels the phage survival rate was between 32.7 and 44%, whilst at the inactive dose levels it was between 60.2 and 100% (Kvelland, 1983).

7.6.2 In vivo

No information available.

7.7 Carcinogenicity

No information available.

7.8 Reproductive toxicity

No information available.

7.9 Effects on the immune system

A study of the possible immunodepressive effect of 1,4-diaminoanthraquinone was carried out in vitro with T-lymphocytes from the spleens of B6C3F1 mice. (The formula given by the authors in this paper is that of 1,2-diaminoanthraquinone, but in the text 1,4-diaminoanthraquinone is always stated). The cytolytic effect of the chemical on P815-mastocytoma cells (from DWA/2-tumours) was studied after 5 days of exposure, at concentrations of 4, 20 and 40 μM (corresponding to about 1, 5 and 10 μg/ml, respectively). Dose-dependent inhibition (by up to 95%) of cytolytic activity occurred (House and Dean, 1987).

7.10 Neurotoxicity

No information available.

7.11 Other effects

The antileukaemic activity of 1,4-diaminoanthraquinone was studied in BDF or CDF1 mice with P388 Ascites leukaemia. On intraperitoneal injection, the highest dose studied (100 mg/kg) showed no curative effect within 60 days, as determined by the survival time of the mice (Murdock et al., 1979).

8. Experience in humans

A retrospective mortality study was conducted of 1975 workers in a Scottish dyestuffs factory. The workers were exposed to substituted anthraquinones for at least 6 months between 1956 and 1965, inclusively. The cohort was followed until 30 June 1980. It cannot be deduced from the study which particular substances were involved. The age-standardized mortality rate revealed no increase in the total number of deaths or in the number of deaths through cancer (Gardiner et al., 1982).

9. Threshold limit values

No information available.

References

BASF AG, Toxicology Department
Gewerbetoxikologische Vorprüfung von 1,4-Diaminoanthrachinon
Unpublished report (1972)

BASF AG
Datenblatt, 1,4-Diaminoanthrachinon (1978)

BASF AG, Toxicology Department
Bericht über die Prüfung von 1,4-Diaminoanthrachinon im Ames-Test
Unpublished report (1982)

BASF AG
DIN-Sicherheitsdatenblatt, 1,4-Diaminoanthrachinon (1990)

Bien, H.S., Stawitz, J., Wunderlich, K.
Anthraquinone dyes and intermediates
in: Ullmann's Encyclopedia of Industrial Chemistry
5th ed., Vol. A 2, 366 (1985)
VCH Verlagsgesellschaft mbH, Weinheim

Brown, J.P., Brown, R.J.
Mutagenesis by 9,10-anthraquinone derivatives and related compounds in *Salmonella typhimurium*
Mutat. Res., 40, 203–224 (1976)

Gardiner, J.S., Walker, S.A., MacLean, A.J.
A retrospective mortality study of substituted anthraquinone dyestuffs workers
Br. J. Ind. Med., 39, 355–360 (1982)

Henry, M.C.
Mutagenic screening of six candidate dyes for colored smoke munitions in the Salmonella reversion assay
US Army Medical Bioengineering Research and Development Laboratory, Fort Detrick, Frederick, MD 21701
Final Report, October 1983

House, R.V., Dean, J.H.
Studies on structural requirements for suppression of cytotoxic T-lymphocyte induction by polycyclic compounds
In Vitro Toxicology, 1 (3), 149–162 (1987)

Kvelland, I.
The mutagenic effect in bacteriophage T4D of a hair dye, 1,4-diaminoanthraquinone, and of two solvents, dimethylsulfoxide and ethanol
Hereditas, 99, 209–213 (1983)

Murdock, K.C., Child, R.G., Fabio, P.F., Angier, R.B., Wallace, R.E., Durr, F.E., Citarella, R.V.
Antitumor agents. 1. 1,4-Bis[(aminoalkyl)amino]-9,10-anthracenediones
J. Med. Chem., 22 (9), 1024–1030 (1979)

Shahin, M.M., von Borstel, R.C.
Comparisons of mutation induction in reversion systems of *Saccharomyces cerevisiae* and *Salmonella typhimurium*
Mutat. Res., 53, 1–10 (1978)

Tamaro, M., Monti-Bragadin, C., Banfi, E.
Mutagenic activity of anthraquinone derivatives used as dyes in a textile factory
Boll. Ist. Sieroter. Milan., 54 (2), 105–107 (1975)

Venturini, S., Tamaro, T.
Mutagenicity of anthraquinone and azo dyes in Ames' *Salmonella typhimurium* test
Mutat. Res., 68, 307–312 (1979)

Yoshikawa, K., Uchino, H., Kurata, H.
Studies on the mutagenicity of hair dye
Bull. Natl. Inst. Hyg. Sci. Tokyo, 94, 28–32 (1976)

2-Mercaptobenzothiazole

1. Summary and assessment

After oral, dermal and parenteral administration, 2-mercaptobenzothiazole (MBT) is rapidly absorbed, is metabolised within 96 hours and is almost completely eliminated, primarily in the urine. Also present in the urine, in addition to the unchanged substance, are the following metabolites: a glucuronide, a mercapturic acid derivative, 2-mercapturic acid benzothiazole sulphate, and the dimer dibenzothiazole disulphide.

MBT is of low acute toxicity and can penetrate the skin (LD_{50} oral rat, mouse, rabbit, guinea-pig 1680–3800 mg/kg; LD_{50} dermal rabbit >7940 mg/kg; LC_{50}, 4 hours, rat >1270 mg/m^3). The symptoms of poisoning in animals include peripheral vasodilation, salivation, lacrimation and tonic/clonic spasms.

The results of animal tests for the irritant activity of MBT on the skin and eyes are contradictory, but in all cases the irritant activity is weak.

In subacute and subchronic tests on rodents, body weight reduction and microscopically visible changes in the liver and kidneys are observed; with repeated inhalation exposure body weight is reduced but no effects are observed on the lung and nervous system. In dogs, the oral administration of about 3 mg/kg per day for 1 year does not result in any adverse effects.

MBT is not mutagenic either in the Salmonella/microsome test (with and without S9 mix) or on *Escherichia coli*. Tests on mammalian cells (CHO, HGPRT and in mouse lymphoma cells) provide contradictory results. In cytogenetic tests on CHO cells, an increased incidence of chromosomal aberrations but no increased sister chromatid exchange rate have been observed at a high concentration, in the presence of a metabolising system (S9 mix). MBT is negative in the mouse micronucleus test, and slightly positive in the rat dominant lethal test. In the DNA covalent binding test, only slight DNA-binding has been observed.

Early long-term oral studies in rats given a low dose of MBT (approx. 6 mg/kg daily) provide no indication of carcinogenic activity, whilst oral administration to mice (50 to 100 mg/kg per day) gives rise to the suspicion of a dose-dependent increase in reticulocarcinomas; after a single subcutaneous injection in mice, followed by observation for 17 months, an increase in reticulocarcinomas is again observed. In neither case is the increased incidence of reticulocarcinomas significant.

In more recent tests involving oral administration of much higher doses (188 to 750 mg/kg per day) by stomach tube for 2 years, increased tumour incidence has been observed in rats of both sexes (male: adrenal gland pheochromocytoma, preputial gland adenomas or carcinomas, glandular cell adenomas in the pancreas, monocytic leukaemia; female: adrenal gland pheochromocytoma, hypophysis adenomas). In female mice, the increased incidence of hepatocellular adenomas or carcinomas in the low-dose group is of questionable significance.

In the cell transformation test in mice, MBT is negative.

In tests on pregnant rats and rabbits MBT is not maternally toxic, foetotoxic or teratogenic. After subcutaneous injection of maternally toxic doses, foetal abnormalities are observed in mice. A three-generation study in rats shows no effect on reproduction or lactation.

Both *in vitro* and *in vivo,* MBT inhibits dopamine-beta-hydroxylase activity, and hence the conversion from dopamine to noradrenaline.

In man, MBT is a skin irritant and a skin sensitizer.

MBT seems to exert a radioprotective effect after intraperitoneal injection in mice.

On the basis of the results obtained in long-term studies, the possibility of MBT being carcinogenic cannot be ruled out. A reproduction toxicity study (2 generations) in rats is currently in progress at NTP. MBT shows a cytotoxic efficiency.

2. Name of substance

2.1	Usual name	2-Mercaptobenzothiazole
2.2	IUPAC-name	2-Mercaptobenzothiazole
2.3	CAS-No.	149-30-4

3. Synonyms, common and trade names

2-Benzothiazolethiol
Captax
MBT
Pennac MBT
Rotax
Sulfadene
Thiotax

4. Structural and molecular formulae

4.1 Structural formula

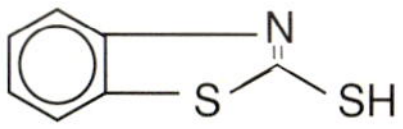

4.2 Molecular formula — $C_7H_5NS_2$

5. Physical and chemical properties

5.1 Molecular mass, g/mol — 167.25

5.2 Melting point, °C — 180.2–181.7
170.0–175.0
(technical grade product)
(Windholz, 1983)

5.3 Boiling point, °C — –

5.4 Vapour pressure, hPa — 253×10^{-4} (at 25 °C)
(Clayton and Clayton, 1981)

5.5 Density, g/cm^3 — 1.42 (at 20 °C)
(Clayton and Clayton, 1981)

5.6 Solubility in water — Insoluble
(Windholz, 1983)

5.7 Solubility in organic solvents — Acetone (10 g/100 ml)
Ether (1.0 g/100 ml)
Alcohol (2.0 g/100 ml)
Benzene (1.0 g/100 ml)
(at 25 °C)
(Windholz, 1983)

5.8 Solubility in fat — No information available

5.9 pH-value — No information available

5.10 Conversion factor — 1 ppm $\hat{=}$ 6.85 mg/m^3
1 mg/m^3 $\hat{=}$ 0.15 ppm
(at 25 °C and 1013 hPa)

5.11 Odour threshold — 1.76 ppm
(Clayton and Clayton, 1981)

6. Uses

Vulcanization accelerator; salts as fungicides (Windholz, 1983).

7. Experimental results

7.1 Toxicokinetics and metabolism

Groups of 20 male and 20 female Fisher-344 rats (8–9 weeks old, weight 153–198 g and 120–140 g, respectively) were given a single dose of 0.592 or 55.5 mg ^{14}C-labelled MBT/kg by stomach tube. 4 males and 4 females from each dose group were killed 8, 24, 48, 72 and 96 hours after administration, and blood, urine and faeces were collected for measurement of the radioactivity (liquid scintillation). Urine from 1 animal per group was collected for 8 hours after administration, and the metabolites were analyzed by HPLC. On average, 83–96% of the radioactivity was excreted in the urine and 4–9% in the faeces within 96 hours of dosing. At this time, 0.4–2% was still detectable in the erythrocytes. The results show that the substance is rapidly absorbed and is essentially eliminated in the urine. Seven metabolites were found in the urine, of which 2 were major metabolites (no further details of the metabolites; Hill, 1986).

Two fasted male rats were given a single oral dose of 50 mg 2-^{35}S-MBT. Their urine and faeces were collected and extracted 24, 48 and 72 hours after administration; 79.4% of the radioactivity was found in the urine and 1.4% in the faeces. Besides unchanged ^{35}S-labelled MBT, the following metabolites were detected: 2-mercaptobenzothiazole sulphate, 2-mercaptobenzothiazole glucuronide, 2,2'-dibenzothiazole disulphide and 2-benzothiazole mercapturic acid; the majority (90%) consisted of the original substance or the metabolite 2,2'-dibenzothiazole disulphide. The authors concluded from the study that the intermediate glutathione conjugate of 2-^{35}S-MBT is metabolized to a cysteine conjugate, which is then cleaved at the C-S bond (Fukuoka and Tanaka, 1987).

The metabolites benzothiazole-2-^{35}S-mercaptoglucuronide and ^{35}S-sulphate, together with non-radioactive benzothiazole-2-mercapturic acid, were detected in the urine of male rats for up to 14 days after a single intraperitoneal injection of 590 mg 2-^{35}S-MBT/kg body weight (Colucci and Buyske, 1965).

In a study involving 28 male and 28 female Fischer-344 rats, a single dose of 0.602 mg ^{14}C-labelled MBT/kg body weight was injected intravenously into the tail vein. The radioactivity in whole blood, blood plasma and in the tail was measured in groups of 4 males and 4 females killed at 5 and 15 minutes, and 1, 2, 4, 24 and 72 hours after administration. Urine and faeces were collected after 8, 24, 48 and 72 hours, from the rats that were kept for 72 hours (4 males and 4 females), and the amount of radioactivity present was measured. After 72 hours, the males had excreted ca. 91% in the urine and ca. 15% in the faeces, and the females ca. 96% in the urine and ca. 4% in the faeces. About 1.5–1.75% of the radioactivity was still present in the erythrocytes. The range of metabolites detected was comparable with that found on oral administration. Unchanged MBT (ca. 10%) was only found in the urine of 1 female (El Dareer et al., 1989).

A single application of ca. 11 mg ^{14}C-labelled MBT/kg body weight to the intact or abraded skin of guinea-pigs showed that absorption through the abraded skin was higher than through the intact skin (37% and 9%, respectively). The substance was almost completely eliminated in the urine and the faeces. Less than 0.1% of the applied dose was found in the blood, the internal organs or the gastro-intestinal tract after 48 hours. The highest specific radioactivity was present in the thyroid gland, followed by the blood and the kidneys (Nagamatsu et al., 1979).

A single dose of 31.1 µg (ca. 5.01 µCi) ^{14}C-labelled MBT in distilled tetrahydrofuran was applied to the skin in male and female Fischer-344 rats (9–10 weeks old, weight 186–199 g and 136–143 g respectively, number not specified) and female guinea-pigs (Hartley, age 9 weeks, weight 398–435 g). The treated area (rats 2 cm^2, guinea-pigs 5 cm^2) was covered with a metal cap for 96 hours. The substance was then washed off the animals. The investigators collected the water used for washing and rinsing, the cloth used for drying, the metal cap, blood plasma and skin from the site of application. In the rats, 16–17% of the applied radioactivity was absorbed, and the majority of this was excreted in the urine (males 91%, females 94%). In the guinea-pigs, 33.4% of the applied radioactivity was absorbed and, as for the rat, the urine was the main excretion route (recovery rate 97% of the absorbed radioactivity; El Dareer et al., 1989).

A single dose of 5 mg 2-^{14}C-labelled MBT/kg body weight was subcutaneously injected into 21 male guinea-pigs. The distribution of radioactivity in the body was measured after 15, 30 and 60 minutes and 3, 6 and 48 hours. The total activity was highest in the blood and internal organs (thyroid gland, lungs, liver, kidneys and adipose tissue) after 15 minutes and then declined rapidly, although a relatively high activity was still present in the thyroid gland after 48 hours. The activity was mainly eliminated in the urine (ca. 64% within 1 hour, and 92% within 6 hours). The metabolites included a glucuronide and a sulphate which accounted for ca. 90% of the administered activity. Up to 7.6% of the dose was excreted in the urine as unchanged MBT. Autoradiographic examination of one guinea-pig revealed that the highest levels of activity were present in the excretory organs (Nagamatsu et al., 1979).

Male and female Fischer-344 rats (weight 147–208 g and 113–153 g, respectively, 8–10 weeks old, number not specified) were given 0.509 mg MBT/kg body weight in corn oil by stomach tube, daily for 14 days, followed by a single dose of ^{14}C-labelled MBT (0.503 mg/kg body weight, ca. 58.6 μCi). The total radioactivity in the urine, faeces, whole blood, kidneys, spleen, lungs, thyroid gland, gonads, liver, brain, fat, heart, muscle, bones and bone marrow was determined. Up to ca. 90% of the radioactivity was excreted in the urine and up to ca. 10% in the faeces. The highest specific radioactivity was measured in the thyroid gland (El Dareer et al., 1989).

7.2 Acute and subacute toxicity

Data on the acute toxicity of MBT are presented in Table 1.

Acute intoxication with MBT in rats caused reduced general activity and muscular weakness. Anatomical and pathological examination of the animals that died during the experiment revealed hyperaemic lungs, pale livers and irritation of the gastro-intestinal tract. These effects were not seen in the surviving rats after the 14-day observation period and were therefore reversible (Monsanto, 1985).

Signs of toxicity which were described in mice after oral or intraperitoneal administration included marked peripheral vasodilation, excessive salivation, lacrimation and tonic-clonic spasms. The maximum tolerated doses were 931 mg/kg by oral administration and 305 mg/kg by intraperitoneal injection (no further details). The authors considered that the salivation and lacrimation might be indicative of cholinergic activity. However, the salivation was not blocked by atropine sulphate (0.2 mg/kg i.p.) and peripheral vasodilation was only slightly reduced, which ruled out strong cholinergic activity. Salivation and convulsions were inhibited by pentobarbital administration (25 mg/kg), from which the authors concluded that the effects were mainly mediated through the central nervous system. The peripheral vasodilation persisted, but the severity was greatly reduced (Guess and O'Leary, 1969).

In a preliminary study to determine suitable doses for a micronucleus test, groups of CD1 mice (2 males and 2 females per

Table 1. Acute toxicity of 2-mercaptobenzothiazole

Species	Sex	Route of administration	Vehicle	LD_{50} (mg/kg) LC_{50} mg/m^3	References
Rat	Male/Female	Oral	–	1680	NIOSH, 1985
Rat	Male/Female	Oral	Powder in corn oil	3800	Monsanto, 1985
Rat	–	Oral	–	1800	Uniroyal, 1985
Rat	–	Oral	–	3000	Vanderbilt, 1985
Rat	–	Inhalation	–	> 722 (7 hours)	Dow, 1985
Rat	Male/Female	Inhalation	–	>1270 (4 hours)	Ciba-Geigy, 1977
Rat	–	i.p.	–	300	NIOSH, 1985
Mouse	–	Oral	–	1851	NIOSH, 1985
Mouse	Male	Oral	Carboxymethylcellulose	2000	Guess and O'Leary, 1969
Mouse	Male	i.p.	Polyethylene glycol	100–200	Doull et al., 1962
Mouse	Male	i.p.	Cottonseed oil	437	Guess and O'Leary, 1969
Rabbit	Male/Female	Dermal	Corn oil	>7940	Younger Labs., 1974
Guinea-Pig	–	Oral	–	1680	Kowalski and Bassendowska, 1965
Guinea-Pig	–	i.p.	–	300	Kowalski and Bassendowska, 1965

– Not specified

group) were given 2 intraperitoneal injections of MBT on 2 consecutive days at doses of 16.6, 50, 166.6, 500 and 1666.6 mg/kg. At the highest dose level, all 4 mice died on the first day. At the next highest level, 500 mg/kg, the 2 females died within 4 hours of the first injection, and the 2 males showed reduced muscle tone, reduced general activity and ptosis. Except for isolated occurrences of reduced muscle tone, doses of 166.6 and 50 mg/kg had no effect. There were no adverse findings in the mice at 16.6 mg/kg (Sorg, 1984).

Autopsy revealed pathological changes in the livers and kidneys of guinea-pigs after oral administration of MBT. This was also seen in guinea-pigs that had received a single lethal intraperitoneal dose of 300 mg MBT/kg body weight (no further details; Kowalski and Bassendowska, 1965).

After a single dermal application of MBT, male and female rabbits showed reduced feed consumption for 3–5 days and lower spontaneous activity (Younger Laboratories, 1974).

Ptosis and reduced movement occurred in rats exposed to 1270 mg MBT dust/m^3 air for 4 hours, but these effects were reversible. No anatomical or pathological changes were seen at autopsy (Ciba Geigy, 1985).

In a range-finding experiment for a study on subchronic and chronic toxicity, 5 male and 5 female rats (F-344/N, 6 weeks old) and 5 male and 5 female mice (Harlan Industry, 5–6 weeks old) were given MBT in corn oil by stomach tube 12 times (on 5 days/week). The following doses were used: 0, 165, 313, 625, 1250 and 2500 mg MBT/kg body weight (rats) and 0, 187.5, 375, 750, 1500 and 3000 mg MBT/kg body weight (mice). Body weight gain was reduced by up to 14% in rats in the highest dose group. No other treatment-related effects were observed in the rats. In the mice, all of the animals in the high-dose group (3000 mg/kg) died, with the exception of 1 male, as did 4/5 females in the 1500 mg/kg group. These animals exhibited lethargy and prostration after treatment by stomach tube (Dieter, 1988).

A range-finding test for a carcinogenicity study in mice established a maximum tolerated dose (MTD, dose which caused no deaths) of 100 mg/kg body weight on single or repeated (daily for 6 or 19 days) oral administration of MBT in 0.5% gelatine (Innes et al., 1969).

Groups of 5 male rats were given feed containing 0, 0.1 or 1% MBT (equivalent to 0, 91 and 866 mg/kg/day) for 11 days. Reductions in body weight gain and feed consumption were observed. The absolute and relative liver weights at the higher dose level were increased at the end of the study. The treatment groups showed no differences from the control group in terms of behaviour, haematological and clinical-chemical parameters, and there were no changes evident on pathological and histopathological examination (Eastman Kodak, 1985).

Daily application of neat MBT to the intact abdominal skin of rabbits for 10 days caused slight hyperaemia after each application (no further details; Dow, 1985).

Male mice (strain and sex not specified) were given a daily intraperitoneal injection of 110 mg MBT/kg (1/4 LD_{50}) for a week. Control mice were treated with the solvent only (cottonseed oil). After 1 week the mice were dissected and histologically examined. A second experiment was carried out with groups of 10 mice (10–20 g) given daily i.p. injections of MBT (either in oil or as a suspension in physiological saline) at a dose of 55 mg/kg (1/8 LD_{50}) for 1 week. The mice were observed and weighed daily. After 1 week, the mice that had been treated with MBT in physiological saline received sodium hexobarbital (75 mg/kg) to measure the sleeping time. Daily administration of 1/4 or 1/8 of the LD_{50} of MBT did not cause any signs of toxicity, nor did it affect body weight gain. Sleeping time was significantly prolonged ($p = 0.05$) in mice in the high dose group. At autopsy there were no macroscopically detectable changes in the organs. Microscopic examination of the mice that had received 1/4 of the LD_{50} revealed damage to the liver (necrosis, cloudy swelling of the cells, fatty degeneration, changes in the cell nuclei, inflammation) and kidneys (diffuse cloudy swelling of the renal tubules) in both experiments (Guess and O'Leary, 1969).

In rats, the inhalation of 350–400 mg MBT/m^3 air for 2 hours daily for 15 days led to weight loss. No adverse effects were found on histopathological examination of the lungs and nervous system (no further details; Vorob'eva and Mezentseva, 1962).

7.3 Skin and mucous membrane effects

MBT was injected into the shaved dorsal skin of albino New Zealand rabbits, either as a carboxymethylcellulose-sodium chloride suspension or as a cottonseed oil suspension, at concentrations of 0.5%, 1%, 2% or 4%. One rabbit was used for each treatment and, in each case, 0.2 ml was injected intradermally at 4 sites on the back.

Visualization of the area and evaluation of the intensity of irritation was accomplished within 30 minutes by injecting 1 ml/kg of a 1% trypan blue solution into the ear vein. The degree of irritation (erythema, oedema, necrosis) was evaluated 24 hours after intradermal application. The rabbits were killed 48 hours after treatment and tissue samples were taken from the application site for microscopic examination. MBT only caused irritation as a 4% suspension in oil. The irritant effect was classified as weak and transient, and was less marked than that caused by a 20% ethanol solution (positive control). After injection of the 4% suspension in oil, slight inflammation was visible on histological examination (Guess and O'Leary, 1969).

In a further experiment, the effect of MBT on the healing of rabbit skin was studied. The clipped dorsal skin of 4 albino New Zealand rabbits was dabbed with 70% alcohol and then superficially scoured with a scalpel 4 times (incisions were 1 cm long, 2 mm deep and 0.5 cm apart). MBT was applied to the entire area (about 1×2 cm) as an oily or aqueous suspension at concentrations of 0.5%, 1%, 2% and 4%. The application site was examined daily for degree of erythema formation, healing, scar formation and the occurrence of other effects. MBT had no observed effect on the healing process. Hair growth and the time required for complete healing were the same in all cases (Guess and O'Leary, 1969).

MBT (500 mg) was applied to the intact or abraded skin of white New Zealand rabbits (24-hour occlusive application, area 2.4×2.4 cm) as a finely-milled powder in water. Evaluations were made 24 and 72 hours after application. MBT did not cause any primary skin irritation (Monsanto, 1985).

Guinea-pigs (age, strain and sex not specified) were treated topically with an aqueous paste of MBT (dose not specified). An evaluation made 24 hours after application revealed no indications of a skin reaction (no further details; Du Pont, 1948).

In another study on skin and eye irritancy in rabbits, 5 mg MBT applied to the skin or instilled into the conjunctival sac produced no irritant effects (no further details; Vorob'eva and Mezentseva, 1962).

The irritant effect of MBT on the eye was tested in New Zealand rabbits. The dry powder (0.1 g) was placed in the conjunctival sac, and evaluations were made 24, 48 and 72 hours later. Slight erythema of the conjunctiva and clouding of the cornea were observed, but these effects were reversible within 24 to 48 hours (Monsanto, 1985; Ciba-Geigy, 1977).

7.4 Sensitization

The sensitizing potential of MBT was studied in a maximization test in guinea-pigs (male and female, mixed breed, weight 250–450 g). At the beginning of the study, 12 guinea-pigs received a subcutaneous injection of MBT (dose not specified) in the neck, followed by an injection of Freund's adjuvant. 8 days later they were pretreated locally with sodium lauryl sulphate, and on the following day MBT was applied topically for 48 hours (dose not specified). Two weeks later a patch test was carried out. Oedema and erythema were observed in 5 out of 12 of the guinea-pigs after 24, 48, 72 and 144 hours. MBT was found to have sensitizing potential in this study (Ziegler et al., 1972).

Similar results have been reported by Magnusson and Kligman (1969), Bourrinet et al. (1979) and Wang and Suskind (1988).

Wang and Tabor (1988) formulated a hypothesis based on in vitro measurements, to explain how MBT acts as a sensitizer. They suggested that the SH-group of MBT reacts with the carboxyl group of free amino acids present in the epidermis by oxidation and/or thioester formation, so that the hapten MBT becomes an allergen (no further details).

7.5 Subchronic and chronic toxicity

Groups of 10 rats of both sexes (age 48–55 days, weight: males 138–180 g, females 110–134 g) and 10 mice of both sexes (age 55–62 days, weight: males 23–30 g, females 18–22 g) received MBT in corn oil (volume administered 5–10 ml/animal) for 13 weeks by stomach tube at the following doses: rats 180, 375, 750, 1500 and 3000 mg/kg body weight; mice 94, 188, 375, 750 and 1500 mg/kg. The rats given 750 mg/kg or more showed reduced body weight gain, and mortality was increased in the highest dose group (3000 mg/kg). Macroscopic and microscopic examination revealed increased liver weights and necrosis of the distal kidney tubules in the highest dose group. In addition, sloughing of the epithelial cells in the seminal vesicles was seen in the males. In the mice, increased mortality was seen in both sexes at the highest dose level (1500 mg/kg). Reduced body weight gain was seen at all dose levels for the last 6 weeks in the females, and from 750 mg/kg body weight in the males. At doses of 750 mg/kg and above, the mice exhibited lethargy, resistance to administration of the chemical and sudden fits (not further defined). Increased liver weight was seen in both sexes at the highest dose level. A no-effect-level of 375 mg/kg body weight was determined for both species (Elsbery, 1981).

Rabbits (age, origin, weight and sex not specified) were treated orally with 20 mg MBT/kg body weight every other day for 2 months and then daily for 1.5 months. Histological examination revealed slight changes in the liver, kidneys and lungs (no further details). There were no effects on general well-being, behaviour, liver function or the blood (Vorob'eva and Mezentseva, 1962).

No effects were seen in dogs (no further details) that received 120 ppm MBT in their feed (ca. 3 mg/kg body weight) daily for 1 year (Lehmann, 1965).

7.6 Genotoxicity

7.6.1 In vitro

MBT was tested in the Salmonella/microsome test in strains TA 1535, TA 1537, TA 1538, TA 98 and TA 100 with and without metabolic activation (S9-mix from the livers of Aroclor 1254 pre-treated Sprague-Dawley rats). As concentrations of 333 μg/plate and above were bacteriotoxic, test concentrations of 3, 10, 30, 100 and 300 μg/plate were used for the mutagenicity study. MBT gave negative results in all strains at these concentrations, with and without metabolic activation. In addition, strains TA 1538 and TA 98 were tested at 450 and 600 μg/plate, with and without metabolic activation, and again the test substance was inactive (Godek, 1984 a).

Similar results were reported in an earlier, comparable study (Bionetics, 1976).

MBT was not mutagenic in *Escherichia coli* (no further details; Szybalski, 1958).

MBT was tested in a forward mutation test in mammalian cells (CHO cells) with and without metabolic activation (S9-mix, no further details). Doses of 0.03 to 1000 μg/ml were used. In the absence of metabolic activation, doses above 100 μg/ml were toxic to the indicator cells, and the survival rate at 33.33 μg/ml was 58%. With metabolic activation, a dose level of 1000 μg/ml was cytotoxic and at 333.33 μg/ml there was a survival rate of 18%. The doses actually selected for the forward mutation test were 10, 25, 75, 150 and 300 μg MBT/ml with metabolic activation and 1, 5, 10, 30 and 50 μg MBT/ml without metabolic activation. Negative results were obtained at all MBT concentrations tested, both with and without metabolic activation (Godek, 1984 b).

In mouse lymphoma cells, both negative (Monsanto, 1982) and weakly positive results (Cifone, 1985) have been reported (no further details).

The ability of MBT to induce chromosomal aberrations was tested in Chinese hamster ovary (CHO) cells. The chemical was tested without the addition of a metabolic activation system at concentrations of 10 to 30.1 μg/ml, and in the presence of a metabolic activation system at concentrations of 351.8 to 500.5 μg/ml. Without metabolic activation there was no indication of chromosomal aberrations, but in the presence of a metabolic activation system there was an increase in chromosomal aberrations at concentrations of 373.5 μg/ml and above (Dieter, 1988; Anderson et al., 1990).

The induction of sister chromatid exchanges (SCE) was studied in CHO cells at the same dose levels. The cells were incubated with the substance, and maintained in culture long enough for at least two metaphase divisions to occur. The cells were then removed, fixed, air-dried and stained. The study was carried out with and without metabolic activation. Bromodeoxyuridine was added as a marker. Without metabolic activation (S9-mix) there was no induction of sister chromatid exchange. The dose-dependent increase of the relative number of SCE/cell with metabolic activation in a first experiment was not observed in a second independent test. In spite of this the authors evaluated the effect as positive (Dieter, 1988; Anderson et al., 1990). The high dose levels of both experiments (501.5 μg/ml and 502.3 μg/ml, respectively), however, exhibited a high cytotoxicity, also visible from the delayed cell-cycle. Therefore the high-dose-level cannot be evaluated as positive for SCE and the described dose-dependency is not given anymore. Since no increase of SCE has been observed in the second experiment, the test has to be evaluated as negative.

The possible induction of mitotic gene conversion by MBT was studied in *Saccharomyces cerevisiae* (strain D4). A plate incorporation test with and without metabolic activation (S9-mix from liver homogenates from Aroclor 1254 pre-treated rats) gave no indications of an increase in the number of revertants (Monsanto, 1985).

7.6.2 In vivo

In a mutagenicity study with *Drosophila melanogaster* the flies were treated at concentrations of 20 to 40 mg/ml in the food for 8 to 10 days. The mutation frequency was 2.5±0.49%, but there are no data on controls (no further details; Revazova, 1968).

In a DNA-binding study, male and female Fischer-344 rats (Charles River, weight 153–211 g, age 9–13 weeks) were given a single dose of 375 mg ^{14}C-labelled MBT/kg body weight (radioactivity ca. 15 mCi) by stomach tube and were killed 8 hours later. The DNA was extracted from the liver, adrenal glands, pituitary gland, pancreas and bone marrow by standard methods, and the DNA-bound radioactivity was determined. Binding to the DNA in the liver was determined by 3 different methods. The binding results were presented as pmol bound MBT/mg DNA and as the so-called "covalent binding index" (CBI). There was only slight binding of radioactivity to the DNA of the liver, pancreas, bone marrow, adrenal glands and pituitary gland. For the liver, a DNA-binding index of ca. 1–3 was determined. The values for the other tissues were all <1. For comparison, the CBI values for potent hepatocarcinogens such as dimethylnitrosamine and aflatoxin were 6000 to >20,000 (Monsanto, 1989).

In a micronucleus test in CD1 mice, a dose of 300 mg MBT/kg was given by intraperitoneal injection on 2 consecutive days, and 1000 polychromatic erythrocytes/mouse were screened for micronuclei. MBT was negative in this study (Sorg, 1984).

Groups of 28 male Sprague-Dawley rats (strain CRr1: COBS CD BR VAF, weight 237 to 238 g) received MBT in their feed at concentrations of 2500, 8750 and 15,000 ppm for 13 weeks before mating and then throughout the 2-week mating period. Each male was paired with 2 nulliparous females for 2 weeks. The females were killed on day 13 of pregnancy, and the number of dead embryos and live foetuses was recorded. A group of 28 males that received only the basal diet during this period served as negative controls. A positive control group of comparable size received the basal diet and, 7 days before the mating period, a single dose (by stomach tube) of 100 mg cytoxan/kg body weight. No dominant lethal effect was found in the MBT-treated groups compared with the controls.

Administration of the medium and high concentrations led to reductions in body weight and food consumption in the males (Springborn Life Sciences, 1989 c).

7.7 Carcinogenicity

Rats that received up to 120 ppm MBT in their feed for 2 years (equivalent to about 6 mg/kg body weight daily) showed no signs of carcinogenesis (no further details; Lehmann, 1965).

Table 2. Tumour incidence after administration of MBT by stomach tube

Species/Tumour		Control	188 mg/kg	375 mg/kg	750 mg/kg
Rat					
Leukaemia of mononuclear cells	♂	7/50		16/50	3/50
	♀	6/50	14/50	9/50	
Pituitary adenomas/carcinomas	♂	14/50		21/50	12/48
	♀	16/49	24/50	25/50	
Phaeochromocytomas of the adrenal	♂	18/50		27/50	24/49
glands	♀	1/50	5/50	6/50	
Acinar cell adenomas of the pancreas	♂	2/50		13/50	6/49
Preputial gland adenomas	♂	1/50		6/50	5/50
Mouse					
Hepatocellular adenomas	♀	3/50		7/49	4/50
Hepatocellular carcinomas	♀	1/50		5/49	0/50

(Significance not reported)

Two groups of 36 mice of different strains (C57BL/6 × C3H/ANF and C57BL/6 × AKR) received 100 mg MBT/kg body weight by stomach tube from day 7 to day 28 of life and then 323 ppm in their feed (ca. 50 mg/kg body weight daily) for 17 months. There was no significant increase in the incidence of tumours in this study (Innes et al., 1979).

In a parallel study, mice were given a single subcutaneous injection of 215 mg MBT/kg body weight on day 28 of life and were then observed for 17 months. This treatment did not produce any significant increase in the tumour incidence (no further details; NCI, 1968).

In a study conducted under the National Toxicology Program, groups of 50 male and 50 female F-344/N rats and the same number of B6C3F1 mice were given MBT in corn oil by stomach tube 5 days/week for 103 weeks. The male and female mice and the male rats received 0, 375 or 750 mg/kg, the female rats 0, 188 and 375 mg/kg. The survival rate was reduced in the male rats at both dose levels and in the female mice at the high-dose level. In the male rats, non-neoplastic effects were observed in the kidneys (nephropathy) and the fore-stomach (ulceration, irritation, epithelial hyperplasia and hyperkeratosis). With regard to neoplastic changes, there was an increase in the tumour incidence in male rats: acinar cell adenomas of the pancreas and mononuclear leukaemias were found at the low-dose level, and preputial gland adenomas/carcinomas and phaeochromocytomas of the adrenal glands were seen at both dose levels. The phaeochromocytomas of the adrenals were also seen dose-dependently in the female rats, as were pituitary adenomas. A low incidence of hepatocellular adenomas and carcinomas was observed in female mice. No tumours were observed in the male mice. The tumour incidence is presented in table 2 (Dieter, 1988).

In a cell transformation test, MBT did not produce any increase in transformed cell foci in BALB-3T3 cells at the 5 graduated concentrations used (survival rates of ca. 100 to 0%). The negative and positive controls (culture medium and 3-methylcholanthrene, respectively) showed the expected results (Litton Bionetics, 1982).

7.8 Reproductive toxicity

The teratogenic activity of MBT (at the maximum tolerated dose) was studied in Sprague-Dawley rats. The rats were given a daily intraperitoneal injection of 200 mg MBT/kg body weight (in oil) from day 1 to day 15 of pregnancy. The animals were killed on day

21 of pregnancy and the foetuses examined. There were no signs of maternal toxicity, foetotoxicity or teratogenicity in this study (Hardin et al., 1981).

In another embryotoxicity study, 26 pregnant Sprague-Dawley rats (strain CrL: COBS CD BR VAF) received MBT (in corn oil) by stomach tube at doses of 300, 1200 and 1800 mg/kg, from day 6 to day 15 of pregnancy. On day 20 of pregnancy, the foetuses were removed by Caesarean section, weighed and assessed for external, visceral and skeletal abnormalities. Maternal toxicity was seen at the medium- and high-dose levels, characterized by salivation, blood-caked mouths, coloured urine and reduced activity. In addition, body weight and feed consumption were reduced. MBT did not cause embryotoxic or teratogenic effects at this dose range (Springborn Life Sciences, 1989 a).

MBT in 1% methyl cellulose (administered volume 2 ml/kg) was given to groups of 20 pregnant rabbits (white New Zealand, nulliparous) by stomach tube from day 6 to day 18 of pregnancy at doses of 50, 150 or 300 mg/kg body weight. A corresponding control group received the vehicle alone over the same period. On day 29 of pregnancy, the foetuses were removed by Caesarean section and examined for external, visceral and skeletal anomalies. There were indications of maternal toxicity, with a slight reduction in body weight at the high-dose level. In addition there was a slight increase in the absolute and relative liver weights. MBT was not embryotoxic or teratogenic at these doses (Springborn Life Sciences, 1989 b).

There were no indications of effects on reproduction or lactation in a 3-generation study in rats that received up to 120 ppm MBT in their feed (ca. 6 mg/kg body weight daily; no further details; Lehmann, 1965).

Mice (no further details) were given daily subcutaneous injections of 464 mg MBT/kg body weight from day 6 to day 14 or 15 of pregnancy. Maternal toxicity, foetal toxicity and an increase in foetal abnormalities were observed (no further details; BRL, 1968).

MBT was tested for embryotoxicity in the course of a dominant lethal assay. One group of female white albino rats (11 animals) received 200 mg MBT/kg body weight orally before pregnancy on days 1 and 3 of oestrus, the second group (15 rats) on days 4 and 11 of pregnancy. Male rats which were mated with the 1st group received the same dose twice before mating, at intervals of 3 days. The second group was mated with untreated males. MBT treatment increased the length of the oestrous cycle of the dams. A significant reduction in foetal weight and fertility (number of live foetuses per dam) occurred, independent of whether the females were treated before or during pregnancy; total embryo mortality increased significantly (Aleksandrov, 1982).

In a dominant lethal assay in rats (described in detail in Sect. 7.6), the administration of MBT at dose levels that covered the maternally toxic range had no effect on the number of live foetuses or dead embryos (Springborn Life Sciences, 1989 c).

The embryotoxicity and teratogenicity of MBT were tested in chicken embryos. The test substance (in acetone) was injected into the heart at doses ranging from 0.1 to 2.0 μmol/egg (9–40 eggs treated per dose level). The number of eggs containing dead embryos was counted 2 days after administration. These were then opened and the embryos examined for external malformations. Incubation was continued for 11 days after administration and the remaining eggs were opened, the survival rate determined, and external malformations evaluated. Malformations were observed at doses of 1 to 2 μmol/egg (smaller eye sockets, open coeloms, defects of the back, neck, wings and legs; Korhonen et al., 1982, 1983).

7.9 Effects on the immune system

No information available.

7.10 Neurotoxicity

Johnson et al. (1970) studied the possible inhibitory effect of MBT on dopamine-β-hydroxylase in vitro and in vivo. Copper ions are important in the oxidative metabolism of dopamine to noradrenaline. The binding of copper ions by chelators, such as MBT, is seen as a possible mechanism for the inhibition of dopamine-β-hydroxylase. The in vitro study was carried out with dopamine-β-hydroxylase isolated from bovine adrenal medulla. MBT inhibited dopamine-β-hydroxylase non-competitively by 72% at a dose of 10^{-5} mol and by 47% at a dose of 5×10^{-6} mol.

Male CF1 mice (18–22 g) were given intraperitoneal injections of MBT (300 mg/kg) and the brain catecholamine concentration was measured after 1, 2 and 4 hours. The noradrenaline content 1 to 2 hours after MBT administration was reduced by ca. 60% compared with controls. After 2 hours the dopamine level was 24% higher than control values. Both the noradrenaline and dopamine levels were within the range of control values after 4 hours. The authors reported that shortly after administration of MBT the mice suffered from extreme weakness, accompanied by ptosis, which lasted for more than 2 hours. The recovery of the mice from their weakness paralleled the return of the catecholamine levels to control values, and the mice appeared normal after 4 hours (Johnson et al., 1970).

Male Sprague-Dawley rats (180–190 g) were treated with metaraminol bitartrate (5 mg/kg i.p.), in order to deplete heart noradrenaline stores. After 18 hours, the rats were given an intraperitoneal injection of MBT (300 mg/kg) or solvent (control group) and after a further 30 minutes an injection of dopamine (35 mg/kg) or solvent. All rats were killed 3 hours after dopamine administration. Dopamine restored the noradrenaline concentration in the myocardium to 60% of the level before metaraminol treatment. The administration of MBT completely blocked the conversion of dopamine to noradrenaline (Johnson et al., 1970).

The effect of MBT (300 mg/kg i.p.) on the motor activity of mice was measured at 30-minute intervals for 4 hours, starting 10 minutes after the administration of MBT or solvent. In the controls, the initial motor activity decreased rapidly within the first hour, and the mice remained relatively inactive until the end of the experiment. The MBT-treated mice lacked the initial explorative activity. However, after about 2 hours spontaneous activity increased, this increase coinciding with the end of inhibition of dopamine-β-hydroxylase activity in the brain by MBT (see above; Johnson et al., 1970).

7.11 Other effects

The toxic effects of MBT on cell cultures in vitro were tested in a mouse fibroblast cell line (strain L 929) and in cells from 10-day-old chicken embryos. The substance was administered as a powder, a suspension in cottonseed oil or a saturated suspension in saline. The cells were stained with a dye, the liberation of which was a sign of cytotoxicity. In all tests MBT was toxic to the mouse cells of the L-line (3–12 mg/ml). It was toxic to chicken embryo cells only when it was added as an oily suspension at a dose of 6 or 12 mg/ml. In a further in vitro study, MBT (0.5 mg/ml) induced marked vacuolization of L 929 cells after 6–14 hours, with subsequent lysis (Guess and O'Leary, 1969).

According to Shinoda et al. (1974) intraperitoneal injection of about 334 mg MBT leads to a radio-protective effect in mice (no further details).

MBT was tested in the cell-culture-test (V79 cells of Chinese hamsters) as a suspension of 1×10^2 cells/ml related to the cytotoxicity. The suspension was incubated at 37 °C for 7 days on culture plates. The colonies then were fixed with formalin, stained with Giemsa and the number of visible colonies counted. 49 µg/ml were determined as IC_{50} (concentration which is cytotoxic for 50% of the cells; Nakamura et al., 1990).

8. Experience in humans

In 1971, skin tests were performed on 1088 workers potentially exposed to MBT (amongst other chemicals). A standard test series was employed which consisted of 16 sensitizing substances including MBT. MBT produced the lowest frequency of positive reactions in these subjects, with 11 reactions (1.0%; Ziegler and Süß, 1974, 1975).

When 145 allergy sufferers were tested with 2% MBT in vaseline, 89 reacted positively (Foussereau and Cavelier, 1977).

Of 106 patients with contact dermatitis due to rubber products, 47% gave a positive reaction in patch tests with MBT (Wilson, 1969).

Fisher (1975) recorded 7 reactions in patch tests carried out on 11 surgeons who had contact dermatitis caused by rubber gloves.

Earlier, Gaul (1957) described the cases of 11 patients (5 females, 6 males) who developed contact dermatitis on repeated contact with MBT.

In a review of further cases, the author stated that men were more frequently affected than women, probably due to a higher incidence of occupationally-related contact (Feinman, 1987).

Dermal application of a 50% suspension of MBT in oil led to redness and irritation which lasted for 2 to 3 days, with subsequent peeling of the skin (Vorob'eva and Mezentseva, 1962).

9. Threshold limit values

No information available.

References

Aleksandrov, S.E.
Effect of vulcanization accelerators on embryonic mortality in rat
Bull. Exp. Biol. Med., 93, 87–88 (1982)

Anderson, B.E., Zeiger, E., Shelby, M.D., Resnick, M.A., Gulati, D.K., Ivett, J.L., Loveday, K.S.
Chromosome aberration and sister chromatid exchange test results with 42 chemicals
Environ. Mol. Mutagen., 16, 55–137(1990)

Bionetics Inc.
Mutagenicity evaluation of Thiotax
Unpublished report to Monsanto Co. (1976)
Cited in: Technical Support Document
Syracuse Research Corporation (1985)

Bourrinet, P., Puchault, P., Sarrasin, G., Berkovie, A.
Etude compareé de quelques substances allergeniques chez l'homme et chez le cobaye
J. Pharm. Bel., 34, 21–26 (1979)

BRL (Bionetics Research Laboratories)
Evaluation of carcinogenic, teratogenic and mutagenic activities of selected pesticides and industrial chemicals
Vol. 2, Pub. No. 223–260 (1968) (cited in Fed. Reg. 1985)

Ciba-Geigy Corporation
Acute heated dust inhalation toxicity study with the intermediate 2-mercaptobenzothiazole dry in albino rats (1977)
Cited in: Technical Support Document, 2-Mercaptobenzothiazole
Syracuse Research Corporation (1985)

Cifone, M.A.
Mutagenicity evaluation of mercaptobenzothiazole in the mouse lymphoma forward mutation assay
Litton Bionetics Inc. for Chemical Manufacturers' Association, FYI-AC-0285-0308, Suppl. Sequence E (1985) (cited in Fed. Reg. 1985)

Clayton, G.D., Clayton, F.E. (eds.)
Patty's Industrial Hygiene and Toxicology
John Wiley and Sons, New York (1981)

Colucci, D.F., Buyske, D.A.
The biotransformation of a sulfonamide to a mercaptan and to mercapturic acid and glucuronide conjugates
Biochem. Pharmacol., 14, 457–466 (1965)

Dieter, M.P.
Toxicology and carcinogenesis studies of 2-mercaptobenzothiazole in F344/N rats and B6C3F1 mice
NTP Technical Report 332 (1988)

Doull, J., Plzak, V., Brois, S.J.
A survey of compounds for radiation protection
NTIS No. DA 277689 (1962)

Dow Chemical Co.
Results of range finding toxicological tests on 2-mercaptobenzothiazole (Captex) (1961)
Cited in: Technical Support Document, 2-Mercaptobenzothiazole
Syracuse Research Corporation (1985)

Du Pont de Nemours & Company, Inc.
Toxicity of Lorol-2-thioazolvinylsulfide (L-2TS) and 2-mercaptobenzothiazole (2-MT), report no. 10-48 (1948)
Cited in: Technical Support Document, 2-Mercaptobenzothiazole
Syracuse Research Corporation (1985)

Eastman Kodak Company
Toxicity and health hazard summary for 2-mercaptobenzothiazole (1985)
Cited in: Technical Support Document, 2-Mercaptobenzothiazole
Syracuse Research Corporation (1985)

El Dareer, S.M., Kalin, J.R., Tillery, K.F., Hill, D.L., Bassett, J.W.
Disposition of 2-mercaptobenzothiazole and 2-mercaptobenzothiazole disulfide in rats dosed intravenously, orally and topically and in guinea-pigs dosed topically
J. Toxicol. Environ. Health, 27, 65–84 (1989)

Elsbery, D.D.
Subchronic test report for mercaptobenzothiazole (78-60-106002)
Physiological Research Laboratories, 1500 Northdale Blod (1981)

Feinman, S.E.
Sensitivity of rubber chemicals
J. Toxicol. Cut. Ocular Toxicol., 6, 117–153 (1987)

Fisher, A.A.
"Hypoallergenic" surgical gloves and gloves for special situation
Cutis, 15, 797 (1975)

Fukuoka, M., Tanaka, A.
The metabolic origin of the sulfur atom in the sulfhydryl group of 2-thiobenzothiazole metabolites derived from benzotriazyl sulfenamide in the rat
Arch. Toxicol., 61, 158–160 (1987)

Foussereau, J., Cavelier, C.
La N-isopropyl-N'-phénylparaphénylénediamine a-t-elle sa place dans la batterie standard d'allergens
Dermatologica, 155, 164–167 (1977)

Gaul, E.
Results of patch testing with rubber antioxidants and accelerators
J. Invest. Derm., 29, 105–110 (1957)

Godek, E.G.
Ames-Salmonella/microsome plate test – Mercaptobenzothiazole
Pharmakon Research International, Waverly, Pennsylvania (1984 a)

Godek, E.G.
CHO/HGPRT mammalian cell forward gene mutation assay – Mercaptobenzothiazole
Pharmakon Research International, Waverly, Pennsylvania (1984 b)

Guess, W.L., O'Leary, R.K.
Toxicity of a rubber accelerator
Toxicol. Appl. Pharmacol., 14, 221–231 (1969)

Hardin, B.D., Bond, G.P., Sikov, M.R., Andrew, F.D., Beliles, R.P., Wiemeier, R.W.
Testing of selected workplace chemicals for teratogenic potential
Scand. J. Work Environ. Health, 7 (4), 66–75 (1981)

Hill, D.L.
Disposition of 2-Mercaptobenzothiazole-ring-UL-^{14}C and 2-Mercaptobenzothiazole disulfide-ring-UL-^{14}C in Fischer-344 male and female rats dosed orally
Southern Research Institute, Birmingham, Alabama, Report 5873-1 (1986)

Innes, J.R.M., Ulland, B.M., Valerio, M.G., Petrucelli, L., Fishbein, L., Hart, E.R., Palotta, A.H., Bates, R.R., Falk, H.L., Gart, J.J., Klein, M., Mitchell, J., Peters, J.
Bioassay of pesticides and industrial chemicals for tumorigenicity in mice: a preliminary note
J. Natl. Cancer Inst., 42, 1101–1114 (1969)

Johnson, G.A., Boukma, S.J., Platz, P.A.
2-Mercaptobenzothiazole, an inhibitor of dopamine-β-hydroxylase
J. Pharm. Pharmacol., 22, 710–712 (1970)

Korhonen, A., Hemminki, K., Vainio, H.
Embryotoxicity of benzothiazoles, benzenesulfohydrazide and dithiodimorpholine to the chicken embryo
Arch. Environ. Contam. Toxicol., 11, 753–759 (1982)

Korhonen, A., Hemminki, K., Vainio, H.
Toxicity of rubber chemicals towards three-day chicken embryo
Scand. J. Work Environ. Health, 9, 115–119 (1983)

Kowalski, Z., Bassendowska, E.
Introductory studies on the toxic action of certain accelerators of vulcanization
Medycyna Pracy, 16, 3–43 (1965)

Lehmann, A.J. (1965)
Cited in: BIBRA, Toxicity Profile (1987)
2-Mercaptobenzothiazole and its sodium salt

Litton Bionetics Inc.
Evaluation of 8048-69-3 (MBT) in the in vitro transformation of BALB/3T3 cells assay
Unpublished report of the Good Year Co. (1982)

Magnusson, B., Kligman, A.M.
The identification of contact allergens by animal assay
The guinea-pig maximization test
J. Inst. Dermatol., 52, 268–276 (1969)

Monsanto
Unpublished information on the production, uses, toxicity, environmental releases and aquatic toxicity of MBT and sodium MBT (1982)
Submitted by J.R. Condray, July 16th (cited in Fed. Reg. 1984)

Monsanto
Toxicologic investigation of Thiotax powder
Unpublished report (1975)
Cited in: Technical Support Document, 2-Mercaptobenzothiazole
Syracuse Research Corporation (1985)

Monsanto
Investigation of the in vivo DNA binding of mercaptobenzothiazole to selected tissues of the rat
Project No. ML-88-06 (1989)

Nagamatsu, K., Kido, Y., Urakulo, G., Aida, Y., Ikeda, Y., Suzuki, Y.
Absorption, distribution, excretion and metabolism of 2-mercaptobenzothiazole in guinea-pig
Eisei Kagaku, 25, 59–65 (1979)

Nakamura, A., Ikarashi, Y., Tsuchiya, T., Kaniwa, M.A., Sato, M., Toyoda, K., Takahashi, M., Ohsawa, N., Uchima, T.
Correlations among chemical constituents, cytotoxicities and tissue responses: in the case of natural rubber latex materials
Biomaterials, 11, 92–94 (1990)

Revazova, Y.A.
Mutagenic activity of some rubber mixture ingredients, preliminary study (1968)
Cited in: Chemical Abstr., 71, 470171 e (1969)

Shinoda, M., Ohta, S., Takagi, Y., Akaboshi, S.
Studies on chemical protectors against radiation
Yakugaku Zasski, 94, 1419–1424 (1974)

Sorg, R.M.
Micronucleus test – mercaptobenzothiazole
Pharmakon Research International, Waverly, Pennsylvania (1984)

Springborn Life Sciences, Inc. (SLS)
Teratology study in rats with MBT
Toxicology and Human Safety Division, Spencerville, OH
SLS study no. 3205.2 (1989 a)

Springborn Life Sciences, Inc. (SLS)
Teratology study in rabbits with MBT
Toxicology and Human Safety Division, Spencerville, OH
SLS study no. 3205.4 (1989 b)

Springborn Life Sciences, Inc. (SLS)
A dominant lethal study in rats with MBT
Mammalian Toxicology Division, Spencerville, OH
SLS study no. 3205.6 (1989 c)

Szybalski, W.
Special microbiological systems: 2. Observations on chemical mutagenesis in microorganisms
Ann. N.Y. Acad. Sci., 76, 475 (1958) (cited in Fed. Reg. 1985)

Uni Royal Inc.
Product safety data sheet (1975)
Cited in: Technical Support Document, 2-Mercaptobenzothiazole
Syracuse Research Corporation (1985)

Vanderbilt
Material Safety Data Sheets
2-Mercaptobenzothiazole and sodium 2-mercaptobenzothiazole
Norwald C.T. (1975 a, b) (cited in EPA, 1976)

Vorob'eva, R.S., Mezentseva, N.V. (1962)
Cited in: BIBRA, Toxicity Profile (1987)
2-Mercaptobenzothiazole and its sodium salt

Wang, X., Suskind, R.R.
Comparative studies of the sensitization potential of morpholine, 2-mercaptobenzothiazole and 2 of their derivatives in guinea pigs
Contact Dermatitis, 19, 11–15 (1988)

Wang, X., Tabor, M.W.
Studies of the reactivity of morpholine, 2-mercaptobenzothiazole and 2 of their derivatives with selected amino acids
Contact Dermatitis, 19, 16–21 (1988)

Wilson, H.T.H.
Rubber dermatitis, an investigation of 106 cases of contact dermatitis caused by rubber
Brit. J. Derm., 18, 175–179 (1969)

Windholz, M. (ed.)
The Merck Index, 10th ed., p. 838
Merck & Co., Rahway, USA (1983)

Younger Laboratories Inc.
Dermal toxicity of 2-mercaptobenzothiazole on rabbits
Project No. Y-73-288
Unpublished report to Monsanto Co. (1974)

Ziegler, V., Süß, E., Standan, H., Hasert, K.
Der Meerschweinchen-Maximationstest zum Nachweis der sensibilisierenden Wirkung wichtiger Industrieprodukte
Allerg. Immunol. (Leipz.), 18, 203–208 (1972)

Ziegler, V., Süß, E.
Die allergene Wirkung der Gummiakzelleratoren
Tetramethylthiuramdisulfid und Mercaptobenzothiazol
Allerg. Immunol. (Leipz.), 20/21, 281–285 (1974/75)

Sodium hypochlorite

1. Summary and assessment

Sodium hypochlorite (NaOCl) is generally tested as an aqueous solution. Under alkaline conditions (pH 9.5 or more) it is relatively stable in aqueous solution. In neutral aqueous solutions, sodium hypochlorite hydrolyses easily to form free hypochlorous acid (HOCl). Under weakly acidic conditions, chlorine is released. For this reason, results with hypochlorous acid are presented when no equivalent studies with sodium hypochlorite are available.

The plasma half-life for hypochlorous acid after oral administration to rats is 44 hours in weaned animals and 89 hours in unweaned animals. Chloride ions are the only metabolites which can be found in the plasma, with no chlorite or chlorate ions detected. Storage in the tissues is not observed after acute oral administration.

The available data indicate that sodium hypochlorite is of low acute oral toxicity (LD_{50} mouse oral 5800 and 6800 mg/kg body weight). Signs of toxicity include reduced general activity, hypothermia, diarrhoea, pilo-erection and mucous membrane irritation and burns.

Aqueous sodium hypochlorite solutions are severely irritating or corrosive to the skin and eyes. The threshold concentration for skin irritancy is 2% for a single 4-hour application. In rabbits' eyes, less than 0.5% is required for a corrosive effect.

Subchronic administration in the drinking water (30–190 mg NaOCl/kg body weight/day for 13 weeks) causes no treatment-related changes in the rat except for marked inhibition of body-weight gain at high doses.

There are a number of studies in the literature which relate to the possible mutagenic activity of sodium hypochlorite, but the test methods do not always comply with modern requirements. The mutagenic potential of sodium hypochlorite in *Salmonella typhimurium* cannot be determined because the data provided do not permit a quantitative or qualitative interpretation. Sodium hypochlorite is mutagenic in the spot test in *Escherichia coli.* In an in vivo assay to detect chromosomal damage, sodium hypochlorite led to an increase in the aberration rate in 2 out of 4 studies, and the sister chromatid exchange rate was increased in a further study. In vivo studies for the detection of chromosome damage (structural aberrations in bone marrow cells and the micronucleus test) give no indications of genotoxic activity.

The available studies on the carcinogenic potential of sodium hypochlorite in mice and rats after oral administration give no indications that sodium hypochlorite is carcinogenic. The results of several long term studies in mice after dermal application are inconclusive.

In mice and rats, sodium hypochlorite does not affect fertility or the incidence of malformations.

Sodium hypochlorite has a weak immunodepressant effect in rats after administration in the drinking water for 9 weeks (30 ppm, calculated as chlorine).

In vivo, sodium hypochlorite chlorinates endogenous organic compounds such as amino acids, peptides and nucleic acids.

In humans, aqueous sodium hypochlorite solutions can be very corrosive and haemolytic, and may lead to metabolic acidosis. A threshold concentration or threshold dose cannot be derived from the numerous cases of acute poisoning described in the literature. Sodium hypochlorite can be sensitizing in humans.

The strongly irritant and corrosive effects of sodium hypochlorite on the skin and eyes are prominent. The systemic toxicity is low. Variable findings have been reported in mutagenicity tests. In humans, severe irritation and burns to the skin and mucous membranes are possible, as well as skin sensitization.

2. Name of substance

2.1	Usual name	Sodium hypochlorite
2.2	IUPAC-name	Sodium hypochlorite
2.3	CAS-No.	7681-52-9 8007-59-8 56172-57-7

3. Synonyms, common and trade names

Hypochlorous acid, sodium salt
Antiformin

B-K Liquid
Carrel-Dakin solution
Caswell No. 776
Chloros
Chlorox
Clorox
Dakins solution
Dan Klorix
Deosan
Domestos
Dazzle
Eau de Labarraque
Hyclorite
Javex
Milton
Na 1701
Neo-cleaner
Surchlor

4. Structural and molecular formulae

4.1	Structural formula	$Na^{+}[OCl]^{-}$
4.2	Molecular formula	NaOCl

5. Physical and chemical properties

5.1	Molecular mass, g/mol	74.44
5.2	Melting point, °C	–20 to –30 (Bayer, 1990) Decomposes at about 180 °C to oxygen and chloride (Vogt et al., 1986)
5.3	Boiling point, °C	–
5.4	Vapour pressure, hPa	–
5.5	Density, g/cm^3	1.22–1.23 (at 25 °C) (Bayer, 1990)
5.6	Solubility in water	Miscible (Bayer, 1990)
5.7	Solubility in organic solvents	No information available

5.8 Solubility in fat	No information available
5.9 pH-value	No information available
5.10 Conversion factor	1 ppm $\hat{=}$ 3.09 mg/m^3 1 mg/m^3 $\hat{=}$ 0.32 ppm (at 25 °C and 1013 hPa)

The data given in Sects. 5.2 to 5.6 apply to an aqueous solution with an active chlorine content of 15%. Disproportionation into sodium chloride and sodium chlorate takes place above 40 °C.

6. Uses

Disinfectant, bleaching agent (in the paper and textile industries), oxidizing agent (Vogt et al., 1986).

7. Experimental results

Pure aqueous solutions of sodium hypochlorite are relatively stable in excess alkali (pH 9.5 and above). In neutral solution, hypochlorous acid (HOCl) forms through contact with carbon dioxide in the air. In weakly acidic solutions, chlorine gas is liberated:

$NaOCl + H_2O \rightleftharpoons HOCl + NaOH$

$2NaOCl + CO_2 + H_2O \rightarrow Na_2CO_3 + 2HOCl$

$NaOCl + 2HCl \rightarrow NaCl + H_2O + Cl_2$

Hypochlorous acid is a weak acid with a dissociation constant of 2.95×10^{-8} at 18 °C (Hollemann and Wiberg, 1971). Accordingly, sodium hypochlorite hydrolyses easily in aqueous solution with the formation of free hypochlorous acid. Results with hypochlorous acid will therefore be referred to when no studies with sodium hypochlorite are available.

7.1 Toxicokinetics and metabolism

4 male Sprague-Dawley rats which had been weaned for 18 hours were each given a single oral dose of 0.75 mg $HO^{36}Cl$/animal (corresponding to 3.3 mg/kg body weight). A further 4 unweaned rats were each given 0.6 mg $HO^{36}Cl$/animal (corresponding to 2.6 mg/kg body weight). Blood samples were taken 10, 15, 20, 30 and 60 minutes and 2, 4, 8, 16, 24, 48, 72 and 96 hours after administration of the chemical. The following toxicokinetic parameters were reported:

Parameter	Weaned rats	Unweaned rats
Dose administered (mg/kg)	3.3	2.6
Time of maximum plasma level (hours)	2	4
Maximum plasma level (µg ^{36}Cl/ml)	7.9	10.7
Absorption half life (hours)	2.2	2.2
Plasma half life (hours)	44.1 (43–46)[a]	88.5 (76–105)[a]

[a] Maximum range for 4 rats in each case

In order to study distribution and excretion, a further group of 4 weaned rats received 0.6 mg HO^{36}Cl/rat. After 96 hours, the following tissue levels were detected (µg ^{36}Cl/g):

Plasma	1.92
Blood	1.59
Bone marrow	1.55
Testes	1.26
Skin	1.20
Kidneys	1.13
Lungs	1.04
Duodenum	0.71
Stomach	0.70
Spleen	0.67
Thyroid gland	0.66
Thymus	0.55
Liver	0.51
Ileum	0.26
Adipose tissue	0.09

Within 24 hours, 7.05% of the administered dose had been excreted in the urine and 7.45% in the faeces. After 96 hours the corresponding figures were 36.43% and 14.80%. No radioactivity could be detected in the expired air. The only metabolite that could be detected in the plasma after 96 hours was the chloride ion ($^{36}Cl^-$).

Chloride ($^{36}ClO_2^-$) and chlorate ($^{36}ClO_3^-$) ions were not detected. In liver homogenates from rats killed 24 hours after administration, 75% of the radioactivity was found in the cytosolic fraction, 2.5% in the microsomal fraction, 1.5% in the nuclear fraction and <0.1% in the mitochondrial fraction. The binding of hypochlorous acid to protein in the blood plasma after 24 hours was 0.30% (Abdel-Rahman et al., 1983, 1985).

3 weaned and 3 unweaned rats received a single dose of 140 mg NaOCl/kg body weight by stomach tube. 6 further animals received water as a control. One hour after administration, dichloroacetic acid (Cl_2CH-COOH), trichloroacetic acid (Cl_3C-COOH) and chloroform ($CHCl_3$) were found in the blood and stomach contents of both the weaned and unweaned animals. In addition, dichloroacetonitrile (Cl_2CH-CN) was found in the stomach of the unweaned rats (Mink et al., 1983).

Sprague-Dawley rats were given 4 ml aqueous sodium hypochlorite solution at concentrations of 200 or 1000 mg/l, equivalent to doses of 2.5 or 12.3 mg NaOCl/kg body weight. After 3–4 minutes, N-chloramino derivatives could be detected in the stomach; more exact identification was not possible. The authors speculated that the amino acids and peptides present in the stomach could have reacted with sodium hypochlorite to form N-chloroamines (Scully et al., 1985).

In vitro, the formation of N-chloroaniline, N-chloroglycine and N-chlorophenylalanine was observed in the gastric juice of weaned rats, following addition of aqueous sodium hypochlorite solution (200–1000 mg Cl_2/l gastric juice, corresponding to 426–2130 mg NaOCl/l; Scully et al., 1986). See also the section on proteins/nucleic acids in Sect. 7.11.

Groups of 8 male Sprague-Dawley rats received hypochlorous acid (HOCl) at concentrations of 1, 10 or 100 mg/l in their drinking water every day for 1 year. This corresponded to doses of about 0.1, 1.0 and 10 mg hypochlorous acid/kg body weight/day, respectively. The chloroform content in the blood after 4, 6, 9 and 12 months was in the range of that of the control group (0.0 to 2.7 ng/ml, n=8; Abdel-Rahman et al., 1984).

7.2 Acute and subacute toxicity

The results of acute toxicity studies are presented in the appendix (Table 1). This shows that the oral LD_{50} in mice was 5800 or 6800 mg/kg body weight (expressed as sodium hypochlorite).

During studies on acute oral toxicity, mice showed reduced activity, hypothermia, diarrhoea, pilo-erection and irritation of the gastro-intestinal tract (Momma et al., 1986).

The acute oral toxicity of a liquid laundry bleach (sodium hypochlorite-based, with a chlorine content of 4.74%) was tested in groups of 5 male and 5 female Osborne-Mendel rats (200–300 g) with an observation period of 14 days. An LD_{50} of >5000 mg/kg was reported (no further details; Osterberg et al., 1977).

A significant increase in haemolysis ($p<0.05$) occurred in male Sprague-Dawley rats 15 minutes after the administration by stomach tube of 0.18, 0.38 and 0.75 mg hypochlorous acid (HOCl)/kg body weight. No further haemolysis was observed after 1 hour. 4 rats were used per dose and time point. The glutathione content of the blood was significantly reduced ($p<0.05$) at all dose levels 60 minutes after administration. The level was within the control range 120 minutes after administration (Abdel-Rahman et al., 1984).

Intradermal injection of a 5.25% aqueous sodium hypochlorite solution (volume not specified) in the clipped backs of rats caused haemorrhages immediately after administration. Concentrations of 1.05, 1.75, 2.63 and 5.25% produced ulceration at the injection site within 24 hours. This cleared up in an unspecified period. Lower concentrations were not tested. Compared with control rats given NaCl, there was roughly a 4-fold increase in vascular effusion of radiolabelled albumin within one hour of intradermal administration of 1.05, 1.75, 2.63 or 5.25% sodium hypochlorite (volume not specified). 3 rats were used at each concentration (Pashley et al., 1985).

Administration of sodium hypochlorite in the drinking water of Fischer-344 rats for 14 days at concentrations of 0.0625, 0.125, 0.25, 0.5, 1.0, 2.0 and 4.0% led to significant decreases ($p<0.05$) in body weight gain and drinking water consumption at concentrations of 0.125% and above. At the highest concentration the average daily drinking water consumption was 3.8% of the control level, and the body weight at the end of the administration period was about 40% of the control level. The body weight at the lowest concentration was within the control range. No macroscopic changes in the organs were revealed at autopsy (Furukawa et al., 1980).

Female Wistar rats were given sodium hypochlorite mixed with milk by stomach tube twice daily for 14 days, at doses corresponding to 8, 40 and 200 mg active chlorine/kg body weight/day (about 17, 85 and 426 mg NaOCl/kg body weight/day, respectively). Water was offered ad libitum. 10 rats were used per dose group and as controls. Body weight gain and relative organ weights (liver, kidney, heart and brain) were in the range of the control values (Cunningham, 1980).

In a further study, groups of 10 male Wistar rats and 10 male guinea-pigs were treated with sodium hypochlorite in the drinking water. The rats were treated for 6 weeks at doses of 4.1, 8.1 or 15.7 mg active chlorine/kg body weight/day (corresponding to about 8.7, 17.3 and 33.4 mg NaOCl/kg body weight/day). The guinea-pigs were treated for 5 weeks at 23.8 mg active chlorine/kg body weight/day (corresponding to about 50.7 mg NaOCl/kg body weight/day). In each case 10 animals served as controls. No significant changes in body weight gain or average drinking water consumption were observed (Cunningham, 1980).

7.3 Skin and mucous membrane effects

The effect of sodium hypochlorite on the skin was studied in rabbits according to OECD Guideline No. 404. Sodium hypochlorite was applied as an aqueous solution to the clipped dorsal skin of groups of 3 rabbits at concentrations of 2, 20, 35 or 50%. The pH-values of these solutions were 11.0, 10.7, 11.4 and 11.4, respectively. The skin was examined after 0.5, 24, 48 and 72 hours. At the lowest concentration (2%), a very slight, barely perceptible erythema was present in 2 rabbits 30 minutes and 24 hours after the end of exposure. After 48 hours, marked or intense erythema and slight oedema were present in 1 animal. After 72 hours, the effects had cleared up in 1 rabbit and diminished in the other, while the third rabbit (which had not yet shown any effects) had pronounced erythema. Concentrations of 20% or more caused moderate to severe erythema and very slight to moderate oedema, 30 minutes after the end of exposure. In addition, 0.3 to 5 cm^2 burns were observed. The effects were unchanged at the end of the 72-hour observation period (Loden et al., 1985).

The primary skin irritancy of a liquid laundry bleach (sodium hypochlorite-based with a chlorine content of 4.74%) was studied in 6 New Zealand rabbits (2–3 kg), in accordance with the specifications in the Federal Hazardous Substances Act. The rabbits were treated with 0.5 ml, applied semi-occlusively to the clipped dorsal skin for 24 hours. Erythema and oedema were evaluated after 24 and 48 hours. The product was not shown to be an irritant (Osterberg et al., 1977).

To assess the histological effects caused by aqueous sodium hypochlorite solution, a lint patch (5×5 cm) soaked in a 0.1% or 0.5% solution was applied occlusively to the shaved dorsal skin of female guinea-pigs for 1, 4, 7 or 14 days. The lint patch was soaked with sodium hypochlorite solution at 8-hour intervals. Histological sections of the skin at the application site taken after 1 and 4 days revealed no morphological changes compared with untreated skin. Epidermal hyperplasia with a cellular reaction in the dermal papillae was observed after 7 days of exposure at the high concentration and also after 14 days at the low concentration. After 14 days of exposure, 15% lower viability was observed in vitro for basal cells isolated from the application site of the guinea-pigs treated with the higher concentration (0.5%). The 0.1% sodium hypochlorite solution had no effect on viability (Cotter et al., 1985).

When Sencar mice with clipped backs were immersed up to their necks in a 1% aqueous sodium hypochlorite solution (pH 8.5) for 10 minutes, there was a significant ($p<0.05$) increase in the thickness of the dorsal epidermal layer after 24 hours. This reached a maximum thickness 10 days after exposure (18.2 μm, control ca. 10 μm). After repeated exposure (10 minutes/day) for 4 days, the dorsal epidermal layer was significantly thicker ($p<0.05$) on day 5 (25.2±6.2 μm, control 15.4±1.5 μm). The ratio of total cells to basal cells was 61:25 cells/μm, compared with 38:24 cells in the control dorsal skin (Robinson et al., 1986).

Groups of 10 albino guinea-pigs received a daily application (0.1 ml) of a 0.125% sodium hypochlorite solution (equivalent to 1.25 mg/ml)or 4 daily applications (0.1 ml each) of a sodium hypochlorite-milk solution (1 part of the above solution to 2 parts ordinary milk), the applications being made to the dorsal side of the ear for 1, 2, 4 or 8 weeks. The other ear served as a control and was treated with water or a mixture of milk and water. The thickness of the epidermal layer, cell size, acanthosis factor and the degree of proliferation, differentiation and cornification of the epidermis were similar for treated and untreated ears (Wohlrab and Wozniak, 1982).

The guinea-pig ear-swelling test was used to study the potential to induce non-immunological urticaria. A positive reaction was observed in 2 out of 10 guinea-pigs within 30 minutes of the application of a 6% aqueous solution (50 μl) of sodium hypochlorite (pH 11.2; Hostynek et al., 1989).

Aqueous sodium hypochlorite solution was irritant to corrosive in rabbit's eyes. The threshold concentration for a corrosive effect may be below 0.5%. The following studies from the literature are arranged in order of increasing concentration. An immediate, slight reddening of the conjunctiva occurred in rabbits (numbers not specified) after a 3-minute (right eye) or 5-minute (left eye) rinse with 0.5% aqueous sodium hypochlorite (pH 9.0) followed by irrigation with physiological saline for 2 minutes. After 6 hours, slight conjunctical oedema was seen, and after 24 hours marked oedema, clouding of the cornea and discharge were observed. The findings were more severe after the 5-minute exposure. While the effects of a 3-minute exposure cleared up completely within the 14-day observation period, slight hyperaemia at the edge of the cornea could be seen 14 days after the 5-minute exposure. Histopathological examination of the mucous membrane immediately after exposure revealed necrosis of the epithelial cells of the conjunctiva and cornea. After 6 hours, sub-conjunctival oedema and an invasion of polynuclear cells into the stromal area of the conjunctiva were also seen. After the 5-minute exposure, infiltration of the stromal region of the conjunctiva was still evident at 24 hours. After 72 hours, cellular regeneration of the epithelium had begun and the sub-conjunctival oedema and leukocyte infiltration were reduced. 14 days after the 3-minute exposure, pathological changes to the tissues could no longer be seen. Very slight conjunctival epithelial erosion, conjunctival stromal oedema and slight sub-conjunctival fibrosis could still be observed 14 days after the 5-minute exposure (van Delft et al., 1983).

A 5% aqueous sodium hypochlorite solution (pH 11.1 to 11.6; volume unspecified) instilled in rabbits' eyes caused marked clouding of the cornea, marked conjunctival oedema and slight haemorrhaging of the conjunctiva. The effects cleared up within a week. If the eye was rinsed within 30 seconds of the instillation, only slight epithelial clouding of the cornea and slight conjunctival oedema occurred, and the eye returned to normal within a day (Grant, 1986).

Instillation of 0.01, 0.03 or 0.1 ml of a 5% aqueous solution of sodium hypochlorite into rabbits' eyes (6 animals/group) caused marked irritation (Draize grade 11, 39 and 40, respectively). The reddening caused by the lowest volume had cleared after 14 days, but the effects in the two remaining groups were only marginally improved at the end of the 21-day observation period (Griffith et al., 1980).

Pairs of albino rabbits were treated with about 0.05 ml of 0.005, 0.052, 0.525 or 5.25% aqueous sodium hypochlorite solution, which was instilled into the conjunctival sac of the left eye. The right eye served as a control and was treated with a sodium chloride solution of the same osmolarity. Within 30 minutes of instillation of the two highest concentrations (0.525 or 5.25%), there was marked palpebral and conjunctival oedema, and bulbar, palpebral and conjunctival hyperaemia. These effects became more pronounced at 2 and 6 hours after exposure. In addition, discharges from the eye were evident. After 24 hours, the effects caused by the 0.525% solution had cleared up, while 7 days after instillation of the higher concentration, conjunctival oedema was still present and the cornea showed slight erosion but no ulceration (time of findings not specified). The corneal thickness remained unchanged. Solutions of 0.005% and 0.052% sodium hypochlorite had no effect (Pashley et al., 1985).

After instillation of 0.1 ml 5.5% aqueous sodium hypochlorite into the conjunctival sac, the observed effects disappeared within 7–35 days in rabbits, and within 2 days in monkeys (no further details; Carter and Griffith, 1965).

One drop of a 15% aqueous solution of sodium hypochlorite (pH 11.2) caused haemorrhages of the conjunctiva and clouding of the corneal epithelium in the eyes of rabbits. Later (time not specified) moderate oedema and discharge occurred. After 2–3 weeks, slight damage to the cornea, scarring of the nictitating membrane and vascularization of the conjunctiva were still present (Grant, 1986).

Instillation of 0.1 ml 50% aqueous sodium hypochlorite (pH 9.0 to 10.3) into rabbits' eyes (n=3) caused marked irritation of the cornea and the conjunctiva (Draize grade 20 and 10) 1 hour later. 7 days after instillation, the respective Draize scores for cornea, iris and conjunctiva were 53.3, 1.7 and 9.3, and 21 days after instillation they were 45.0, 1.7 and 1.3. If the eyes were rinsed 4 seconds after application, the marked irritation of the cornea and conjunctiva disappeared within 14 days; if they were rinsed 30 seconds after application, no normalisation of the effects occurred within the 21-day observation period. The Draize scores at the end of the 21-day observation period were 25.0 for the cornea, 2.0 for the conjunctiva and 0 for the iris (Momma et al., 1986).

The eye irritancy of a liquid laundry bleach (sodium hypochlorite-based, with a chlorine content of 4.74%) was studied in accordance with the specifications in the Federal Hazardous Substances Act. 6 New Zealand rabbits (2–3 kg) had 0.1 ml instilled into the conjunctival sac of one eye; evaluation took place 24 hours later and after 2 and 3 days, and again after 7 days where necessary.

Severe eye irritation occurred (no further details; Osterberg et al., 1977).

Anaesthetized cats (n=30 or 37) were treated with 10 ml bleach (including Chlorox, Linco Purex; containing ca. 5% NaOCl; pH ≤11) instilled into the oesophagus which had been closed off by a cotton wool plug towards the stomach. After 3 minutes the fluid was aspirated by means of a catheter (7–8 ml) and the cotton wool plug was removed after a further 7 minutes. The animals were divided into groups of 5 or 6, and killed 10 minutes to one month after treatment. In all cases, the mucous membrane and the deeper-lying tissue layers of the oesophagus were damaged. As the gastric mucosa was also affected to some extent, the authors assumed that small quantities of the bleach must have passed the cotton wool barrier. Sodium hypochlorite caused oedema, haemorrhages, ulceration of the mucosa, muscularis and submucosa, necroses with granulation tissue (7–14 days after treatment), fibrosis and oesophageal strictures (Weeks and Ravitch, 1969, 1971).

3 months after the instillation of 3 or 10 ml Clorox containing 5.25% NaOCl into the oesophagus of 1 and 2 rabbits, respectively, no macroscopic pathological changes could be detected in the oesophagus (Landau and Saunders, 1964).

To study the irritant effect on the upper gastro-intestinal tract, groups of 6 New Zealand rabbits (2–3 kg) were treated with 0.3, 1.0 or 3.0 ml/kg of a liquid laundry bleaching agent with a chlorine content of 4.74%. The liquid was applied to the base of the tongue with a syringe and was swallowed spontaneously by the animals. Control rabbits received distilled water. After 24 hours the rabbits were killed and macroscopically examined. A dose of 0.3 ml/kg was non-irritant (score <1.0), while 1.0 and 3.0 ml/kg were irritating (score 1.0 to 3.0). Irritation of the stomach was prominent (no further details; Osterberg et al., 1977).

Clorox (25–100 ml) containing 5.25% NaOCl was instilled into the upper oesophagus of 12 dogs by catheter. 10 of the 12 dogs vomited as soon as ca. 5 ml Clorox reached the stomach. The oesophageal mucosa was diffusely haemorrhagic and the stomach was hyperaemic. Bleeding of the stomach did not occur. Macroscopic examination after 3 months revealed no substance-related effects in the mouth, pharynx, larynx, oesophagus or stomach. In a further 15 dogs, the oesophagus was clamped off towards the stomach and completely filled with Clorox for 2, 5 or 10 minutes. Eight dogs died immediately from oesophageal perforation into the pleural cavity. No substance-related effects were seen in the remaining 7 animals at autopsy 3 months later (Landau and Saunders, 1964).

Rinsing of the gut for 3 hours with 0.1 or 0.5 mM solutions of hypochlorous acid (equivalent to 5.25 and 26.25 mg/l, respectively), led to a significantly increased ($p<0.05$) mucous membrane permeability in 1-day-old piglets. The parameter measured was the blood-intestinal clearance capacity for ^{51}Cr-EDTA. The treatment did not affect permeability in 1-month-old piglets (Clark et al., 1989).

7.4 Sensitization

No information available.

7.5 Subchronic and chronic toxicity

Fischer-344 rats received sodium hypochlorite in their drinking water at concentrations of 0.025, 0.05, 0.1, 0.2 or 0.4% for 13 weeks. This corresponded to doses of about 30, 60, 100, 165 and 190 mg/kg body weight/day, respectively. Ten animals of each sex were used per dose group and as controls. Body weight gain was significantly reduced ($p<0.05$) in the males in the upper two dose groups, but only in the high-dose group in the females. Water consumption was reduced at 0.05% and above in both sexes. At the highest dose, the average daily drinking water consumption was about 35% of the control value, and at the end of the study body weight was 53% of the control value in males and 69% in females. The absolute organ weights of the lungs, liver, thymus and spleen in males and the salivary glands, lungs, thymus, heart and brain of females in the high-dose group were significantly reduced ($p<0.05$). No data were given on relative organ weights. The pituitary gland, adrenals, kidneys, testes and ovaries were unaffected. Biochemical assays revealed significantly increased blood urea levels ($p<0.05$) in males in the higher dose groups and, in the females, significantly increased aspartate aminotransferase activity ($p<0.05$) and significantly reduced triglyceride levels ($p<0.05$). Alanine aminotransferase, alkaline phosphatase, lactate dehydrogenase and cholinesterase activities were unaffected, as were the levels of total bilirubin, total cholesterol, total protein and creatinine, the albumin-globulin quotient, and the sodium, potassium and chloride concentrations. No macroscopic effects were observed, although a few animals, particularly in the high dose group, were very cachectic. Histological examination of the brain, thyroid gland, salivary glands, lungs, heart, liver, spleen, adrenals, kidneys, testes and ovaries revealed no substance-related effects. The maximum tolerated dose was between 100 and 165 mg/kg body weight in male rats, and 165 and 190 mg/kg body weight in female rats (Furukawa et al., 1980; Hasegawa et al., 1986).

Hypochlorous acid (HOCl) was administered daily in the drinking water to groups of 4 male Sprague-Dawley rats at concentrations of 1, 10 and 100 mg/l water for 12 months. These levels were equivalent to about 0.1, 1.0 and 10 mg/kg body weight/day, respectively, at an assumed drinking water intake of 100 ml/kg body weight/day. Four rats served as controls in each case. Haematological and biochemical studies after 2, 3, 4, 6, 8, 10 and 12 months included leukocyte and erythrocyte counts, haemoglobin content, mean corpuscular volume (MCV), mean corpuscular haemoglobin content (MCH), mean corpuscular haemoglobin concentration (MCHC), haematocrit, osmotic resistance of the erythrocytes and glutathione content of the blood. After 3 months of exposure to hypochlorite, the erythrocyte count and the haematocrit level were significantly reduced ($p<0.05$) in the high dose group. The glutathione content of the blood had significantly decreased ($p<0.05$) after 10 and 12 months in the middle- and high-dose groups. The parameters were within the range of the control group values at the remaining time points (Abdel-Rahman et al., 1984).

7.6 Genotoxicity

7.6.1 In vitro

The mutagenic properties of sodium hypochlorite were studied in the *Salmonella typhimurium* strains TA 92, TA 94, TA 98, TA 100, TA 1530, TA 1535, TA 1537 and TA 1538. The study (standard plate test) was conducted with and without metabolic activation (S9-mix from Aroclor 1254-induced rat liver). Without metabolic activation, no induction of point mutations by sodium hypochlorite could be detected in strains TA 92, TA 94, TA 98, TA 100, TA 1535, TA 1537 or TA 1538 (Ishidate et al., 1984; Kawachi et al., 1980 a, 1980 b; Rosenkranz et al., 1976; Wlodkowski and Rosenkranz, 1975), although other investigators observed a concentration-dependent increase in reverse mutations in strains TA 1530 (maximum 3.7-fold increase) and TA 1535 (maximum 2.7-fold increase; Wlodkowski and Rosenkranz, 1975). With metabolic activation, sodium hypochlorite caused a 3.4-fold increase in the number of reverse mutations at 5 mg/plate in strain TA 100, but not in strains TA 92, TA 94, TA 98, TA 1535 or TA 1537 (Ishidate et al., 1984; Kawachi et al., 1980 a,

1980 b). No detailed information was given in the publications on whether the concentrations tested covered the cytotoxic range.

In 3 further publications, sodium hypochlorite was classified as mutagenic in *Salmonella typhimurium*. However, no information was given on the conditions under which a mutagenic effect occurred (Ishidate and Yoshikawa, 1980; Ishidate et al., 1981, 1988).

In a spot test in *Escherichia coli* pol A^+/pol A^- (differential inhibition), sodium hypochlorite was mutagenic at concentrations of 0.26 and 0.74 µg/plate (Rosenkranz, 1973; Rosenkranz et al., 1976).

There were no indications of genotoxic activity in the rec-test in *Bacillus subtilis* with or without metabolic activation (no further details; Kawachi et al., 1980 a, 1980 b).

In studies to assess chromosome damage in Chinese hamster lung (CHL) fibroblasts in vitro, sodium hypochlorite caused a significant increase in aberrations at 0.5 mg/ml without metabolic activation. This dose caused 50% cytotoxicity. With metabolic activation (Kanechlor 400) the findings were not clear (no further details; Ishidate et al., 1981, 1984, 1988; Matsuoka et al., 1979).

An increased aberration rate in CHL cells due to sodium hypochlorite was also observed in another study. The study was carried out without metabolic activation (no further details; Kawachi et al., 1980 a, 1980 b).

No treatment-related increase in the aberration rate was seen in human fibroblasts (HE 2144) tested up to a concentration of 148.8 µg/ml. In contrast, there was a concentration-dependent increase in the sister chromatid exchange rate. At 148.8 µg/ml the value was doubled. It was not specified whether the highest concentration in the study covered the cytotoxic range. No metabolic activation system was used (Kawachi et al., 1980 a, 1980 b; Sasaki et al., 1980).

No genotoxic effect was observed in human lymphocytes (no further details; Shaw, 1970).

7.6.2 In vivo

In a micronucleus test, groups of 5 male and 5 female CD1 mice received aqueous solutions of sodium hypochlorite by stomach tube 5 times at 24 hour intervals. The doses used were 1.6, 4.0 and 8.0 mg chlorine/kg body weight/day (equivalent to 3.4, 8.4 and 16.8 mg sodium hypochlorite/kg body weight/day, respectively). Whether the doses covered the maximum tolerated range was not specified. Two different aqueous sodium hypochlorite solutions were used in this study (pH 8.5, mainly present as OCl^-; pH 6.5, mainly present as HOCl). Bone marrow preparations from the femur were obtained from 5 mice per sex, dose group and sodium hypochlorite solution, 6 hours after the last treatment. In addition, positive and vehicle controls were used. For each mouse, 1000 polychromatic erythrocytes were examined for the presence of micronuclei. A significantly increased ($p<0.05$) occurrence of micronuclei in polychromatic erythrocytes was observed after administration of OCl^- solution. The view of the authors, however, was that this was an artifact caused by the low micronucleus levels in the control group (0.01±0.01%). The values for the treated groups (0.04–0.12%) were within the range of the historical control values of the Institute (Meier et al., 1985).

In a further micronucleus test, groups of 6 male mice were given single intraperitoneal injections of 312.5, 625, 1250 or 2500 mg sodium hypochlorite/kg body weight. 6 other mice were used as controls. Bone marrow preparations from the femur were obtained 24 hours after administration of the chemical. For each mouse, 1000 polychromatic erythrocytes were examined for the presence of micronuclei. All of the animals in the high-dose group died. At 1250 mg/kg body weight, the ratio of polychromatic to normochromatic erythrocytes was reduced by 48%. There were no indications of a treatment-related increase in the number of micronuclei (Hayashi et al., 1988).

In a cytogenetic test to screen for structural chromosomal aberrations in bone marrow in vivo, CD-1 mice were given an aqueous solution of sodium hypochlorite by stomach tube once or 5 times at 24 hour intervals. The doses used were 1.6, 4.0 and 8.0 mg chlorine/kg body weight/day (equivalent to 3.4, 8.4 and 16.8 mg sodium hypochlorite/kg body weight/day, respectively). Details of whether the doses covered the maximum tolerated dose range were not provided. Again, two different aqueous sodium hypochlorite solutions were used in the study (pH 8.5, mainly present as OCl^-; pH 6.5, mainly present as HOCl). Bone marrow preparations were obtained 6, 24 and 48 hours after acute administration. With repeated administration, they were obtained 6 hours after the last dose was given. 4 mice were used per sex, dose and sodium hypochlorite solution. Fifty metaphases per mouse were evaluated. There were no indications of a treatment-related increase in the aberration rate, either after single or repeated administration (Meier et al., 1985).

Two further studies also found that sodium hypochlorite was not mutagenic in the bone marrow of the rat (no further details; Kawachi et al., 1980 a, 1980 b).

7.7 Carcinogenicity

Groups of 50 male and 50 female B6C3F1 mice received sodium hypochlorite in their drinking water for 103 weeks at concentrations of 0.05 or 0.1%, equivalent to about 63 or 105 mg NaOCl/kg body weight/day in the males and 54 or 108 mg/kg body weight/day in the females. The control group consisted of 73 males and 72 females. The observation period was 3 weeks. The upper concentration was equivalent to the maximum tolerated dose, which was determined in a preliminary 13-week study. Behaviour was monitored every day, body weight and water consumption at regular intervals. At the end of the study, biochemical, haematological, macroscopic and histopathological investigations took place. Further details on the study design were not provided. Body weight gain in males and females in the high-dose group was 10% below control values from week 20 of the study, while that of the low-dose group was within the control range. After 106 weeks, the following mortality rates were recorded:

Concentration in drinking water % NaOCl	Number of surviving mice week 0	Number of surviving mice week 106	Mortality (%) week 106
Males			
0	73	48	34
0.05	50	39	22
0.1	50	37	26
Females			
0	72	56	22
0.05	50	40	20
0.1	50	39	22

There were no indications of a treatment-related increase in the tumour rate (no detailed information on the statistical methods or on the extent of histopathological examination; Kurokawa et al., 1986).

Sodium hypochlorite was administered in the drinking water of Fischer-344 rats for 104 weeks at concentrations of 0.05 or 0.1% (males) and 0.1 or 0.2% (females). These doses were equivalent to about 37 or 74 mg/kg body weight/day in males (average body weight 340 g; drinking water consumption 25 ml/day) and about 100 or 200 mg/kg body weight/day in females (average body weight 200 g; drinking water consumption 20 ml/day). Groups of 50 males and 50 females were used, with a further 50 rats per sex as controls. The observation period was 8 weeks. The two higher concentrations were equivalent to the maximum tolerated dose, which was established in a preliminary 13-week study (see Sect. 7.5). Behaviour was observed daily, and body weight was recorded weekly for the first 6 weeks and then monthly. Drinking water consumption was monitored regularly (no further details). At the end of the study, brain, pituitary gland, salivary glands, lungs, heart, liver, spleen, adrenal glands, kidneys, testes and ovaries were weighed. Histopathological examination was made of the adrenal glands, bone marrow, clitoris, ear canal (Zymbal glands), eyes, forestomach, heart, kidneys, liver, lungs, mammary glands, nasal passages, nervous tissues, ovaries, pancreas, parathyroid glands, peritoneum, pituitary gland, prostate gland, salivary glands, skin, small and large intestines, spleen, stomach, subcutaneous tissues, testes, thyroid gland, tongue, trachea, uterus and vagina. From week 16 of the study, the body weight of all of the treated groups was slightly below the control values (dose-dependently). At the end of 104 weeks, the body weights at the low and high concentrations were 96% and 93%, respectively, of control values for the males, and 89% and 80%, respectively, for the females. The body weight gain returned to normal during the observation period. Water consumption in the females was within the range of the control group, but in the males it was 10–20% above the control values during the last 20 weeks of the study. The following survival and mortality rates were reported (see Table on page 301).

Biochemical and haematological investigations at the end of the study revealed no treatment-related effects on erythrocytes, on alkaline phosphatase, gamma-glutamyl transpeptidase, aspartate aminotransferase, alanine aminotransferase, or lactate dehydrogenase activities, on levels of total bilirubin, creatinine, uric acid, triglyceride, urea, β-lipoprotein or total cholesterol, or on the albumin-globulin ratio. The relative weight of the salivary glands was significantly reduced ($p<0.01$) in females in the low-dose group, as

Concentration in drinking water % NaOCl	Number of surviving rats			Mortality (%)
	week 0	week 104	week 112	week 112
Males				
0	50	43	30	40
0.05	50	39	26	48
0.1	50	37	31	38
Females				
0	50	40	31	38
0.1	50	39	36	28
0.2	50	40	35	30

was the relative heart weight in males in the high-dose group. Under these experimental conditions there were no indications that sodium hypochlorite increased the tumour rate (χ^2-test; no information on confidence limits). The number and types of tumours were similar to the controls. The remaining histopathological findings were also of a similar nature to those of the control group, and occurred to a similar extent (Hasegawa et al., 1986; Kurokawa et al., 1986).

A 1% sodium hypochlorite solution (0.2 ml) was applied twice weekly to the clipped dorsal skin of 20 female Sencar mice (4 weeks old), for 51 weeks. Acetone was used as the vehicle and was also applied to a further 15 animals as a control. The doses were determined in a preliminary 4-week study (no further details). The animals were clipped once a week, and examined for tumours; body weight was recorded monthly. After 51 weeks of treatment, no skin tumours or skin hyperplasia could be observed histopathologically, in either the control or experimental groups (Kurokawa et al., 1984).

In a further dermal study, 40 female ddN mice were treated with 0.05 ml sodium hypochlorite solution (with an active chlorine content of >10%), which was dropped onto the shaved dorsal skin 60 times over 300 days (no further details). The observation period was 150 days. No skin tumours were found in the 27 surviving mice. There was no indication of how the doses were selected (Hayatsu et al., 1971).

Sodium hypochlorite was studied in a 2-stage carcinogenicity experiment with 9,10-dimethyl-1,2-benzanthracene (DMBA) as the initiator. 20 4-week-old female Sencar mice received a drop of 20 nmol DMBA (dissolved in 0.2 ml acetone) on the dorsal skin, which had been clipped 48 hours earlier. After an interval of 7 days, 0.2 ml 1% sodium hypochlorite solution was then applied twice weekly for 51 weeks. The total duration of the study was thus 52 weeks. A control group of 15 mice was treated with DMBA and the vehicle in the same manner. The doses used were determined in a preliminary 4-week study (no further details). The animals were clipped once a week and examined for tumours; body weight was recorded every week. Three out of 20 mice developed skin tumours (15%), one of which was a squamous epithelial carcinoma which had metastasized in the lungs. Hyperplasia was not observed. No skin tumours were found in the control group. Statistical evaluation (Fischer's Exact Test, χ^2-test, $p<0.01$) revealed no significance. In a further control group, all 20 animals treated with 0.2 ml of a 10 µg/ml 12-O-tetradecanoylphorbol-13-acetate (TPA) solution developed skin tumours and epidermal hyperplasia (Kurokawa et al., 1984).

In another 2-stage carcinogenicity study, 40 female ddN mice each had 0.05 mg of an initiator, 4-nitroquinoline-1-oxide (dissolved in benzene), painted onto the clipped dorsal skin 20 times in 50 days. Six days after the end of the initiator treatment, 0.05 ml sodium hypochlorite solution (with an active chlorine content of >10%) was applied to the shaved dorsal skin 45 times over a period of 245 days. A group of 40 control animals received 60 applications of 0.05 mg 4-nitro-quinoline-1-oxide over 300 days (no further details). In the 32 mice that survived sodium hypochlorite treatment, 4 malignant and 5 benign skin tumours and 1 leukaemia were found. No skin tumours were detected in the 29 surviving mice in the control group. There was no information on choice of doses and no indication of whether the solution induced skin irritation (Hayatsu et al., 1971).

A 1% solution of sodium hypochlorite (in acetone) was applied to the shaved dorsal skin of NMRI mice, twice a week for 10 weeks. In 6 groups of mice, sodium hypochlorite was applied either before, during or after treatment with a 0.22 or 0.44% solution of 3,4-benzopyrene (in acetone) which was also applied twice a week for 10 weeks (no information on dose or group size). The control groups were as follows: one untreated group, one group that received acetone, one group that received sodium hypochlorite, and three groups that were treated with acetone before, during or after NaOCl application. The mice were examined for skin tumours in week 124 of the study (they were apparently not examined earlier). Treatment with sodium hypochlorite before, during and after administration of benzopyrene apparently reduced benzopyrene-induced tumour development by about 5–35%. The reduced tumour development was expressed as a reduction in the total number of tumours and in the number of carcinoma-bearing mice (no information was given on the number of mice affected per group). No association with the benzopyrene dose was established. In the control groups treated exclusively with sodium hypochlorite or acetone, 2 and 5 mice, respectively, had tumours (total number of mice used not specified; Pfeiffer, 1978).

The existing studies on the tumour-promoting and co-carcinogenic potential of sodium hypochlorite on dermal application do not permit a conclusive evaluation.

In the in vitro C3H/10T1/2 cell transformation test, sodium hypochlorite (concentration not specified) with or without the addition of 0.25 µg 12-O-tetradecanoylphorbol-13-acetate did not increase the transformation rate, while N-methyl-N'-nitro-N-nitrosoguanidine showed marked transforming properties (Abernethy et al., 1983).

7.8 Reproductive toxicity

In an experiment to detect sperm-head anomalies, male B6C3F1 mice were given aqueous sodium hypochlorite solution 5 times at 24-hour intervals by stomach tube. The doses used were 1.6, 4.0 and 8.0 mg chlorine/kg body weight/day (equivalent to 3.4, 8.4 and 16.8 mg sodium hypochlorite/kg body weight/day). It was not stated whether the doses cover the maximum tolerated range. In this study, 2 different aqueous sodium hypochlorite solutions were again used (pH 8.5, mainly present as OCl^-; pH 6.5, mainly present as HOCl). Sperm were obtained from 10 mice at each dose, 1, 3 and 5 weeks after the last administration. Vehicle controls and positive controls (ethyl methane sulphonate) were also set up. For each mouse, 1000 sperm-heads were evaluated for anomalies. Each dose of the OCl- solution caused a significant dose-dependent increase ($p \leq 0.01$) in the number of anomalies, 3 weeks after the last administration. At the high dose, the malformation rate was 3.68±0.47% (vehicle control 2.12±0.19%; positive control 18.35±4.47%). Examination of the sperm 1 and 5 weeks after the last administration did not reveal any increase in the number of malformations. These results were confirmed in an independent experiment. In contrast, the HOCl solution did not cause an increase in the number of anomalies at any time. This result was also confirmed in an independent experiment (Meier et al., 1985).

Male Long-Evans rats received 1.0, 2.0 or 5.0 mg hypochlorous acid (HOCl)/kg body weight/day by stomach tube for 56 days before mating and then throughout the 10-day mating period. Females were treated with the same doses for 14 days before mating, throughout the mating period and until the end of lactation. Each group, including a control group, consisted of 24 females mated with 12 males. The pH-value of the solution used was 8.5. The behaviour and body weight gain of the rats of the F_0-generation were unaffected. Similarly, the fertility rate, number of litters, number of pups per litter, perinatal loss to the end of the lactation period, body weight gain of the pups and behaviour of the pups (eye opening) were within the range of the control group values. Histopathological examination of the rats in the F_0-generation revealed no treatment-related effects on the testes, epididymides, prostate gland, seminiferous tubules or uterus. The number of sperm and their motility were within the range of the control group, as was the differential blood count in males and females (Carlton et al., 1986).

In another fertility study, C3H/HeJ and C57BL/6J mice received sodium hypochlorite in the drinking water at a concentration of 10–13 ppm chlorine (pH 2.5) for 6 months. This was equivalent to about 2.1–2.8 mg NaOCl/kg body weight/day. During the 6 months, 1 male was kept in a cage with 1 or 2 females for mating. The control group received tap water (pH 9.6). The number of dams used was 168 and 291 per strain, respectively. The number of offspring per dam and the number of pups at the end of the lactation period were within the range of the control group values in both strains (Les, 1968).

Groups of 6 female Sprague-Dawley rats received 1, 10 or 100 mg hypochlorous acid (HOCl)/l water daily in their drinking water for 2.5 months before mating, throughout the mating period and up to day 20 of pregnancy. These doses were equivalent to about 0.1, 1 and 10 mg/kg body weight/day at an assumed water intake of 100 ml/kg body weight/day. The males were not treated. Six further animals served as controls. Laparotomy was performed on day 20 of pregnancy. Half of the foetuses were used to detect skeletal malformations, the other half to detect soft-tissue malformatiions. There was no indication whether the chosen doses were toxic to the dams. Foetal weight and the number of resorptions were within the range of control group values. A slight increase in the number of foetuses with skeletal and visceral abnormalities was seen in the middle- and high-dose groups (27.1 and 38.5% in the treated animals, control 21.1%). In the high-dose group, this increase was statistically significant ($p<0.05$; χ^2-test). The number of incomplete or missing sternebrae was increased in the high-dose group; in addition there were 3 adrenal ageneses, 1 dextrocardia and 1 enlarged atrio-ventricular valve, abnormalities or malformations which also occurred or could have occurred in the control group (Abdel-Rahman et al., 1982).

7.9 Effects on the immune system

Groups of 12 male 3-week-old Sprague-Dawley rats received sodium hypochlorite (chlorine content 6.05%) in their drinking water until the age of 12 weeks. The concentrations used were 5, 15 and 30 ppm, calculated as chlorine. The rats were then killed and several immunological parameters were studied, including spleen and thymus weight, antibody production, delayed-type hypersensitivity (DTH) reactions, natural killer cell (NKC) cytotoxicity, oxidative metabolism response (i.e. chemiluminesence – CL), phagocytic activity of macrophages and production of interleukin (IL2) and prostaglandin E_2 (PGE_2). In the high-dose group (30 ppm) there was a significant reduction ($p\leq0.05$) in spleen weight, DTH reactions and oxidative metabolism by macrophages, while PGE_2 production was increased. On the basis of these results, the authors concluded that sodium hypochlorite was not a particularly strong immunodepressant (Exon et al., 1987).

7.10 Neurotoxicity

In male Sprague-Dawley rats (n=12) acute oral administration of an aqueous sodium hypochlorite solution with a free chlorine content of 1% caused a reduction in hypothalamic noradrenaline content by more than 25% ($p<0.05$), 3 and 24 hours after treatment. The level had returned to normal after 7 days. The histamine and dopamine levels in the hypothalamus were slightly, but not significantly, reduced. The authors did not rule out the possibility that stress could have caused the change in transmitter levels (Vogt et al., 1982).

7.11 Other effects

Cloths soaked with buffered 0.5% sodium hypochlorite solution (pH 9.0) were surgically placed in the abdominal cavities of 6 dogs. Liver alkaline phosphatase activity and blood urea content were increased by a maximum of 1.4-fold on the first and second day after treatment. There were no effects on the levels of bilirubin and uric acid in the serum or on thymol turbidity in comparison with the controls during the 5-week observation period (Zwaveling, 1963).

Male Sprague-Dawley rats received hypochlorous acid (HOCl) at concentrations of 1, 10 or 100 mg/l daily in the drinking water for 3 months. This was equivalent to doses of about 0.1, 1.0 and 10 mg/kg body weight/day at an assumed water intake of 100 ml/kg body weight/day. Four animals were used per dose and as controls. At the high dose, there was a significant increase ($p<0.05$) in DNA synthesis in the nuclei of the kidneys and testes. The parameter measured was the incorporation of radio-labelled thymidine, which had been administered by intraperitoneal injection 8 hours previously. No effect on DNA synthesis was observed in the nuclei of the spleen, liver or gut mucosa (Abdel-Rahman et al., 1984).

A sodium hypochlorite concentration of 60 µg/ml medium influenced thymidine incorporation in vitro in the following cell lines (Wohlrab and Wozniak, 1982):

Cell line	Inhibition of thymidine incorporation (%)
Lymphocytes human	0
Epidermal cells	
human	0
guinea-pig	0
Bone marrow cells	
golden hamster	51
Melanoma	
human	15
golden hamster M Mel 1	41
golden hamster A Mel 3	77

The threshold values and LC_{50} values for non-specific cytotoxicity in various cell lines are given in the following table:

Cell line	Threshold concentration	LC_{50} value	References
	µg/ml Medium		
Human			
Lymphoblasts	–	200	Koskinen et al., 1981
Fibroblasts	–	50	Koskinen et al., 1981
Hepatoma cells (Hep G2)	159	–	Borenfreund and Borrero, 1984
Mouse			
Fibroblasts (Balb/c 3T3)	79	–	Borenfreund and Borrero, 1984
Macrophages (RAW 264.7)	37.2	–	Borenfreund and Borrero, 1984
Fibroblasts (C3H/10T1/2)	–	12	Abernethy et al., 1983
Hamster			
Lung fibroblasts (V 79)	52.9	–	Borenfreund and Borrero, 1984
Rabbit			
Leukocytes (migration)	0.25	–	Kazol et al., 1988
Fibroblasts	25	–	Kozol et al., 1988
Corneal epithelial cells	20.8	–	Borenfreund and Borrero, 1984
Cow			
Endothelial cells	25	–	Kozol et al., 1988

It can be inferred from the table that rabbit cells are the most sensitive and human cells the least sensitive.

At 50 µg/ml and above, sodium hypochlorite caused reduced liberation of plasminogen activator in vitro in rabbit corneal epithelial cells after short-term exposure (no exact details; Chan, 1985).

In vitro, aqueous sodium hypochlorite solution caused hydrolysis of human and animal serum proteins (albumins, globulins), followed by oxidation of the resulting amino acids and peptides. The threshold concentration would be about 0.5 mg NaOCl/ml protein nitrogen (pH 9.4, 37 °C; Baker, 1947; Bartmann et al., 1952; Gehrmann and Remmer, 1952; Herken and Schunk, 1949 a, 1949 b).

An aqueous 42 μM sodium hypochlorite solution (equivalent to 3.13 μg/ml) caused 50–100% chlorination of cytosine, thymine and uracil in *Escherichia coli* $6_3.86U^-$ after 6 hours of incubation at 37 °C (Prat et al., 1967).

At room temperature, aqueous solutions of hypochlorous acid reacted in equimolar proportions with cytosine to form 4-N-chlorocytosine. The yield was 76% (Patton et al., 1973).

8. Experience in humans

Sodium hypochlorite solution is strongly corrosive in humans. In the following section, the information from the literature is organized according to the route of exposure. Often it was not possible to deduce whether the observed effects were caused by sodium hypochlorite, by chlorine released from aqueous sodium hypochlorite solutions, and/or by other components of the solution.

A 6% sodium hypochlorite solution (pH 11.2; 0.1 ml) was applied to the foreheads of 10 volunteers. Slight, but definite erythema and small wheals formed in 4 volunteers within 20 minutes (Hostynek et al., 1989).

Onycholysis occurred in an 18-year-old woman who was temporarily working as a swimming pool attendant, after exposure to aqueous sodium hypochlorite solution. Among other things, her duties included the daily addition of 16% NaOCl solution to the water in the swimming pool. 1 to 2 months after finishing her employment, the fingernails had grown back normally (Coskey, 1974).

Exposure to the vapours that developed from a sodium hypochlorite-containing cleaning fluid caused acute reversible alopecia (depilatory-type) in 2 people, with a trichogram revealing signs of hair dystrophy. In both cases, a wash basin had been intensively cleaned with a sodium hypochlorite-containing product, and the head had been immersed in the resulting vapours. Fourteen days after exposure, hair loss occurred in 1 subject, and the hair on the head was diffuse and thin in irregular patches. On the right upper arm there was a single patch of subacute eczema (diameter 3 cm). Diffuse hair loss continued 1 month after exposure. In the second subject the cleaning fluid splashed onto the forearms and neck, and because she felt the skin burning where it had been splashed, she wiped her hand and arm on the hair on the side of her head. Hair loss began after 3 days. After 20 days, diffuse hair loss was visible, which was less marked at the front and over the crown. In the parietal region isolated strands remained, and hairs with roots could be painlessly pulled out. At the back of the head, the covering of hair remained. The skin of the head was normal, as were the lymph nodes, and the body hair and nails were unaffected. Isolated subacute patches of eczema were present on the forearms and the neck, and there were clear signs of eczema in the area of the left ear. A biopsy from the parietal region revealed intercellular oedema in the lower part of the epidermis with moderate round cell infiltration, erythrocyte diapedesis, fibrous decomposition of the hair structure in the follicle, epidermal loosening in the follicular region and detachment of the epidermis. The stratum granulosum was no longer present in the normal form. In both subjects, new hair growth could be seen after 4 weeks, and after 1 year the hair was completely restored (Stüttgen et al., 1982).

A patient who got chlorox spray (containing 5% NaOCl) in the eye, rinsed it out several minutes later because of a burning sensation. On the same day, slight surface damage to the corneal epithelium was observed, which healed up after 1 or 2 days without further treatment (no further details; Grant, 1986).

In another patient who also got chlorox spray in the eye (which was immediately rinsed with water), reddening of the conjunctiva developed on the same day, with numerous small grey spots in the corneal epithelium which were joined together in parts (no further details). These effects had cleared up completely the next day (Grant, 1986).

Ingestion of aqueous sodium hypochlorite solution can cause vomiting and severe burning and ulceration of the mouth, throat, oesophagus and stomach. Isolated cases of strictures of the oesophagus have been described (information on the volume ingested could often not be established retrospectively). Out of 31 children who ingested a bleach containing 5% sodium hypochlorite, 11 developed burns in the mouth, 17 developed slight oesophageal burns, 9 developed severe oesophageal burns, and 2 had oesophageal stenosis (no further details; Yarington, 1965).

Out of 80 children (aged 11 months to 8 years) who had accidentally ingested sodium hypochlorite solution used as bleach (5.5% NaOCl, 0.5% NaCl), 40 were reported to have ingested between 10 and 200 ml. 36 children vomited, 12 coughed and 10 had lung infiltration. Oesophageal burns were seen in 3 children who had taken 30 ml, 75 ml and an unknown quantity of bleach. Oesophageal strictures were seen in 2 further children (no further details). The quantity consumed by the remaining patients could not be determined (Tanyel et al., 1988).

In 23 patients who had been taken a 3–5% sodium hypochlorite solution (quantity unspecified), oesophageal burns were seen in only 1 case, and this healed up after 2 weeks (von Mühlendahl et al., 1978).

Oesophageal damage (erythema, oedema and localized ulceration) occurred in 2 out of 129 children who had swallowed an unknown quantity of Clorox (5.25% NaOCl, 0.2% Na_2CO_3, 0.0015–0.005% NaOH, pH 10.5–11.0; Pike et al., 1963).

In a 2-year-old girl and a 38-year-old women who had swallowed about 100 ml of a sodium hypochlorite-containing bleach (no further details), severe burns of the mouth, throat, oesophagus and stomach occurred, and after about 3 weeks, oesophageal strictures developed (5 and 25 cm long, respectively). These could not be dilated, and a bypass made from a section of the colon was necessary. A further 158 patients investigated over 10 years had no oesophageal injuries of this nature after ingestion of bleach (French et al., 1970).

A 7-month-old boy vomited after swallowing a sterilizing tablet. He had acute difficulty in breathing, with stridor on inspiration and intercostal and sternal constriction. He also developed marked oedema around the pharynx and epiglottis, which turned into an ulcer within 48 hours. The patient was discharged from hospital after 12 days. The tablet consisted of dichloroisocyanurate, which liberates sodium hypochlorite on contact with water (Williams, 1985).

In a 3-week-old premature baby which suffered from slight RDS (respiratory distress syndrome), massive Heinz body formation and haemolysis occurred after oral intake of sodium hypochlorite. The haemoglobin level fell from 16.8 g% to 4.7 g%, and the erythrocyte count from $4.5\times10^6/mm^3$ to $1.63\times10^6/mm^3$. The reticulocyte value increased from 6.0% to 11.7%, and the number of Heinz bodies from 0.0% to 40%. The activity of glucose-6-phosphate dehydrogenase was 10.4 μMol/minute/10^{11} cells (normal value for newborn infants

38.2±8.6 μMol/minute/10^{11} cells). It was later reported that every day for 5 consecutive days the premature baby had received 8×0.4 ml aqueous sodium hypochlorite solution (Milton solution), orally by means of a feeding tube. This tube had been filled with diluted Milton solution for sterilization, but had not subsequently been emptied and rinsed. As this report provided no details on concentration, it could not be established how much NaOCl the premature baby had ingested. The neat Milton solution contained 23.3 g NaOCl/l. In order to clarify the signs of toxicity, 10 premature babies were treated orally with 0.4 ml of the dilute aqueous NaOCl solution, 8 times a day from day 3 to day 7 of life (concentration not specified). 10 more premature infants served as controls. On day 2 of life, the Heinz body value was 5±1% (control 4±6%), and on day 8 it was 26±11% (control 3.5±5%; Schuchmann and Steinitz, 1974).

It was suggested that frequent sucking on socks that had been bleached with sodium hypochlorite (no further details) since the 14th month of life was responsible for chronic gastroduodenitis, a localized stomach ulcer and pneumonia in a 7-year-old girl. When the socks were no longer bleached with sodium hypochlorite, the symptoms cleared up completely (Loeb and King, 1974).

An 18-month-old girl died 19 hours after ingesting a few spoonsful of bleach containing 5% sodium hypochlorite. Ten minutes after the NaOCl ingestion, the stomach was rinsed with dilute acetic acid solution. The patient then became sedated, and eventually comatose. Autopsy revealed focal necroses, haemorrhages and surface erosion of the gastric mucosa. The cause of death was reported to be acute tracheo-bronchitis and secondary obstructive atelectasis (Done, 1961).

Ingestion of about 1.0 l Clorox (5.25% NaOCl, pH 10.8) by a 49-year-old man caused severe corrosion of the stomach region. After 3.5 months there was no change in the oesophagus, and the stomach lumen was reduced by scars and fibrosis to a 3 mm-wide fissure in the middle section. The haemoglobin level, leucocyte count, albumin, globulin and non-protein nitrogen content were all in the normal range. The stomach had to be completely removed. The stomach wall was ulcerated and almost completely scarred, the serosa was raised into thick folds, the mucosa and submucosa were fibrotic, the epithelial tissues were extensively destroyed and the normal histological appearance was markedly changed (Strange et al., 1951).

A 72-year-old man died after suicidal oral ingestion of a sodium hypochlorite-containing bleach (no further details). Autopsy revealed strongly alkaline gastric juice (pH 10). The Na^+ content was increased 2.73-fold, and the Cl^- content 1.25-fold. Overlapping necroses, haemorrhages and oedema were observed from the lips to the upper section of the digestive tract. Oedema of the glottis and lung emphysema were also found (Kamiyama and Beppu, 1979).

A 66-year-old woman with severe endogenous depression attempted suicide by drinking 500 ml of a strong bleaching agent containing 10% NaOCl. Two hours previously she had taken 8 Flurazepam tablets. On admission to hospital she was very drowsy, was breathing with difficulty and had reduced blood pressure. Surface corrosion was found in the mouth. Examination revealed metabolic acidosis. The sodium content in the serum was measured as 150 and 169 mmol/l, the chlorine content as 130 mmol/l. After intravenous treatment with 5% dextrose the electrolyte balance improved, and after 5 days the patient was free of symptoms except for dysphagia resulting from oesophagitis (Ward and Routledge, 1988).

In a suicide attempt, a 27-year-old man who was dependent on amphetamines ingested 300 mg diazepam and 60 ml of a 5.25% sodium hypochlorite solution (equivalent to 3150 mg), and also injected himself intravenously with 0.3 ml of the sodium hypochlorite solution (equivalent to 16 mg). No painful reaction occurred at the site of injection. The patient was lethargic but arousable. The haemoglobin level, leucocyte count, and values for serum electrolytes, serum urea nitrogen and glucose were in the normal range (Froner et al., 1987).

During routine haemodialysis in a 61-year-old woman with end-stage kidney disease and pheripheral neuropathy, the blood returning to the patient was accidentally contaminated with sodium hypochlorite solution (5.25% NaOCl, 4.00% NaCl, 0.20% NA_2CO_3, 0.01% NaOH). The sodium hypochlorite solution, which was put into the dialysis machine for cleaning purposes, entered the blood-carrying section of the dialyser by means of a valve which was inadvertently left open. The sodium hypochlorite-soaked membrane was in contact with the blood returning to the patient for less than 2 minutes. The patient developed massive haemolysis and hyperkalaemia, was comatose and cyanotic, and the cardio-respiratory activity was minimal. The patient recovered after medical treatment (Hoy, 1981).

During treatment of the root canal of the upper right eye-tooth in a 23-year-old woman, about 0.5 ml of a 5.25% sodium hypochlorite solution was accidentally injected into the root canal and the periapical tissues. This led immediately to severe pain, bleeding in the root canal and swelling of the right side of the face. Following alternating cold and warm compresses and medical treatment the patient recovered in 4 weeks (Becker et al., 1974).

Inadvertent administration of 1.8 ml of a 5.25% sodium hypochlorite solution instead of a local anaesthetic into the medial pterygoid muscle during routine dental treatment of a 21-year-old woman led to severe pain, oedema which extended to the throat, and trismus. The patient was admitted to hospital because of possible obstruction of the airways from oedema. Following medical treatment, the patient had almost returned to normal after 4 days, and after 2 weeks she was free of symptoms (Herrmann et al., 1979).

A 46-year-old vet had suffered from itchy skin lesions on the hands and forearms for 3–4 years. He had occasionally washed his hands and forearms with an undiluted antiseptic containing 4–6% sodium hypochlorite. A patch test with 0.25–2% sodium hypochlorite solution was positive, while 3 control subjects gave negative results (Eun et al., 1984).

Two female patients aged 28 and 30 years old, who for several years had used a bleaching agent containing 10% sodium hypochlorite, developed chronic itchy dermatitis of the hands (particularly on the backs of the fingers) and severe chronic hand eczema, respectively. Patch tests with 0.1–2% aqueous sodium hypochlorite were positive in both women. No reactions were seen with a 0.01% solution. Twenty control subjects gave negative results at concentrations of 0.5% or 1%. At a concentration of 2%, 15 out of 69 controls showed a weak or moderate irritant reaction (Habets et al., 1986).

2 out of 40 housewives who suffered from allergic hand dermatitis developed sensitization reactions in patch tests with a 1% sodium hypochlorite solution (Van Joost et al., 1987).

A 36-year-old women developed blisters after 4 hours of cleaning with a hypochlorite-containing bleach (no further details). The blisters took 2 weeks to heal. Subsequent use (time not specified) of a hypochlorite-containing product provoked a marked allergic reaction of the left foreleg, as well as a very itchy, maculopapular erythema of the body and extremities, watering eyes, shortness of breath and swelling of the face. The skin at the site of the lesions on the extremities was spongiotic with sparse perivascular lymphocytic infiltration in the upper dermis. The complete and differential blood count, the liver and kidney function, and the blood sugar level were within normal limits. The reaction to a 1% sodium hypochlorite solution was immediately positive in an open application test (Hostynek et al., 1989).

In a 43-year-old woman who for 1 year had suffered repeated episodes of severe dermatitis on the arms, and milder dermatitis on the thighs, legs and face, a patch test with 0.5% aqueous sodium hypochlorite solution produced a strongly positive reaction after 48 and 96 hours. During an abortion, 15 years previously, the patient had been treated with a sodium hypochlorite-containing disinfectant, after which severe dermatitis had developed in the genital area. Out of a further 225 patients tested for hypersensitivity to sodium hypochlorite, 3 showed a positive reaction. One subject was a 53-year-old man who had cleaned windows for several months with a sodium hypochlorite-containing bleach. The second subject, a 73-year-old woman, had a stasis dermatitis which had been treated with sodium hypochlorite-containing disinfectant. No previous exposure to sodium hypochlorite was known in the third subject, a 28-year-old women (Osmundsen, 1978).

In a 28-year-old man a cylindrical carcinoma of the thoracic oesophagus was detected 4 years after the ingestion of concentrated sodium hypochlorite. The caustic burr followed by carcinoma was of special significance in this case owing to the development of an adeno-carcinoma (Cornet et al., 1976).

In vitro, sodium hypochlorite had haemolytic properties from about 5.25 μg/ml erythrocyte suspension (Pashley et al., 1985).

9. Threshold limit values

No information available.

Table 1. Acute toxicity of sodium hypochlorite

Species (strain)	No. of animals/ dose	Sex	Route	Observation period (days)	LD_0 (mg/kg body weight)	LD_{50} (95% confidence level; mg/kg body weight)	Reference
Mouse (ddY)	5	Male	Oral	14	4950–5700	6800[a] (6200–7400)	Momma et al., 1986
Mouse (ddY)	5	Female	Oral	14	4300–4950	5800[a] (5300–6350)	Momma et al., 1986
Mouse	Σ 17	n.s.	i.p.	n.s.	120– 240	n.s.	Taylor and Austin, 1918
Guinea-pig	Σ 6	n.s.	i.p.	n.s.	30– 63	n.s.	Taylor and Austin, 1918
Guinea-pig	Σ 6	n.s.	s.c.	n.s.	130– 240	n.s.	Taylor and Austin, 1918

n.s. Not specified
Σ Total
[a] In the publication the values were given as ml/kg, however, based on table 4 of the paper, they should have been mg/kg on administration of a 50% solution

References

Abdel-Rahman, M.S.
Pharmacokinetics of chlorine obtained from chlorine dioxide, chlorine, chloramine, and chloride
Water Chlorination: Chem. Environ. Impact Health Eff., Proc. Conf. 5th, 281–293 (1985)

Abdel-Rahman, M.S., Berardi, M.R., Bull, R.J.
Effect of chlorine and monochloramine in drinking water of the developing rat fetus
J. Appl. Toxicol., 2, 156–159 (1982)

Abdel-Rahman, M.S., Waldron, D.M., Bull, R.J.
A comparative kinetics study of monochloramine and hypochlorous acid in rats
J. Appl. Toxicol., 3, 175–179 (1983)

Abdel-Rahman, M.S., Suh, D.H., Bull, R.J.
Pharmacodynamics and toxicity of chlorine in drinking water in the rat
J. Appl. Toxicol., 4, 82–86 (1984)

Abernethy, D.J., Frazelle, J.H., Boreiko, C.J.
Relative cytotoxic and transforming potential of respiratory irritants in the C3H/10T1/2 cell transformation system
Environ. Mutagen., 5, 419 (1983)

Baker, R.W.R.
Studies on the reaction between sodium hypochlorite and proteins
Biochem. J., 41, 337–342 (1947)

Bartmann, K., Gehrmann, K., Remmer, H.
Die Reaktion von Natrium-Hypochlorit mit verschiedenen Serumproteinen
Arch. Exp. Pathol. Pharmakol., 215, 433–442 (1952)

Bayer AG
Grunddatensatz für Altstoffe (1990)

Becker, G.L., Cohen, S., Borer, R.
The sequelae of accidentally injecting sodium hypochlorite beyond the root apex
Oral Surg. Oral Med. Oral Pathol., 38, 633–638 (1974)

Borenfreund, E., Borrero, O.
In vitro cytotoxicity assays. Potential alternatives to the Draize ocular allergy test
Cell Biol. Toxicol., 1, 55–65 (1984)

Carlton, B.D., Barlett, P., Basaran, A., Colling, K., Osis, I., Smith, M.K.
Reproductive effects of alternative disinfectants
Environ. Health Perspect., 69, 237–241 (1986)

Carter, R.O., Griffith, J.F.
Experimental bases for the realistic assessment of safety of topical agents
Toxicol. Appl. Pharmacol., 7, 60–72 (1965)

Chan, K.Y.
Alternative to the Draize test
Altern. Methods Toxicol., 3, 407–422 (1985)

Clark, E.S., Crissinger, K.D., Granger, D.N.
Increased mucosal permeability induced by hydrogen peroxide and hypochlorous acid in the developing piglet
Gastroenterology, 96, A 89 (1989)

Cornet, A., Barbier, J.P., Grenier, G., Elhadad, A., Breaute, H., Carnot, F.
Brûhre caustique et adénocarcinome de l'oesophage
Semaine Hopitaux de Paris, 52, 1999–2003 (1976)

Coskey, R.J.
Onycholysis from sodium hypochlorite
Arch. Dermatol., 109, 96 (1974)

Cotter, J.L., Fader, R.C., Lilley, C., Herndon, D.N.
Chemical parameters, antimicrobial activities, and tissue toxicity of 0.1 and 0.5% sodium hypochlorite solutions
Antimicrob. Agents Chemother., 28, 118–122 (1985)

Cunningham, H.M.
Effect of sodium hypochlorite on the growth of rats and guinea-pigs
Am. J. Vet. Res., 41, 295–297 (1980)

Done, A.K.
Personal communication (1961)
In: Gosselin, R.E., Smith, R.P., Hodge, H.C., Braddock, J.E.
Hypochlorite
Clinical Toxicology of Commercial Products, 5th ed.
Williams and Wilkins, Baltimore/London, III-202–205 (1984)

Eun, H.C., Lee, A.Y., Lee, Y.S.
Sodium hypochlorite dermatitis
Contact Dermatitis, 11, 45 (1984)

Exon, J.H., Koller, L.D., O'Reilly, C.A., Bercz, J.P.
Immunotoxicologic evaluation of chlorine-based drinking water disinfectants, sodium hypochlorite and monochloramine
Toxicology, 44, 257–269 (1987)

French, F.J., Tabb, H.G., Rutledge, L.J.
Esophageal stenosis produced by ingestion of bleach: report of two cases
South. Med. J., 63, 1140–1144 (1970)

Froner, G.A., Rutherford, G.W., Rokeach, M.
Injection of sodium hypochlorite by intravenous drug users
JAMA, 258, 325 (1987)

Furukawa, F., Kurata, Y., Kokubo, T., Takahashi, M., Nakadate, M.
Oral acute and subchronic toxicity studies for sodium hypochlorite in F-344 rat
Bull. Natl. Inst. Hyg., 98, 62–69 (1980)

Gehrmann, K., Remmer, H.
Die Oxydation von Menschenserumalbumin durch wechselnde Mengen an Natriumhypochlorit
Arch. Exp. Pathol. Pharmakol., 215, 342–353 (1952)

Grant, W.M.
Toxicology of the eye
3rd ed., p. 838–839
Thomas, C. Publisher, Springfield, Illinois, USA (1986)

Griffith, J.F., Nixon, G.A., Bruce, R.D., Reer, P.J., Bannan, E.A.
Dose-response studies with chemical irritants in the albino rabbit eye as a basis for selecting optimum testing conditions for predicting hazard to the human eye
Toxicol. Appl. Pharmacol., 55, 501–513 (1980)

Habets, J.M.W., Geursen-Reitsma, A.M., Stolz, E., van Joost, T.
Sensitization to sodium hypochlorite causing hand dermatitis
Contact Dermatitis, 15, 140–142 (1986)

Hasegawa,R., Takahashi, M., Kokubo, T., Furukawa, F., Toyoda, K., Sato, H., Kurokowa, Y., Hayashi, Y.
Carcinogenicity study of sodium hypochlorite in F-344 rats
Fd. Chem. Toxicol., 24, 1295–1302 (1986)

Hayashi, M., Kishi, M., Sofuni, T., Ishidate, M., jr.
Micronucleus tests in mice on 39 food additives and eight miscellaneous chemicals
Fd. Chem. Toxicol., 26, 487–500 (1988)

Hayatsu, H., Hoshino, H., Kawazoe, Y.
Potential cocarcinogenicity of sodium hypochlorite
Nature, 233, 495 (1971)

Herken, H., Schunk, J.
Untersuchungen an Eiweißkörpern mit Natriumhypochlorit
Arch. Exp. Pathol. Pharmakol., 206, 102–116 (1949 a)

Herken, H., Schunk, J.
Über den Nachweis von Strukturveränderungen der Serumproteine mit Hypochlorit
Arch. Exp. Pathol. Pharmakol., 206, 302–313 (1949 b)

Herrmann, J.W., Heicht, R.C.
Complications in therapeutic use of sodium hypochlorite
J. Endodont., 5, 160 (1979)

Hollemann, A.F., Wiberg, W.
X. Gruppe der Halogene
In: Lehrbuch der Anorganischen Chemie, p. 248
Walter de Gruyter, Berlin (1971)

Hostynek, J.J., Patrick, E., Younger, B., Maibach, H.I.
Hypochlorite sensitivity in man
Contact Dermatitis, 20, 32–37 (1989)

Hoy, R.H.
Accidental systemic exposure to sodium hypochlorite (clorox) during hemodialysis
Am. J. Hosp. Pharm., 38, 1512–1514 (1981)

Hummelsberger, P.
Vergiftungen durch hypochlorithaltigen Sanitärreiniger
Dtsch. Med. Wochenschr., 110, 398 (1985)

Ishidate, M., jr., Harnois, M.C., Sofuni, T.
A comparative analysis of data on the clastogenicity of 951 chemical substances tested in mammalian cell cultures
Mutat. Res., 195, 151–213 (1988)

Ishidate, M., jr., Sofuni, T., Yoshikawa, K.
Chromosomal aberration tests in vitro as a primary screening tool for environmental mutagens and/or carcinogens
GANN Monogr. Cancer Res., 27, 95–108 (1981)

Ishidate, M., jr., Sofuni, T., Yoshikawa, K., Hayashi, M., Nohmi, T., Sawada, M., Matsuoka, A.
Primary mutagenicity screening of food additives currently used in Japan
Fd. Chem. Toxicol., 22, 623–636 (1984)

Ishidate, M., jr., Yoshikawa, K.
Chromosome aberration tests with Chinese hamster cells in vitro with and without metabolic activation – a comparative study on mutagens and carcinogens
Arch. Toxicol., Suppl. 4, 41–44 (1980)

Kamiyama, S., Beppu, K.
A fatal suicidal case by drinking of liquid bleach
Nippon Hoigaku Zasshi, 33, 13–19 (1979)

Kawachi, T., Komatsu, T., Kada, T., Ishidate, M., Sasaki, M., Sugiyama, T., Tazima, Y.
Results of recent studies on the relevance of various short-term screening tests in Japan
Appl. Meth. Oncol., 3, 253–267 (1980 a)

Kawachi, T., Yahagi, T., Kada, T., Tazima, Y., Ishidate, M., Sasaki, M., Sugiyama, T.
Cooperative programme on short-term assays for carcinogenicity in Japan
IARC Int. Agency Cancer Res., 27, 323–330 (1980 b)

Koskinen, K.P., Rahkamo, A., Tuompo, H.
Cytotoxicity of some solutions used for root canal treatment assessed with human fibroblasts in lymphoblasts
Scand. J. Dent. Res., 89, 71–78 (1981)

Kozol, R.A., Gillies, C., Elgebaly, S.A.
Effects of sodium hypochlorite (Dakin's solution) on cells of the wound module
Arch. Surg., 123, 420–423 (1988)

Kurokawa, Y., Takamura, N., Matsushima, Y., Imazawa, T., Hayashi, Y.
Studies on the promoting and complete carcinogenic activities of some oxidizing chemicals in skin carcinogenesis
Cancer Lett., 24, 299–304 (1984)

Kurokawa, Y., Takayama, S., Konishi, Y., Hiasa, Y., Asahina, S., Takahashi, M., Maekawa, A., Hayashi, Y.
Long-term in vivo carcinogenicity tests of potassium bromate, sodium hypochlorite, and sodium chlorite conducted in Japan
Environ. Health Perspect., 69, 221–235 (1986)

Landau, G.D., Saunders, W.H.
The effect of chlorine bleach on the oesophagus
Arch. Otolaryngol., 80, 174–176 (1964)

Les, E.P.
Effect of acidified-chlorinated water on reproduction in C3H/HeJ and C57BL/6J mice
Lab. Anim. Care, 18, 210–213 (1968)

Loden, M., Larsson, R., Häggqvist, I., Karlsson, N.
Dermal irritancy/corrosion of 20 compounds in aqueous solution
NTIS PB 86-129913, p. 1–30, 53–54 (1985)

Loeb, F.X., King, T.L.
Chronic gastroduodenitis due to laundry bleach
Am. J. Dis. Child., 128, 256–257 (1974)

Matsuoka, A., Hayashi, M., Ishidate, M., jr.
Chromosomal aberration tests on 29 chemicals combined with S9 mix in vitro
Mutat. Res., 66, 277–290 (1979)

Meier, J.R., Bull, R.J., Stober, J.A., Cimino, M.C.
Evaluation of chemicals used for drinking water disinfection for production of chromosomal damage and sperm-head abnormalities in mice
Environ. Mutgen., 7, 201–211 (1985)

Mink, F.L., Coleman, E.W., Munch, J.W., Kaylor, W.H., Ringhand, H.P.
In vivo formation of halogenated reaction products following peroral sodium hypochlorite
Bull. Environ. Contam. Toxicol., 30, 394–399 (1983)

Momma, J., Takada, K., Suzuki, Y., Tobe, M.
Acute oral toxicity and ocular irritation of chemicals in bleaching agents
J. Food Hyg. Soc. Japan, 27, 553–560 (1986)

Mühlendahl, von, K.E., Oberdisse, U., Krienke, E.G.
Local injuries by accidental ingestion of corrosive substances by children
Arch. Toxicol., 39, 299–314 (1978)

Okonek, S., Reinecke, H.J., Krienke, E.G., Oberdisse, U., Brambach, U., Smend, J., Gädeke, R., Fabricius, W., Preußner, K.
Vergiftungen durch hypochlorithaltige Sanitärreiniger
Dtsch. Med. Wochenschr., 109, 1874–1877 (1984)

Osmundsen, P.E.
Contact dermatitis due to sodium hypochlorite
Contact Dermatitis, 4, 177–178 (1978)

Osterberg, R.E., Bierbower, G.W., Van Seabaugh, M., Porter, W.K., jr., Lowther, D., Hoheisel, C.A.
Potential biological hazards of commercially available cleansers of dentures
J. Toxicol. Environ. Health, 3, 969–977 (1977)

Pashley, E.L., Birdsong, N.L., Bowman, K., Pashley, D.H.
Cytotoxic effects of NaOCl on vital tissue
J. Endodont., 11, 525–528 (1985)

Patton, W., Bacon, V., Duffield, A.M., Halpern, B., Hoyano, Y., Pereira, W., Lederberg, J.
Chlorination studies. I. The reaction of aqueous hypochlorous acid with cytosine
Biochem. Biophys. Res. Commun., 48, 880–884 (1972)

Pfeiffer, E.H.
Zur Frage der Cocancerogenität von Chlor
WaBoLu-Ber., 129–141 (1978)

Pike, D.G., Peabody, J.W., jr., Davis, E.W., Lyons, W.S.
A re-evaluation of the dangers of clorox ingestion
J. Pediatr., 63, 303–305 (1963)

Prat, R., Nofre, C., Cier, A.
Effects de l'hypochlorite de sodium, de l'ozone et des radiations ionisantes sur les constituants pyrimidiques d'*Escherichia coli*
Ann. Inst. Pasteur, 595–606 (1967)

Robinson, M., Bull, R.J., Schmer, M., Long, R.E.
Epidermal hyperplasia in mouse skin following treatment with alternative drinking water disinfectants
Environ. Health Perspect., 69, 293–300 (1986)

Rosenkranz, H.S.
Sodium hypochlorite and sodium perborate: preferential inhibitors of DNA polymerase-deficient bacteria
Mutat. Res., 21, 171–174 (1973)

Rosenkranz, H.S., Gutter, B., Speck, W.T.
Mutagenicity and DNA-modifying activity: a comparison of two microbial assays
Mutat. Res., 41, 61–70 (1976)

Sasaki, M., Sugimura, K., Yoshida, M.A., Abe, S.
Cytogenetic effects of 60 chemicals on cultured human and Chinese hamster cells
La Kromosomo, II-20, 574–584 (1980)

Schuchmann, L., Steinitz, H.
Toxische Heinzkörperbildung durch Desinfektionsmittel bei Frühgeborenen
Klin. Pädiat., 186, 436–440 (1974)

Scully, F.E., jr., Mazina, K., Sonenshine, D., Daniel, F.B.
Reactions of hypochlorite and organic N-chloramines in stomach fluid
NTIS Report PB 85-225050 (1985)

Scully, F.E., jr., Mazina, K., Sonenshine, D., Kopfler, F.
Quantitation and identification of organic N-chloramines formed in stomach fluid on ingestion of aqueous hypochlorite
Environ. Health Perspect., 69, 259–265 (1986)

Shaw, M.W.
Human chromosome damage by chemical agents
Annual Review of Medicine, 21, 409–432 (1970)

Strange, D.C., Finneran, J.C., Shumacker, H.B., jr., Bowman, D.E.
Corrosive injury of the stomach
Arch. Surg., 62, 350–357 (1951)

Stüttgen, G., Haas, N., Mittelbach, F., Zesch, A.
Toxischer akuter reversibler Haarausfall durch Dampf/Dunst-Kontakt mit Natriumhypochlorit bzw. Natriumhydroxid enthaltenden Abfluß- und Sanitärreinigern
Wien. Klin. Wochenschr., 94, 479–484 (1982)

Tanyel, F.C., Byüyükpamukcu, N., Hicsönmez, A.
Chlorine bleach ingestion in children: A review of 80 cases
Turk. J. Pediatr., 30, 105–108 (1988)

Taylor, H.D., Austin, J.H.
Toxicity of certain widely used antiseptics
J. Exp. Med., 27, 635–646 (1918)

Van Delft, J.L., De Wolff-Rouendaal, D., Oosterhuis, J.A.
Irrigation with mercury chloride and sodium hypochlorite to prevent local recurrence after excision of conjunctival melanoma – an experimental study
Doc. Ophthalmol., 56, 61–67 (1983)

Van Joost, T., Habets, J.M.W., Stolz, E., Geursen-Reitsma, A.M.
Sodium hypochlorite sensitization
Contact Dermatitis, 16, 114 (1987)

Vogt, H., Balej, J., Bennett, J.E., Wintzer, P., Sheikh, S.A., Gallone, P.
Chlorine oxides and chlorine oxygen acids
In: Ullman's Encyclopedia of Industrial Chemistry
5th ed., A6, p. 483–525
VCH Weinheim (1986)

Vogt, C.R., Kapila, S., Chang, J.S., Sun, A.Y.
Effect of acute administration of chlorinated water on hypothalamic norepinephrine content
Pergamon Ser. Environ. Sci., 7, 163–167 (1982)

Ward, M.J., Routledge, P.A.
Hypernatraemia and hyperchloraemic acidosis after bleach ingestion
Human Toxicol., 7, 37–38 (1988)

Weeks, R.S., Ravitch, M.M.
Esophageal injury by liquid chlorine bleach: experimental study
J. Pediatr., 74, 911–916 (1969)

Weeks, R.S., Ravitch, M.M.
The pathology of experimental injury to the cat esophagus by liquid chlorine bleach
Laryngoscope (St. Louis), 81, 1532–1541 (1971)

Williams, D.C.
Acute respiratory obstruction caused by ingestion of a caustic substance
Br. Med. J., 291, 313–314 (1985)

Wlodkowski, T.J., Rosenkranz, H.S.
Mutagenicity of sodium hypochlorite for Salmonella typhimurium
Mutat. Res., 31, 39–42 (1975)

Wohlrab, W., Wozniak, K.D.
Untersuchungen zur Wirkung von Natriumhypochlorit als Modellsubstanz auf die Haut und verschiedene Zellsysteme
Derm. Beruf Umwelt, 30, 79–83 (1982)

Yarington, C.T., jr.
Ingestion of caustic: a pediatric problem
J. Pediatr., 67, 674–677 (1965)

Zwaveling, A.
Local application of a buffered solution of sodium hypochlorite in cancer surgery
Ned. Tijdschr. Geneeskd., 107, 351–357 (1963)

Compound chemical index vol. 1–4